HATHA YOGA

ACKNOWLEDGMENTS

I would like to extend a warm thank you to the VTF Hamburg's training and education department. For the past 15 years, we have worked continuously and successfully on yoga instructor training at the VTF's Gym Academy.

I would like to thank Winshape (www.winshape.de) for providing the functional yoga attire,

Winshape®

our yoga model Sara Lyn Chana, and our photographer Sonja Lesinski (www.sonjalesinski.com). Working with you and doing the photo shoot was an absolute pleasure. The beautiful malas in the photos were provided by Chandra Gems (www.chandra-gems.com).

I would also like to express my gratitude to all of my students, participants, and yoga instructors from whom I was allowed to learn. I would like to thank my trainer Ortwin Schulz (Integrale Yogaschule Hamburg) for the many perspectives and drives I was able to experience during the four years of my training under him, and my very first yoga teacher and mentor Kirti Peter Michel.

And last but not least, I would like to thank Meyer & Meyer Sport for their support in realizing the book project and the fantastic teamwork.

MARTINA MITTAG

HATHA YOGA

THE COMPLETE BOOK

Meyer & Meyer Sport

WHERE EXERCISE IS FUN

Author's Note: This book is part of the DTB (German Gymnastics Association) series "Where Exercise is Fun". It provides a complete introduction to the fundaments of DTB yoga training, and it also serves as a reference work. We are aware that terms like "sport" and "training" with regard to yoga may cause some confusion and may seem contradictory to the yoga philosophy. While Hatha Yoga is considered a "physical practice", the practice of yoga is neither competitive, nor is it a form of athletic training or a method for increasing athletic performance.

British Library Cataloguing in Publication Data

A catalogue record for this book is available from the British Library

Hatha Yoga

Maidenhead: Meyer & Meyer Sport (UK) Ltd., 2020

ISBN: 978-1-78255-185-0

Aachen, Auckland, Beirut, Dubai, Hägendorf, Hong Kong, Indianapolis, Cairo, Cape Town, Manila, Maidenhead, New Delhi, Singapore, Sydney, Tehran, Vienna

 Member of the World Sport Publishers' Association (WSPA)), www.w-s-p-a.org

Printed by Print Consult, GmbH, Munich, Germany

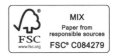

ISBN 978-1-78255-185-0

Email: info@m-m-sports.com

www.thesportspublisher.com

CONTENTS

Preface 12

Introduction 16

1 Yoga – Significance and History 20
    1.1 Evolution of yoga as reflected in Indian spirituality 20
        1.1.1 High civilization in the Indus valley: 3000-1800 BC 21
        1.1.2 Vedism: 1500–1000 BC 21
        1.1.3 The Upanishads 22
        1.1.4 Brahmanism: 800–500 BC 22
        1.1.5 Sankhya: 800 BC–700 AD 22

    1.2 Time of the epics: 400 BC–400 AD 24
        1.2.1 Mahabharata, Ramayana, Bhagavadgita, Gita 24

    1.3 Classical yoga according to Patanjali: 200 BC–200 AD 25

    1.4 Tantrism: from 500 AD 25

    1.5 Hatha Yoga: from 900 AD 27

2 Classical yoga according to Patanjali 30
    2.1 Yoga Sutra 31
    2.2 Vrittis – mental waves 32
    2.3 Abhyasa and Vairagya – practice and letting go 32
    2.4 The five Kleshas – origins of grief and sorrow 33
    2.5 Ashtanga Marga 34
    2.6 Yamas and Niyamas 36

3 Hatha Yoga 42
    3.1 Western Hatha Yoga 43

4   The Gunas – basic forms of energy 46

     4.1   Nama Rupa – from essence to form 47

     4.2   The Mahabhutas – the five elements 48

         4.2.1 Maha = great / Bhuta = ghost 48

         4.2.2 The element earth (Prithlvi) 49

         4.2.3 The element water (Ap) 50

         4.2.4 The element fire (Tejas) 51

         4.2.5 The element air (Vayu) 52

         4.2.6 The element space / Ether (Akasha) 53

     4.3   Gunas – basic properties of nature 54

         4.3.1 Rajas Guna: fire, water, air 55

         4.3.2 Tamas Guna: earth, water 55

         4.3.3 Sativa Guna: space, air, fire (light) 56

     4.4   Triguna – interplay of the three Gunas 57

     4.5   The Gunas and the yoga practice 58

5   The chakra system 62

     5.1   Pancha Kosha – the five sheaths 62

     5.2   Pranamaya Kosha – the energy sheath 64

     5.3   Nadis – the energy pathways 66

     5.4   Kundalini Shakti 67

     5.5   The chakras 68

     5.6   The seven main chakras 69

         5.6.1 Muladhara chakra – root chakra 74

         5.6.2 Svadhisthana chakra – sacral chakra 77

         5.6.3 Manipura chakra – solar plexus chakra 80

         5.6.4 Anahata chakra – heart chakra 83

         5.6.5 Vishuddha chakra – throat chakra 86

         5.6.6 Ajna chakra – third eye chakra 89

         5.6.7 Sahasrara chakra – crown chakra 91

6   Significance and practice of Asana 96

     6.1   Significance 96

     6.2   Basic poses 98

     6.3   Directions of spinal movement 99

6.3.1 Based on their form and orientation in space 99
6.3.2 Based on their function 100
6.3.3 Based on the spine's direction of movement 102

6.4 General effects of Asanas 105

6.5 Structure and effects of Asanas 107
6.5.1 Structure and effects of the forward bend 107
6.5.2 Structure and effects of backbends 109
6.5.3 Structure and effects of side bends 110
6.5.4 Structure and effects of twists 110
6.5.5 Structure and effects of inversions 111

6.6 The practice of Asanas (alignment criteria) 112

6.7 The quality of Asanas 114

6.8 Static and dynamic Asana practice 114

6.9 To build up an Asana (from dynamic to static practice) 115

6.10 Importance of preparatory and introductory exercises 118

6.11 Karana – movement sequences 121

6.12 The three Bandhas – the body locks 121
6.12.1 Mula Bandha – root lock 121
6.12.2 Uddiyana Bandha – abdominal lock/upward lock 123
6.12.3 Jalandhara Bandha – throat lock 123

6.13 Injury risks/contraindications 124
6.13.1 Neck 126
6.13.2 Shoulders 128
6.13.3 Lumbar spine 128
6.13.4 Knees 130

7 The Asanas 134

7.1 Asana practice and props 134

7.2 About Asana descriptions 134

7.3 Individual Asanas 135
7.3.1 Adho Mukha Svanasana – Downward-Facing Dog 135
7.3.2 Alanasana – High lunge 141
7.3.3 Anjaney Asana – Low lunge 142
7.3.4 Apanasana – Knees-to-chest pose 146
7.3.5 Eka Pada Apana Asana – (Single) knee-to-chest pose 149
7.3.6 Ardha Matsyendrasana – Half Lord of the Fishes pose 152

7.3.7 Balasana – Child's pose/Utthita Balasana......................................156

7.3.8 Baddha Konasana – Bound Angle pose and ....
Upavistha Konasana – Wide-angle Seated Forward Bend 159

7.3.9 Bhujangasana – Cobra...163

7.3.10 Chaturanga Dandasana – Plank (Phalakasana) 167

7.3.11 Dandasana – Staff pose 171

7.3.12 Dhanurasana – Bow pose 174

7.3.13 Janu Shirsasana – Head-to-Knee Forward Bend 178

7.3.14 Makarasana – Crocodile pose 182

7.3.15 Marjaryasana – Cat pose 187

7.3.16 Navasana – Boat pose 191

7.3.17 Paschimottanasana – Seated Forward Bend 195

7.3.18 Prasarita Padottanansana – Standing Straddle Forward Bend........199

7.3.19 Setu Bandha Sarvangasana – Bridge pose 203

7.3.20 Shalabhasana – Locust pose 208

7.3.21 Shavasana – Corpse pose...212

7.3.22 Sukhasana – Easy pose 214

7.3.23 Supta Padangusthasana – Reclining Hand-to-Big-Toe pose...........218

7.3.24 Tadasana – Mountain pose...221

7.3.25 Urdhva Hastasana – Upward Hands pose...................................224

7.3.26 Urdhva Prasarita Padasana – Table pose....................................226

7.3.27 Uttanasana – Standing Forward Bend..229

7.3.28 Utthita Parshvakonasana – Extended Side Angle pose..................233

7.3.29 Utthita Trikonasana – Triangle pose..238

7.3.30 Utkatasana – Chair pose 244

7.3.31 Ustrasana – Camel pose...248

7.3.32 Vrikshasana – Tree pose 251

7.3.33 Virabhadrasana II – Warrior II pose...256

7.3.34 Viparita Karani – Legs-up-the-wall pose (Half shoulder stand).......261

8   Significance of Karana and Surya Namaskar....................................268

8.1   Karana/Vinyasa Flow 268

8.2   Surya Namaskar – Sun Salutation..269

8.2.1 Sun Salutation and mantras 270

8.2.2 Surya Namaskar modifications 272

9   Yogic breathing 280

9.1   Importance of breathing..280

9.2   The breath in everyday life 281

9.2.1 Breath awareness..282

9.2.2 Watching your breath..282

9.2.3 Awareness of breathing space...283

9.2.4 Directing the breath to different breathing spaces........................284

9.3 Complete breathing in yoga...286

9.4 Finding your own pace – breath flow practice.....................................288

9.5 Lengthening the breath..288

9.6 The Ujjayi breath...290

10 Relaxation...294

10.1 From absentmindedness to composure...294

10.2 The nervous system..295

10.2.1 Voluntary and vegetative nervous system..295

10.2.2 Performance state – sympathetic nervous system..............................295

10.2.3 Recovery state – parasympathetic nervous system...........................296

10.3 Stress...297

10.3.1 Eustress...298

10.3.2 Distress..299

10.4 Relaxation..299

10.5 Perception..300

10.6 Pratyahara – sense withdrawal...303

10.7 Samyama – the three higher paths...304

10.7.1 Dharana – concentration...305

10.7.2 Dhyana – meditation...306

10.7.3 Samadhi – fusion...306

11 Teaching yoga...310

11.1 What is yoga?...310

11.2 Planning a class...312

11.3 Structured and planned yoga instruction..313

11.3.1 Classroom conditions...313

11.3.2 Goal setting...315

11.3.3 Didactics and methods..316

11.3.4 Vinyasa Krama..317

11.4 Design and advantages of themed classes..319

11.5 Building a yoga class..320

11.6 Planning class content: guide to creating a lesson plan............................321
    11.6.1 Theme: "Improving breath and body awareness".................................321
    11.6.2 Classroom conditions...322
    11.6.3 General preparation...322
    11.6.4 Learning objectives..323
    11.6.5 Didactic considerations..323
    11.6.6 Methodological considerations...324
    11.6.7 Practice progression based on the principle of Vinyasa Krama.............325

12 Themed sample classes..334

12.1 Lesson plan 1: Finding your own pace..334

12.2 Lesson plan 2: The Muladhara chakra – grounding and stability.................339

12.3 Lesson plan 3: The Svadhisthana chakra – water, flow of movement, letting go..........348

12.4 Lesson plan 4: The Manipura chakra – fire, transformation, willpower.........355

12.5 Lesson plan 5: The Anahata chakra – air, expanse, spiritual center.............366

12.6 Lesson plan 6: The Vishuddha chakra – space, vibration, sound, voice, communication..........374

12.7 Lesson plan 7: The Ajna chakra – intuition, superior wisdom, polarities, inner center, light..........379

12.8 Lesson plan 8: The Sahasrara chakra – superior knowledge, superior consciousness.....387

13 Deep relaxation and visualization techniques...392

13.1 Suggestive and non-suggestive forms of relaxation.................................392
    13.1.1 Non-suggestive forms of relaxation...392
    13.1.2 Suggestive forms of relaxation...393

13.2 Imagination techniques..394

13.3 Yoga Nidra – yoga's healing sleep...395

13.4 Guide to relaxation and visualization techniques....................................396

13.5 Relaxation texts..398
    13.5.1 Whole-body relaxation based on body awareness...............................398
    13.5.2 Whole-body relaxation (autosuggestive guidance)..............................399
    13.5.3 Whole-body relaxation (suggestive guidance)....................................400
    13.5.4 Breathing relaxation...401
    13.5.5 Tree (Muladhara chakra)..402

13.5.6 Waterfall (Svadhisthana chakra)..404

13.5.7 Golden Temple (Manipura chakra)..405

13.5.8 Light in the Heart (Anahata chakra)...406

13.5.9 Cleansing exercise for the throat chakra (Vishuddha Chakra)..............407

13.5.10 Yoga Nidra (short form)...409

13.5.11 Journey through the chakras...411

Appendix

1 References...416

2 Credits..418

3 Portrait: Sara Lyn Chana (yoga model)...420

PREFACE

Yoga – the "gentle way of working the body and finding relaxation".

That is how the teaching about the oneness of all life has gained popularity in the West over the past 20 years.

This millennia-old practice from India has been credited with many positive effects on health and wellbeing, vitality, and mobility. The benefits are obvious. Interest in yoga classes at fitness studios and athletic facilities is correspondingly large. New styles of yoga have been and are constantly being created for the various target groups and their respective needs.

Inevitably, there are many misunderstandings as to the actual meaning and purpose of yoga. The interpretations and objectives of the different yoga styles are as varied as there are physical, emotional, social, creative, and spiritual needs.

The holistic teachings of YOGA facilitate many objectives. By definition, the term yoga indicates that ONENESS is the path and the goal.

Thus, the desire to stay healthy and fit and relax through simple movements that are conducive to rehabilitation and regeneration is just as valid as the urge to occasionally burn off energy through dynamic exercise sequences. To some extent, this already demonstrates yoga's intent to integrate polar opposites.

In doing so the actual intention of yoga, namely "quieting the cognitive-mental activity" (Patanjali, Yoga Sutra: *citta-vrtti-nirodha*) and practicing in the spirit of "detachedness" (*vairagya*), can easily be forgotten. After all, detachedness means that one practices yoga absent of concern for the past and future achievements. The centuries-old, even millennia-old yoga tradition was always about reconciling the intention of practicing and the lack of intention, two seemingly irreconcilable opposites. If we fail to question the performance that we find so often on the mats, the practice of yoga can no longer live up to its original meaning of ONENESS.

Yoga is not a random form of "trendy exercise" for the masses as the media likes to portray it. In fact, yoga is based on a mindset that should be cultivated and refined in silence so that its beneficial effects can truly take effect.

Ultimately, yoga's effectiveness does not depend on specific Asanas (physical poses) but primarily on mindfulness, inner calm, precision of execution, and the intention of the practitioner. Aspiring yoga instructors should focus in particular on developing their sense of sensitivity.

In this sophisticated foundational work, Martina Mittag has set herself to meeting all of these requirements. The book *Hatha Yoga* unveils the traditional teaching that from a philosophical point of view is often difficult for Westerners to understand.

In fact, yoga is a holistic empirical science with the goal of reconciling the seemingly opposite poles of body and consciousness, intellect and emotion, matter and spirit, and harmonizing them.

Hatha Yoga – the family name or umbrella term for all types of yoga based on the body's energy and the respective poses – begins with the physical experience, but while quietly holding an external pose, an inner mindset can develop that is focused, alert, and extremely sensitive.

Based on this understanding, the "body" in yoga isn't just the body but something comprehensive that includes subtle levels of energy, the mental and the spiritual. Thus, the integral approach of the Hatha Yoga practice goes well beyond the "modern", functional understanding of a "body workout".

In the 1970s/1980s, when yoga had not yet found its way into fitness studios and athletic facilities, this holistic view was still met with a complete lack of understanding in the West. It had an air of the exotic and mysterious. Staying in seemingly acrobatic poses without moving reminded many of the images of Indian ascetics on a bed of nails, an absurd image for modern man. Yoga enthusiasts were often met with suspicion as if they were followers of religious cults or at best they were derided as eccentric weirdoes.

But over the past 20 years, the image of yoga has gradually changed in the western world. Yoga became socially acceptable in Germany when adult education centers began to offer Hatha Yoga classes as part of their regular course schedule to promote and protect health.

At that time – in 1989 – I was asked to teach a yoga class at Club Meridian (later MeridianSpa) that would provide a balance between strictly physical exercise and a spiritual orientation. It was the first fitness business in Hamburg to place an unusually high degree of importance on medical fitness and ambience to provide its membership with the best conditions for regeneration and wellbeing.

Martina, dance instructor and fitness trainer, as well as area director of classes at MeridianSpa Wandsbek, attended my weekly yoga classes. Her unbiased, open attitude towards yoga and other alternative disciplines such as the Feldenkrais Method, Shiatsu, Tai Chi, and Qigong became apparent when she took over responsibility for conceiving, managing, and developing the "Spirit Center" in Wandsbek.

An active exchange took place over the course of increasing collaboration with Martina. After several yoga instructor training courses, she became a trainer for yoga instructors for the German Sports Association's VTF (Association for Gymnastics).

As a consultant and co-examiner, I had the opportunity to witness the superior quality she demanded from her aspiring yoga instructors.

Meanwhile, the demand for responsible health practices has increased in many businesses, whereby great importance is attached to the functionality of training methods. Detailed knowledge of anatomy is not only required of PE teachers but also of yoga instructors so that they are better able to assess their participants' abilities and capacities.

Martina has given lots of consideration to the active interplay between physical and cognitive-mental processes and thoroughly addressed the important aspects of the composition and effect of a pose, muscle function, the importance of breathing, and the inner attitude with respect to directing energy and consciousness. She also formulated the careful preparation, introduction, and execution of each Asana, its release, and follow-up sensation after each pose.

⧫ HATHA YOGA

In the opening chapters, Martina offers a philosophical overview of the sources of yoga, points out its major spiritual demands in terms of self-discovery and self-awareness, and offers a detailed description of the basic energy requirements within the Kosha system, the subtle body regions or realms of experience, and the chakras, the energy transformers within the etheric body.

In her description of the origin of individual Asanas, she takes into account the different key aspects of lines of tradition and thereby confirms a very generous, impartial view that makes it possible to assess the advantages and disadvantages of the effects of an exercise.

The precise, plainly illustrated instructions for 34 classic Asanas and different lesson plans that have been compiled from many different teaching units, offer extensive material to highly motivated yoga instructors for years of study, whereby both the scientific analytical side as well as intuitive creative abilities are being nurtured.

The reader is given detailed guidelines for structuring his classes that leaves nothing to be desired with respect to inspiration for different exercise sequences and specific analysis of all relevant aspects.

This primarily practice-oriented book is intended as a companion to yoga instructor training. Knowing full well that participants can't remember the entire training content of 200-500 hours of instruction, this book can also serve as a reference work to deepen knowledge on certain topics and provide the reader with the opportunity to incorporate the knowledge, in appropriate doses, into the respective class situations.

Kirti Peter Michel

Yoga instructor, instructor of psychosomatic health education, author

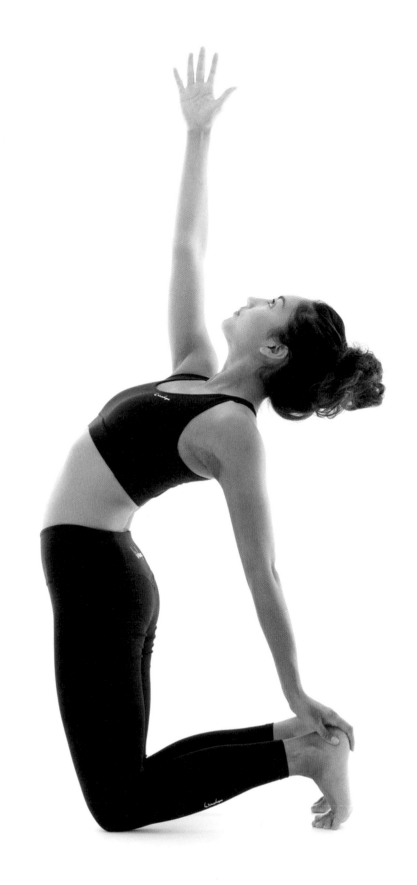

INTRODUCTION

This book provides an introduction to the fundaments of yoga for aspiring yoga instructors but also works as a well-researched reference work for those interested in all yoga traditions.

The content of this book includes the first 100 hours of the German Gymnastics Association yoga instructor training. It is based on classical yoga according to Patanjali and uses the *Ashtanga Marga*, the eightfold yoga path, as a guideline. This book also forms the basis for subsequent levels of the 500 total training hours, over the course of which additional philosophical systems and concepts are taught.

Since 2006, I have been the director of the VTF/DTB's yoga instructor training in Hamburg, which since its inception, I have played a decisive role in its design and conception. During my now nearly 12 years of yoga training experience, it has become obvious to me that during the process participants develop an increasingly deeper interest in living the yoga practice. Sometimes they start out with only cautious curiosity. Over the course of their training they tend to develop a deep affection for yoga combined with a desire to learn more. The individual training modules are very dense in terms of theoretical and practical content and require processing of and immersion in the material between modules. It was from these circumstances that this book emerged.

This guide focuses on Hatha Yoga's energy concept and its practical implementation. The reader will receive an introduction in the chakra system, and complete lesson plans provide the readers with opportunities to personally experience and implement the content. The 34 most common yoga poses are explained with respect to their correct alignment, symbolism, execution, as well as preparatory and introductory exercises, which in turn provides a sound background for the lesson plans.

This book provides aspiring yoga instructors with a detailed manual on how to create a lesson plan, taking into account didactic and methodological aspects. The participant and his needs take priority at all times. People do not have to adapt to yoga, rather yoga is adapted to the respective target groups. A beginning yoga practitioner does not require certain prerequisites such as flexibility, motor skills, or strength. The practice is not oriented to yoginis and yogis with perfect bodies who accomplish seemingly impossible feats in breathtaking "poses", but it wants to encourage people to feel comfortable attending a yoga class, especially if they don't feel particularly fit or feel very stressed.

Teaching is a dynamic process. Every teacher is also a student. The longer you do yoga, the deeper you immerse yourself in the contents and always discover new aspects. As I was writing the individual chapters, I became aware over and over again how varied, profound, and insightful engaging with the individual topics really is. The book is an invitation to take a look at yourself in the mirror of the millennia-old and still highly relevant wisdom of yoga, and to recognize and embrace your own needs, essential features, and qualities in the yoga light.

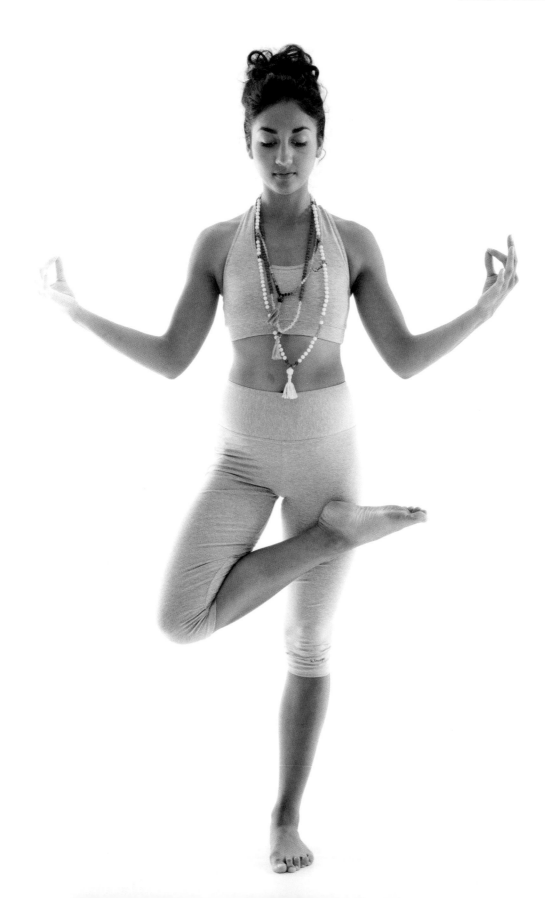

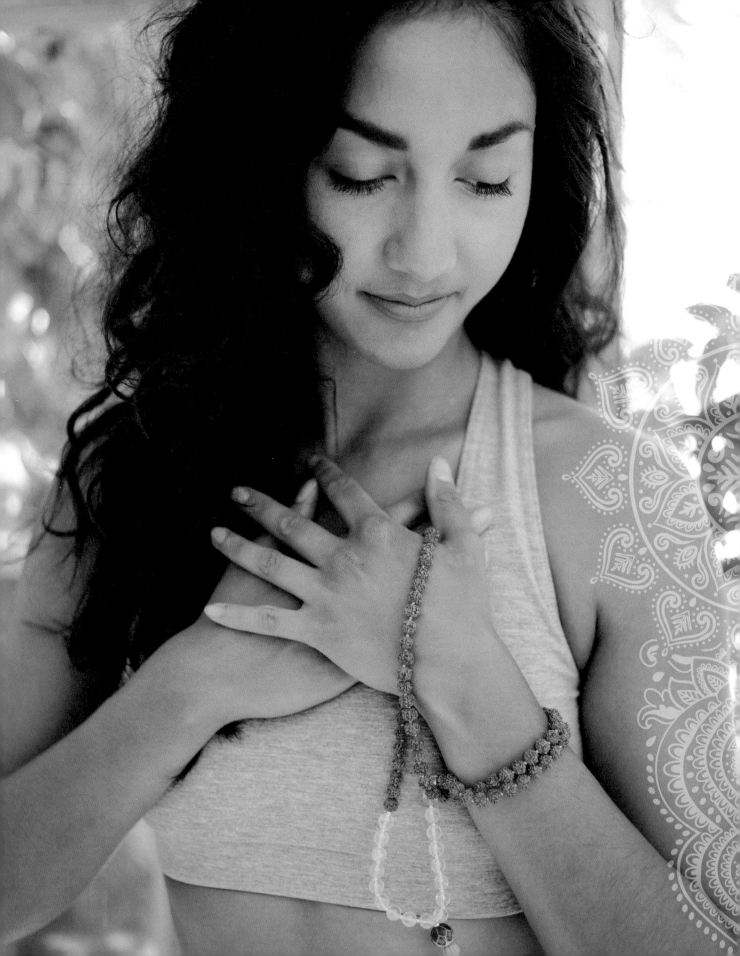

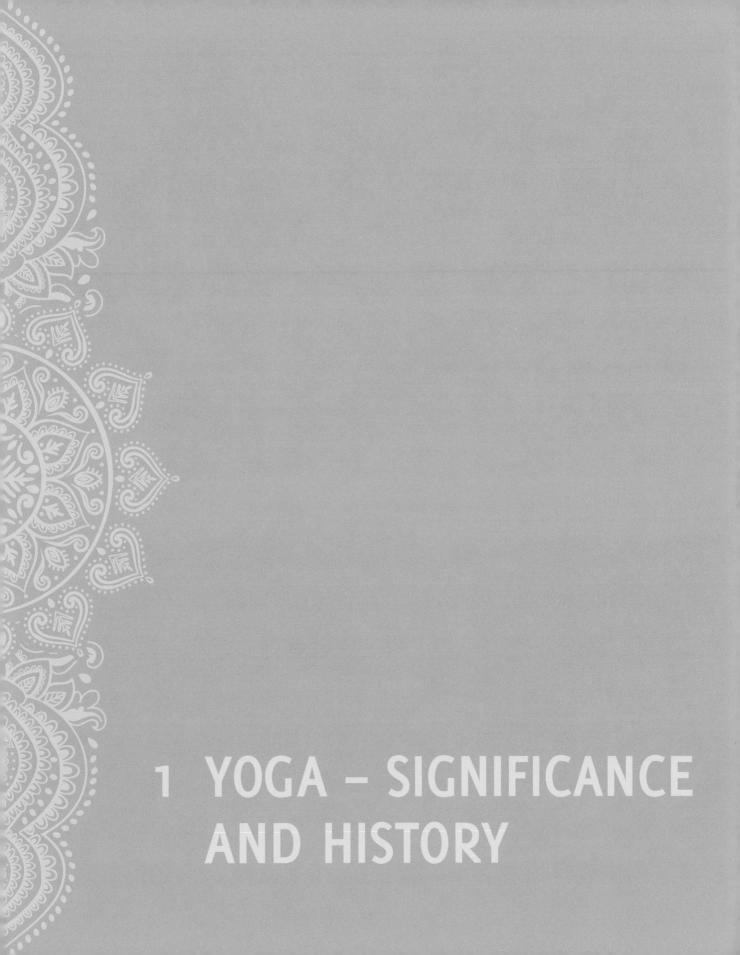

1 YOGA – SIGNIFICANCE AND HISTORY

1 YOGA – SIGNIFICANCE AND HISTORY

"THE STATE OF ONENESS"

"AS I WAS WRITING THE INDIVIDUAL CHAPTERS, I BECAME AWARE OVER AND OVER AGAIN HOW VARIED, PROFOUND, AND INSIGHTFUL ENGAGING WITH THE INDIVIDUAL TOPICS REALLY IS."

Yoga is considered one of the oldest practice regimens in human history still being practiced today. Yoga is comprised of different spiritual paths and systems intended to help people achieve the yogic state, oneness.

The Sanskrit word *yoga* means *unification, connection*. It comes from the root word *yui*, which means to *harness, unite, connect*, but also to yoke. Etymologically, yoga refers to the German word "Joch"[1] (yoke). It refers to the individual's connection and unification with his universal primal force. The universal primal force is also referred to as "the Absolute", "the One", "the Source of all Being", or the "Divine Source".

Yoga means an individual's state that is rooted in his true existence. The yoga practice focuses exclusively on achieving awareness that involves the integration of heart, mind, body, and spirit.

1.1 EVOLUTION OF YOGA AS REFLECTED IN INDIAN SPIRITUALITY

The evolution of yoga is a process that stretches over centuries and millennia. Summarizing it in just a few sentences does not even remotely do justice to the topic's complexity. Since this reference and practice book focuses on Hatha Yoga, the following overview includes only basic information to provide a rough outline of the overall system and its contexts. The book's appendix provides and overview of the more detailed literature on the evolution of yoga.

---

1 Huchzermeyer, W. (2006, 6th edition. 2015). The Yoga Dictionary, Sanskrit terms and definitions, practice styles, biographies. (Pg. 226) Karlsruhe: W. Huchzermeyer Publishing

1.1.1 HIGH CIVILIZATION IN THE INDUS VALLEY: 3000-1800 BC

The history of yoga can be traced back to approx. 3000-5000 BCE. There is debate about the exact date. Some writings estimate the age of seals discovered in the Indus valley (today's Northwest India) as approx. 3500 BCE, others even as far back as 5000 BCE.

The seals show symbols that depict yoga poses (seated poses). One of the most famous images is "Muhlabandhasana", an Asana that affects the root center (Muladhara) in the lower pelvic area and is said to direct energy.

During the early Indus culture, people revered the female energy (Shakti force) as the Mother of all Life, placed the feminine principle above the male. The invasion of Indo-Aryans beginning around 1500 BCE, in Northwestern India ended Shaktism.

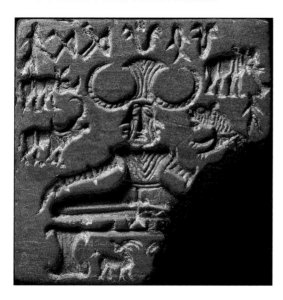

Fig. 1: This seal from the Indus valley shows yoga poses (seated poses), here the "Muhlabandhasana".

1.1.2 VEDISM: 1500-1000 BC

India's oldest texts are the Vedas. They are considered the source texts of yoga, as well as the foundation of Hinduism. *Veda* means *knowledge*. According to tradition, the "Rishis" (wise, holy men) received these texts during meditation. They are referred to as "Shruti" texts, which means "not created by man". These collections of texts (Samhitas) consist largely of hymns and mantras of which the *Rigveda-Samhita* is the oldest and most famous. For centuries, these texts were passed down orally.

The era of Vedas was characterized by deep religious beliefs and a close relationship with nature. Deities like Indra (king of the gods, thunder), Agni (fire), Surya (sun) and Vayu (wind) were worshipped and were presented with different sacrificial rituals, and loving veneration was expressed in the form of chants, sacrifice sayings, and sacred actions. But the Rigveda also says:

"Truth is ONE, though the wise men refer to it in many different ways." (Rigveda,1.164.46).

1.1.3   THE UPANISHADS

The *Upanishads* are the most recent and the final portion of the Vedas. The era of external, sacred, and ritual actions ended with the beginning of the Upanishads. *Upanishad* means *to sit close, to be close to the truth*, intending to sit at the feet of an enlightened teacher and receive guidance.[2]

The Upanishads are part of the Shruti texts, but they have a distinctly different character. While the Vedas emphasize the external physical world, the Upanishads focus on internalization and the meditative experience of the reality that is the basis of life.

"Hidden within the heart of every living creature there exists the Self, subtler than the most subtle, greater than the greatest." (Katha Upanishad, I.2.20[3]).

1.1.4   BRAHMANISM: 800-500 BC

Old Vedic poems, the Brahmanas, are thought to be the basis. The Brahmans, the caste of priests and scholars, played an important role. As experts on sacrifices and rituals, the occupied a key position and were considered intermediaries between humans and gods. But in Brahmanism the Vedic gods, like Agni, Indra, Vayu, lost their importance.

Brahman means *growing*, stretching, that which stretches, bursting into growth[4]. Brahmanism is based on the teaching of *Atman* and *Brahman*, which was already couched in the Upanishads. *Atman* is the individual soul, man's true self. Brahman is the world soul, the dynamic principle that is behind all appearances. Brahman is not an individual god but the cosmic substance, the source of everything. Atman is the cosmic, divine spark in a human being.

Significant groundwork for the Indian religions was laid during this time, like the concepts of *Maya* (the world as we know it is an illusion), *Karma* (consequence of an action), *Samasara* (flow, cycle of reincarnations), and *Moksha* (redemption, spiritual relief).

"The Self is truly Brahman, but out of ignorance people identify it as the intellect, the mind, the senses, passions, and the elements earth, water, air, space, and fire". (Brihadaranyaka-Upanishad, 4.5).[5]

1.1.5   SANKHYA: 800 BC-700 AD

The original *Sankhya system* (pronounced Sum-khya) is traced back to the wise man Kapila. It is a spiritual-cosmic evolutionary theory that has greatly influenced a large part of Indian spirituality.

---

2 Easwaran, E. (2008, 4th edition). *The Upanishads* (pg. 16) Munich: Goldmann
3 Easwaran, E., pg.125.
4 Easwaran, E., pg. 419.
5 Easwaran, E., pg. 70.

Sankhya means *number*. The universe and everything in it is listed via 25 Tattvas (guiding principles, existence factors). The Purusha principle (pure consciousness, amorphous mind) and *Prakriti* (the sum of all tangible and ethereal natural appearances) are important parts of Sankhya philosophy. Classic, systematized Sankhya implies a dualistic worldview.

THE 25 TATTVAS ARE:

1) **Purusha** – amorphous mind, the silent witness, the Self,

2) **Prakriti** – active, primordial nature,

3) **Buddhi** – cosmic, higher intelligence,

4) **Ahamkara** – "ego maker", awareness of the Self,

5) **Manas** – the thinking intellect, tied to the senses,

6-10) **Jnanendriyas** – the perceiving and cognitive senses: smell, taste, sight, touch, hearing,

11-15) **Karmendriyas** – working senses: walking, excretion, procreation, grasping, speaking,

16-20) **Tanmatras** – the ethereal elements: sound, touch, form, taste, smell,

21-25) **Mahabhutas** – the great elements: space, air, fire, water, earth.

The systematic listing is meant to facilitate better understanding of the structure of the universe and the mind. Apprehending all of these aspects of reality requires acute observation combined with an extremely refined perception.

Anna Trökes describes three major stages in the evolution of the Sankhya theory:[6]

» **Early Sankhya precursor from 800-100 BC**
The early forms of Sankhya have a theistic focus. According to Trökes, the principal goal of liberating knowledge is for the individual to understand his innermost reality as a reflection of and sharing in the absolute or the divine, and most of all, to experience himself in this sharing.

» **Systematic Sankhya and classic Sankhya from 500 BC-450 AD**
This way of thinking is atheistic. Classic Sankhya does not include reciprocal penetration of Purusha (the essence) and Prakriti (nature). It is a dualistic worldview.

One of the key assertions of classic Sankhya philosophy is: "The innermost being should not be confused with nature, the world of appearances."[7]

6 Trökes, A. (2013). *Die kleine Yoga Philosophie.* (pg. 150-166). Munich: O. W. Barth.
7 Michel, K. P. & Wellmann, W. (2003). *Das Yoga der Fünf Elemente.* (pg. 45.) Bern: Scherz Verlag.

According to the Sankhya perspective, sorrow and pain exist only on the Prakriti level. Identifying with Prakriti is a delusion, and it is important to realize that Purusha and Prakriti are not one.

» **Vedantization of Sankhya and its end as a separate system**
During the final phase, the original idea of oneness comes into effect once more.

The basic elements of Sankhya theory are found in the *Bhagavadgita*, in Patanjali's *Yoga Sutra*, and also in *Tantrism*, each in modified form.

1.2   TIME OF THE EPICS: 400 BC – 400 AD

1.2.1   MAHABHARATA, RAMAYANA, BHAGAVADGITA, GITA

The *Mahabharata* and the *Ramayana* are India's great national epics. The Ramayana describes the life of the hero Rama and his wife Sita[8] in 24,000 double verses. *Maha* means great. The *Mahabharata* tells the story of the Bharatas in 10,000 double verses.

The *Bhagavadgita* (the song of the sublime) is embedded in the *Mahabharata* as a sixth chapter. It is a spiritual poem and a timeless teaching document consisting of 18 chapters with 701 verses.

The *Gita* is a spiritual instruction in which *Krishna* (the sublime) explains the yoga pathways to the warrior Arjuna, who is floundering. Krishna came to earth during a dark time as a friend to men to lead the to a new consciousness.

The Gita's narrative framework is an imminent fight between two related families, which is preceded by a long-standing conflict. This conflict represents the conflict of a person inside of whom the enlightening mental faculties fight the dark forces of the ego for supremacy. The highly symbolic story reveals that light and shadow are not neatly separated from each other. There is always an aspect of darkness in light, and an aspect of light in darkness.

The different yoga pathways Krishna shows are not mutually exclusive. They imply that it is possible for every person to also follow the yoga pathways in everyday life according to their individual predisposition.

» Jnana Yoga as the path of knowledge, wisdom, enlightenment;
» Dhyana Yoga as the path of meditation, immersion;
» Karma Yoga as the path of action, acting selflessly;
» Bhakti Yoga as the path of love, reverence, devotion.

8 Huchzermeyer, W. (2015, pg. 157).

"It is better to fulfill one's own law of action (swadharma) even if it is flawed, than the law of another even if it is perfect. Suffering death while abiding by one's own essential law is preferable. Following another's essential law is dangerous."[9] *(Yoga des Handelns, chapter III, verse 35)*.

1.3 CLASSICAL YOGA ACCORDING TO PATANJALI: 200 BC-200 AD

The *Yoga Sutras* by Patanjali are combinations and restatements of philosophical source texts. The sutras are considered a guideline and one of the most important standard works of modern yoga. In chapter 2 the yoga sutras are explained in more detail.

"Yoga is that inner state in which emotional-cognitive processes come to rest."[10]
(YS, I, 2).

1.4 TANTRISM: FROM 500 AD

Tan means *stretching, stretching oneself*. The term *Tantra* is translated as *fabric* or *mesh*. On the one hand this could refer to the spreading of the Tantric theory as a major movement that stretches across entire segments of society such as low castes or women. This applies particularly to groups of people who had previously been denied an active role in spirituality without a participating priest (Brahmans).

But it is more likely that the term *Tantra* refers to the supposed inseparable connection between macrocosm (the world at large, the entire universe) and microcosm (small world in its tiny components). The Tantric theory assumes that everything is inseparably connected via the energy plane. The small mirrors the large, and vice-versa. Thus everything that happens in the universe affects the whole since everything is interwoven.

In Indian spirituality Tantrism is considered a revolutionary movement. Tantrism was preceded by long phases of asceticism during which everything worldly had to be defeated. As a result, the human body with all its functions was seen as impure, particularly the female body, and sexuality.

Anna Trökes says about the Tantric revolution: "An important part of the theory was the acknowledgement that the divine can reveal itself in all its perfection in every possible form. Under this point of view the old categories of pure/impure, in which the social order and caste system had solidified over centuries, broke down."[11]

9   Aurobindo, S. (1981). *Bhagavadgita*. chapter. III, verse 35. Gladenbach: Hinder + Deelmann Publishing.
10 Bäumer, B. & Deshpande, P. Y. (1976, 6th edition, 1990). *Patanjali. Die Wurzeln des Yoga*. (pg. 21). Bern: Scherz Verlag.
11 Trökes, A. (2013, pg. 236).

One of Tantrism's basic principles is to revere nature with all its diverse appearances and to experience it with all of one's senses. Instead of strict asceticism, Tantrism now advocated for joy, ritual pleasure, sensuality, and an attitude that embraces life and nature as a basis for spiritual growth.

The many physical rituals and practices are spiritual means on the path to liberation. The core of the theory is to unite the cosmic consciousness (*Shiva/Purusha*, the male principle) with the cosmic energy (*Shakti/Prakriti*, the female principle). The significance of Shakti as both a dynamic creative principle and the divine mother plays a central role in Tantrism. The knowledge surrounding the subtle energy centers (chakras), energy pathways (Nadis), Mudras (energy seals with the body), directing of energy (the rise of the Kundalini Shakti), breath control, reciting mantras (vibration and sound), and visualization techniques are principal elements of Tantrism.

There are different Tantric directions such as *white*, *red*, and *black Tantra*. The *white Tantra*, also referred to as the *right path*, consists of the above-mentioned elements of the cosmic principle and devotion to the divine primal force, the theory of energy and its practices to raise energy levels.

The *red Tantra*, also referred to as the left path, includes energy practices for the sublimation of sexual energy. In the western world, this Tantra arm is often erroneously reduced to sexual pleasure and thought to be the entire teaching.

The *black Tantra* works with magical formulas and mantras and is about manipulation and control, similar to black magic.

When someone enters into the state of divine energy, a meditation that knows no distinction, he becomes one with the nature of Shiva, because the opening of Shiva is called Shakti. Much as one recognizes parts of a room by the light of a lamp or the rays of the sun, one recognizes Shiva by his energy."[12]
(Vijnana Bhairava, verse 20-21).

12 Bäumer, B. (2013, third edition). *Vijnana Bhairava. Divine Consciousness.* (pg. 67). Frankfurt: Insel Publishing.

1.5 HATHA YOGA: FROM 900 AD

Until the beginning of Tantrism, yoga in all its forms was viewed as world renunciation. Most important was to overcome suffering. Hatha Yoga that focuses on the body during the spiritual practice historically came from the Tantric tradition. Instead of overcoming the body as was done previously, the body now became the focus of the practice. See chapter 3.

"Wearing a special dress is not a way to achieve perfection, and neither is talking about yoga: the exercises alone are the means to achieving perfection; that is without a doubt true."
(Hatha-Yoga-Pradipika, verse 66). [13]

---

13 Svatmarama, S. (2009). *Hatha-Yoga-Pradipika. Light on Hatha Yoga.* (pg. 47). Hamburg: Phänomen Publishing.

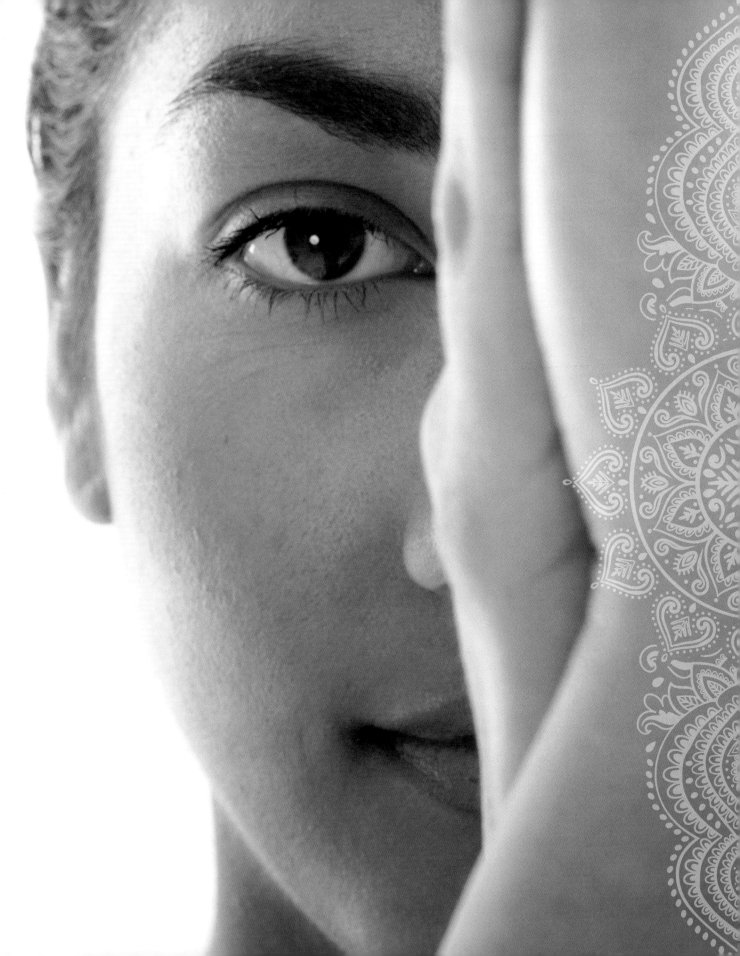

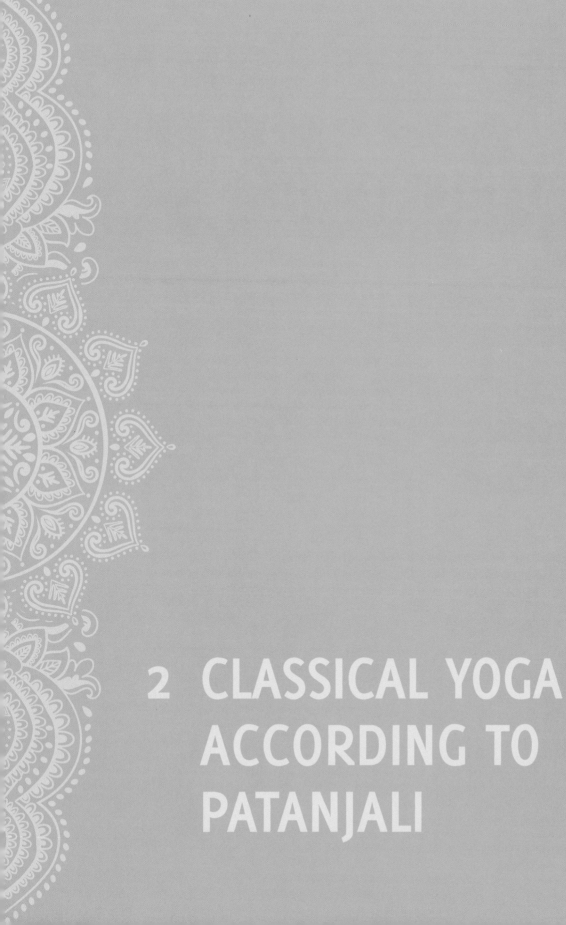

2 CLASSICAL YOGA ACCORDING TO PATANJALI

2 CLASSICAL YOGA ACCORDING TO PATANJALI

Often people initially associate the word yoga with certain body postures. One might imagine an Indian yogi doing a headstand or sitting deep in thought in a meditative pose. Or one thinks of relaxation exercises, breathing exercises, or a sweat-inducing practice on the yoga mat. Hardly anyone thinks of it as psychological work that explains the function of the human mind and mentions only one yoga pose.

The *Yoga Sutra* of *Patanjali*, on whose content much of this book is based, is a summary of significant pathways from yoga philosophy and also their essence. The Sutras include elements and concepts from Sankhya philosophy as well as from Vedanta, Buddhism, and tantric philosophy.

The *Yoga Sutra* of Patanjali is the basis for classical yoga and is considered the foundational work. We don't know who Patanjali really was. It is assumed that he was active somewhere between 200 BCE and 200 CE.[14] His aphorisms have been summarized in the form of verses, in the so-called *Sutras*. *Sutra* means *thread* or *guideline*. The Sutra style is an extremely compact form of a text with a very large body of content. Since these texts and their tradition were handed down for centuries via memorization, due to their volume, they were written down in the form of short memorable theorems. Over time, reading the Sutras has resulted in a plethora of interpretations, explanations, and commentaries. Most commentators refer primarily to the Sutra interpretations by the wise man Vyasa, who lived in the fifth century CE.

Patanjali is also called the "father of classical yoga". At the South Indian Nataraj temple in Chidambaram, which is dedicated to the dancing god Shiva, there is a sacred place that is revered as Patanjali's work site. Here Patanjali is depicted as a hybrid creature, part snake and part human, whereby the coiled up snake forms the lower body. In Hindu mythology the snake is a symbol for wisdom and healing. The spiral shape is a reminder that all of human and spiritual history is like a spiral. We continuously pass through cycles of becoming and passing, the snake's shedding of its skin.

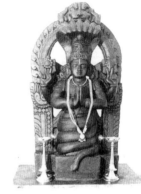

Fig. 2: Patanjali

---

14 Trökes, A. (2013, pg. 167).

2.1   YOGA SUTRA

The *Yoga Sutra* consists of a total of 195 verses divided into four chapters.

The first four Sutras are among the most quoted because their content summarizes the essence of Patanjali's entire treatise.

It is typical for the Sutra style to place the essence of the entire tenet at the beginning.

Sutra I.1 "atha yoga anusasam"
Here now follows the yoga discipline.

Sutra I.2 "yogas chitta-vritti-nirodhah"
"Yoga is that inner state in which emotional-cognitive processes come to rest" (Bäumer & Deshpande)".[15]
"Yoga is the coming to rest of the constantly changing mental patterns". (Skuban).[16]

Sutra I.3 "tada drashtuh svarupe avasthanam"
"The sighted one then rests in his essential identity" (Bäumer & Deshpande).
"The sighted one then rests within himself: this is self-realization" (Skuban).

Sutra I.4 "vritti-saruyam itarata"
"All other inner states are caused by identifying with the emotional-cognitive processes" (Bäumer & Deshpande).

"At other times, when we are not in a state of self-realization, the sighted one takes on the shape of the mental patterns (vrittis); It seems as though they are identical" (Skuban).

At the outset, Patanjali explains the state we could be in. He places the goal, meaning the result of the practice, right at the beginning. Yoga means being in the "now" (atha), in a mental state (chitta) in which the everyday, constantly present and ever changing mental patterns (vrittis) dissolve and give way to a state of powerful stillness.

But since this is not easy for most people to do, in what follows the Sutras give a very plausible explanation of how the human mind works, which obstacles there are along the way and how to deal with them. Engaging with the Yoga Sutras is supposed to help us better understand ourselves and act accordingly.

15 Bäumer & Deshpande (1990, pg. 37).
16 Skuban, R. (2011). *Patanjalis Yoga Sutra. The Regal Path to a Wise Life.* (pg. 18). Munich: Arkana.

2.2 VRITTIS – MENTAL WAVES

Vritti – roles, swirl, wave, mental-cognitive activity

The Vrittis are a part of Chitta (spirit, psyche). They are part of the workings of our mind, but when the Vrittis are unconsciously or unintentionally working inside us –and that is generally the case – they can become distressing. That is when we find ourselves in an endless string of internal actions and reactions.

Patanjali explains five types of mental patterns that can either be full of anguish or devoid of anguish.

1. *Pramana* – real knowledge (perception of reality, logical derivation, passed down through reliable sources).

2. *Viparyaya* – false knowledge (fallacy, delusion, perceiving that which does not exist).

3. *Vikalpa* – imaginings (a perception that is not in line with reality, imagination).

4. *Nidra* – Deep sleep (lethargic mental state, absence of any impressions).

5. *Smriti* – memories (impressions that were created in the past and are still present).

We are unable to completely escape the movements of the mind, but we can learn to observe them and to differentiate, and learn to become aware of the unconscious Vrittis, so they will lose their power over us.

The Indian scholar and Hindu monk Swami Vivekananda (1836-1902), who was the first Hindu to give an attention-getting speech in front of the Word's Parliament of Religions in Chicago in 1893, summarizes the link between Chitta, Vritti, and the Self as follows:

"We cannot see the bottom of a lake when the surface is moving. Only when the little waves have subsided and the water is still are we able to see the bottom. When the water is muddy and in constant motion we cannot see the bottom, but we can when the water is clear and there are no waves. The bottom of the lake is our true self, the lake is Chitta and the waves are Vrittis." (Swami Vivekananda).

2.3 ABHYASA AND VAIRAGYA – PRACTICE AND LETTING GO

Abhyasa = continuous practice, repetition / *Vairagya* = letting go, not being held

Becoming aware of our Vrittis, perceiving and observing them to finally let them go, requires practice. *Abhyasa* means that we regularly practice achieving a state of mental stillness. Closely linked is *Vairagya*, the conscious letting go of thoughts, impressions, wishes, or dislikes that keep our mental experiences in motion.

There are many different obstacles on the yoga path. Patanjali attributes them to "Vasanas", "Samskaras", and the "five Kleshas" among other things.

Vasanas (imagination, impression, memory) are latent impressions in our subconscious in the form of hidden desires and ambitions.[17]

Closely linked are the Samskaras, the countless impressions our daily thoughts, actions and emotions leave behind in our mind. The Samskara can be compared to paths or trails that run every which way in our consciousness, though most of them are hidden in our subconscious. The more often we think a certain thought, complete a certain action, or certain emotions manifest themselves in us, the bigger and wider these paths grow until finally they are broad streets. When new thoughts, emotions, or actions are added they initially are only individual tracks in the sand that peter out if they are not repeated. If we want to develop new habits or behavior patterns it requires regular repetition so we form new impressions, Samskaras.

2.4 THE FIVE KLESHAS – ORIGINS OF GRIEF AND SORROW

Klesha = evil, pain, torment, plague

Patanjali names five different causes of inner tension or grief. Ultimately all conflicts and problems can be attributed to these five Kleshas.

1. **Avidya**
   Ignorance or lack of understanding, lack of knowledge. Avidya is the main cause of all suffering. This means that man is not aware of his true nature, the essence of his Self. We see what is real as unreal, and the unreal (the impermanent) as truth.

2. **Asmita**
   Self-attachment. We identify with the impermanent, the body, thoughts, emotions, our abilities and inclinations, our character and possessions. And aspects of our personality that we learn about through our education and feedback from others (family, teachers, friends). This also includes roles we take on over the course of our life, e.g. the successful one, the loser, the diligent one, the lazy one, the intelligent one, etc.

3. **Raga**
   Passion, intense longing, wants, desire, greed. The more we want something, the more restless the mind gets. When we desperately wish for something, it can completely permeate our spirit. At the same time the joy that results from fulfillment of purely material desires is usually short-lived. And subsequently the desire becomes increasingly greater and the wants bigger. Here true joy is easily confused with quickly fading pleasures.

---

17 Huchzermeyer, W. (2015, pg. 210).

4. **Dvesha**

   Dislike, rejection, not wanting, hate. The human spirit constantly vacillates between the polarities of good and bad, pleasant and unpleasant, sorrow and no sorrow. At the same time we also often reject things that are unfamiliar to us, and which we assume to be uncomfortable because the known is more familiar and gives us a sense of security.

5. **Abhinivesha**

   Clinging to life, mortality, thirst for life, self-preservation. Ultimately Abhinivesha is the primal fear all fears are based on, the fear of physical death and the process of dying, which is deeply rooted in the human spirit. Making ourselves aware of the nature of impermanence and remembering that all life is a process of becoming and ceasing to be, and that our true, cosmic self is immortal can help us mitigate the fear.

According to Patanjali, the Kleshas are the cause for accumulated karma that was accumulated in a previous or in this life. Patanjali advises dissolving the distressing tensions by focusing on the opposite as well as meditation.

Viveka – differentiation

To remove the Kleshas, it is necessary to develop *Viveka*, the ability to differentiate, to recognize when a Klesha is at work. It is about distinguishing what is real from what is not real.

Sadhana

The term *Sadhana* comes from the root word *sadh*, which means moving straight towards a goal. *Pada* means *foot*, but also *step*, *stride*, or *footprint*. Sadhana is the spiritual discipline that leads us incrementally towards our higher goals. In the course of the Yoga Sutra, Patanjali shows us a methodical path that we can effectively follow, step-by-step, rung-by-rung.

2.5 ASHTANGA MARGA

Ashta = eight / *Anga* = link / *Marga* = way, path

Yogasutra, 2.29 >yama-niyama-asana-pranayama-pratyahara-dharana-dhyana-samadhi<

In this brief sutra lies a complete and practical path intended to help us manage obstacles and the causes of sorrow to achieve "yogash-chitta-vritta-nirodha".

What is often referred to as the *eightfold way* or *path* can also be viewed as a circle or chain, because it is not imperative to begin with the Yamas and the Niyamas (yoga ethics).

Yoga practitioners in the West usually find their path to the yoga practice via the *Asanas*, the *physical poses*. As focus, perception, mindfulness, and breath awareness develop over time, so does one's behavior with respect to environment and one's own life evolve. It is therefore not necessary and actually rather more of a hindrance to strictly follow an external set of rules when the inner self is not yet ready. The deeper understanding, regardless of where one's path begins, will set in once all of the steps or links have been integrated into the practice at the same pace as the evolution of the inner self.

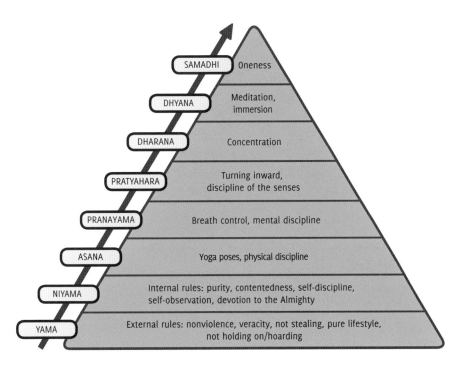

Fig. 3: The eightfold plan

1. Yama – dealing with our environment

2. Niyama – dealing with ourselves

3. Asana – body posture

4. Pranayama – breath control

5. Pratyahara – pulling back (controlling) the senses

6. Dharana – working on the ability to focus

7. Dhyana – meditation, internalization

8. Samadhi – superconsciousness

The first four levels are referred to as the outer links, and the subsequent steps are the inner links.

Samyama (concentration, taming, domination) refers to the mastering of the final three levels Dharana, Dhyana, and Samadhi.

2.6 YAMAS UND NIYAMAS

Each of the five *Yamas* and *Niyamas* are considered to be a code of conduct for dealing with our environment and ourselves. Here it is not about blindly adhering to rules but rather about developing behaviors based on inner knowledge that keep the likelihood of external and internal conflict as low as possible.

1. YAMA – DEALING WITH OUR ENVIRONMENT

Yama means *repression*, and the term is also equated with external discipline. The Yamas are ethical guidelines and mean "to act responsibly with respect to our environment."

» **Ahimsa = not causing injury, non-violence**
In many yoga traditions, *Ahimsa* is equated with not killing and eating animals. Furthermore Ahimsa also means not causing harm to humans, be it through deed, words, or thoughts.

» **Satya = veracity, authenticity**
Satya refers to an honest and authentic lifestyle. It means to forego deliberate lying, cheating, and dishonesty, and to act according to the inner truth.

» **Asteya = not stealing, being content with what one has**
Taking possession of material or spiritual things that belong to other people results in sorrow and conflict, and it is important to avoid this, as well as desire with respect to the property of others.

» **Aparigraha = not hording, lack of possessions**
Hoarding or amassing possessions can, on the one, hand trigger desires in other people and, on the other hand, much of the accumulated property can turn out to be baggage that consumes energy.

» **Brahmacharya = austerity, chastity**
Brahmacharya means a lifestyle in accordance with Brahman. Traditionally this refers to sexual abstinence for Swamis (monks). An overly sexual or hedonistic lifestyle (or the respective fantasies) severely disrupts inner peace.

2. NIYAMA – DEALING WITH OURSELVES

Niyama is translated as *self-control* or *repression* and refers to inner discipline. They are guidelines that facilitate inner clarity and focus on the yoga path.

» **Sauca = cleanliness, inner purity**
In addition to external physical cleanliness, *Sauca* refers to the release of impure energy or thoughts. The practice of Asana and Pranayama as well as self-observation and all forms of concentration and meditation facilitate inner purity.

» **Santosha = contentedness**
Contentedness means accepting life conditions as they are. Getting lost in complaining and discontent creates an inner climate of rejection and separation. A content, grateful, and accepting inner attitude facilitates spiritual growth.

» **Tapas = discipline, transformation, inner fire**
Tapas means *cleansing*, *transformation*, but also *discipline*. Tapas refers to a steady, gently smoldering inner fire which provides the strength to stay on the spiritual path, particularly in difficult situations or phases of life. Tapas also means discipline. We need discipline to liberate ourselves especially from stubborn habits or identifications that impede inner growth.

» **Svadhyaya = self-observation, self-exploration**
To feel the effects of the Vrittis, it is necessary to gain some inner distance. That means learning self-observation, to recognize the automatic inner action-reaction patterns. But *Svadhyaya* also means reading and engaging with educational spiritual texts.

» **Ishvara Pranidhana = devotion to the Highest/to God**
Ishvara means the *highest Lord*. Different spiritual systems agree that "the Highest" is present in the spiritual heart. This could refer to the inner light or a power that is greater than oneself. Contrary to classical Sankhya philosophy, which does not subscribe to this principle, Patanjali explicitly mentions devotion to the Highest.

3. ASANA – BODY POSITION

➔ This level will be explained in detail in chapters 6 and 7.

4. PRANAYAMA – BREATH CONTROL

➔ See explanations in chapter 9.

5. PRATYAHARA – PULLING BACK (CONTROLLING) THE SENSES

➔ See chapter 10.

6. DHARANA – WORKING ON THE ABILITY TO FOCUS

➔ See chapter 10.

7. DHYANA – MEDITATION, INTERNALIZATION

→ See chapter 10.

8. SAMADHI – STATE OF ABSORPTION, MEDITATIVE PEAK EXPERIENCE[18]

Samadhi is the highest level of the eightfold path of the Ashtanga Marga. *Samadhi* is referred to as *superconsciousness*, *absorption*, *ecstasy*, or *conscious oneness*.

In the first chapter of the Yoga Sutras, verses 1.17 and 1.18 (Samadhi), Patanjali explains the two levels of Samadhi, which are subdivided into different aspects. A more detailed explanation of the aspects can be found in chapter 3 (Vibhuti Pada/ disengagement) and chapter 4 (Kaivalya Pada/liberation).

---

18 Skuban, R. (2011, pg . 342).

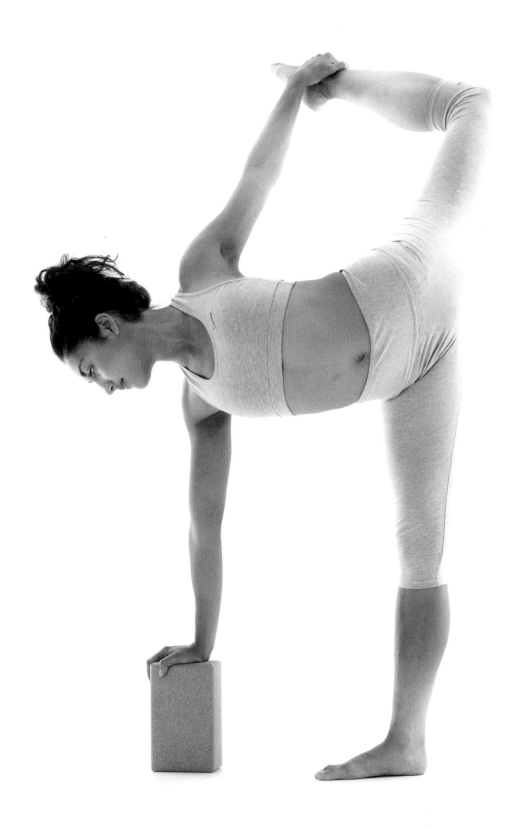

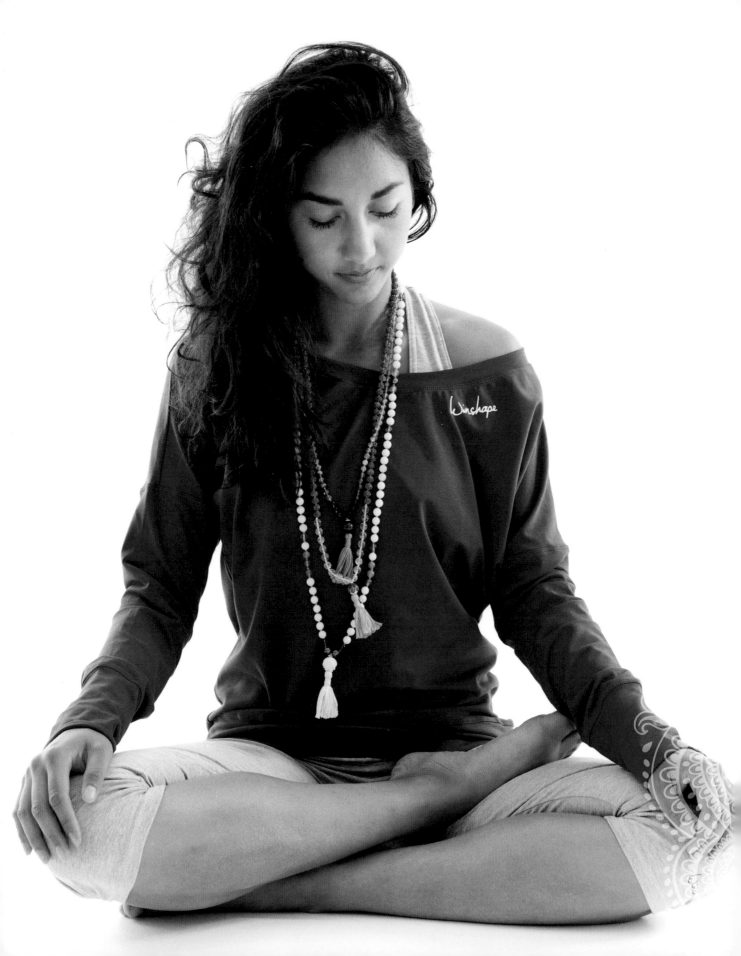

3 HATHA YOGA

3　HATHA YOGA

"Whether young or grown, very old or sick or weak, he who is indefatigable in all yoga exercises will find perfection through the practice". (Hatha-Yoga-Pradipika, verse 64).[19]

Hatha Yoga refers to the physical practice that historically came from the Tantric philosophy. An Indian yogi by the name of *Goraksha*, who presumably lived between the seventh and ninth centuries AD, is considered the creator and innovator of Hatha Yoga. He authored the *Goraksha Shataka*, whose verses are considered the source texts of Hatha Yoga.

The most important and most famous foundational work of Hatha Yoga is the *Hatha Yoga Pradipika*[20] (Hatha Pradipika). It was authored in the 14th century, by Svatmarama and is comprised of four chapters with descriptions of the Asana practices (body postures), Pranayama (breath control), Kumbhaka (breath retention), and Bandha (energy lock).

The term *Hatha* is translated as *strength*, *force*, *endurance*, *persistence*, and *energy*. Common translations of Hatha Yoga are *strength-based yoga* or *energy-based yoga*.

The definition "strength-based yoga" suggests that the Hatha Yoga system's methods require a lot of endurance combined with vigorous exertion and self-control. In fact, there have been and are orientations within Hatha Yoga that heavily emphasize the physical body or the body's resistance in their practice.

Hatha Yoga orientations that emphasize "energy-based yoga" are based on the world-, life-, and body-affirming views of Tantrism. One famous school is "Kashmir Shaivism", which is similar to Hindu Tantra but considers Shiva the uncreated absolute consciousness.

Another very common translation of Hatha, one that is not documented in the Sanskrit yoga texts and is considered esoteric, interprets the syllable Ha as sun and the syllable *Tha* as *moon*. This means that the polar energies inside us are brought into harmony with each other and need to be balanced. The moon signifies the thoughtful, cooling, emotional and intuitive aspects within us. The sun represents the active forces such as light, warmth, fire, activity, and determination.

19 Svatmarama, S. (2009, pg. 47).
20 Svatmarama, S. (2009.

3.1 WESTERN HATHA YOGA

Nowadays the term *Hatha Yoga* is often used colloquially to express that it is a gentle form of yoga in contrast to physically intensive orientations like Ashtanga Vinyasa yoga, Vinyasa Flow yoga, Jivamukti yoga, or power yoga. In fact, all of these styles are in the Hatha Yoga category, but they have been given a specific designation within the Hatha Yoga system.

Some designations of Hatha Yoga styles relate to a yoga master or guru like, for instance, Shivananda Yoga or Iyengar Yoga. Other designations refer to the spiritual orientation, like Ashtanga Yoga, and are directly related to the Ashtanga Marga, or the yoga path's ultimate goal like Jivamukti, which refers to the spiritual liberation inside the body during one's life.

Over the past few years, new names have been derived to designate certain content and directions within the Hatha Yoga system, such as Yin Yoga, Chi Yoga, Fasciae Yoga, Detox Yoga, Slow Down Yoga, Elements Yoga, Ayurveda Yoga, Hot Yoga, or meditative yoga.

In some types of yoga, Hatha Yoga is merely of secondary importance like, for instance, in integrated yoga according to Sri Aurobindo. In his comprehensive work, *The Synthesis of Yoga*, the famous Indian yogi, philosopher, and poet who coined the phrase, "All life is yoga", explains that it is possible to either completely forgo the Hatha Yoga methods or that the Hatha Yoga methods can be used for beginning or occasional assistance but are not essential.[21]

All subsequent chapters in this book are dedicated to different aspects of Hatha Yoga and use Patanjali's *Yoga Sutra* as a guideline.

---

21 Aurobindo, S. (2008). *The Synthesis of Yoga*. chapter 27, pg. 539. Gladenbach Publishing Hinder + Deelmann.

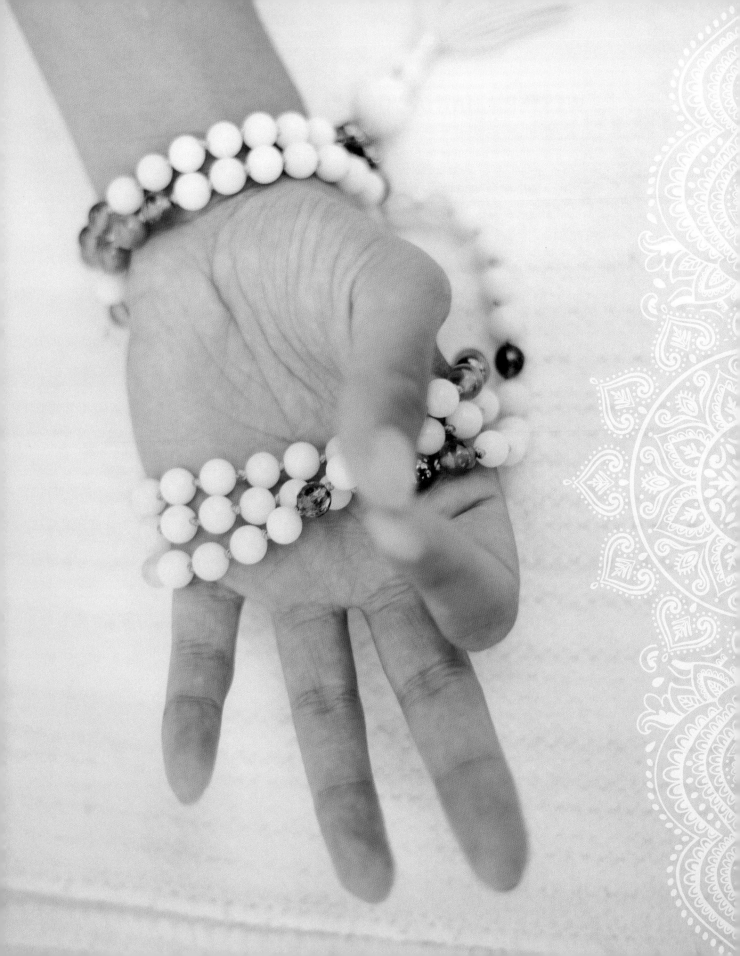

4 THE GUNAS – BASIC FORMS OF ENERGY

4   THE GUNAS – BASIC FORMS OF ENERGY

The concept of Purusha, Prakriti, and the Gunas

Purusha = pure, absolute consciousness, Shiva, Brahman

Prakriti = primordial matter, manifest creation, Shakti

Guna = cord, string, trait, quality

The *Gunas* are basic forms of energy. To understand the concept of Gunas, it helps to take a look at the spiritual model of Purusha and Prakriti, in which the Gunas are embedded.

Purusha refers to pure, absolute consciousness that is unchanging, steadfast, and eternal. *Prakriti* refers to all natural appearances, everything variable, changeable, anything that is subject to becoming and passing away. Prakriti is characterized by the three Gunas, which represent forces that are responsible for anything changeable.

The Vedas and the Upanishads already mentioned the relationship between the amorphous absolute (Purusha) and the manifest creation (Prakriti). The *Mundaka Upanishad* states:

"Purusha is the radiant, yet amorphous, cosmic spirit, the Self of the universe. It is in everything and also beyond it, unsullied by the breath and the intellect. It is even beyond the impulse of taking shape. It brings the breath, the intellect, and the senses into being, and during the further course ether, air, light, water, and finally earth are created – as a basis of everything."[22]

In the *Bhagavadgita*, the god Krishna explains these relationships as he instructs the prince and warrior Arjuna in the yoga paths. And in the first part of the Yoga, Sutra Patanjali explains the significance of Purusha, Prakriti, and the Gunas, which refer to Samkhya philosophy.

---

22 Michel & Wellmann (2003, pg. 57).

4.1   NAMA RUPA – FROM ESSENCE TO FORM

Nama = Name / Rupa = Form

The *Ashwattha tree*[23], the Hindu upside-down world tree that represents the entire cosmos, shows how creation evolves from the ethereal essence.

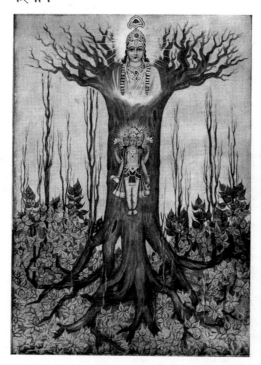

Fig. 4: The Ashwatta tree

All living things, all of creation, originate from the ethereal, the pure, absolute consciousness (Purusha, Shiva), symbolized by the tree's roots at the top of the picture.

From there the manifest creation/Shakti force gradually develops over many intermediate stages and increasingly solidifies into the tangible levels (Prakriti). This cosmic principle is referred to as *Nama Rupa*, from essence to form.

All the way at the bottom, in the tree's branches, the world we live in manifests itself with its many small branches and leaves. Here is the level of the five elements. The more creation grows into the tangible world, the more varied become, on the one hand, the forms and the expression, and on the other hand, the tree's foliage is very far away from its origin so that the pure consciousness is still present, but for the human everyday consciousness it is not, or only barely perceptible. When we meditate and focus on the

23 http://rapunzelturm.blogspot.de/2016/06/der-weltenbaum-teil-2-kabbala-ashwatta.html

infinite, clear consciousness, we can gain access to the higher levels. That is the real reason for pursuing a spiritual practice.

People are fundamentally capable of developing a spiritual consciousness, but it can only happen in connection with the material body.[24] The model of the world tree and the knowledge of the Gunas and the elements provide us with a kind of spiritual energy map as well as road signs that can help us find our way back to the essence.

4.2   THE MAHABHUTAS – THE FIVE ELEMENTS

4.2.1   MAHA = GREAT / BHUTA = GHOST

In yoga and Ayurveda philosophy, the universe along with all things and all living organisms, including humans, consists of five elements.

These elements are called Mahabhutas. They are:

Earth (Prithivi),

Water (Ap),

Fire (Tejas),

Air (Vayu), and

Space/ether (Akasha).

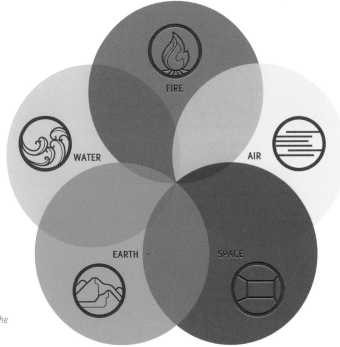

Fig. 5: All of life originates from the interplay of the five elements. [25]

24 Also see: Thode, E. (2015). *Die göttliche Shakti. Die Kraft des Weiblichen im Yoga*. (pg. 128). Bielefeld: Theseus Publishing.
25 Graphic illustrations courtesy of Kirti Peter Michel.

Based on the point of view that all of creation evolved from the ethereal to the tangible, Prakriti is dynamic, subject to change, and characterized by the three attributes of nature that also represent the basic qualities of human consciousness.

To understand the Gunas' dynamics and effect, it helps to first take a closer look at the five elements and their special attributes, which characterize the individual Gunas.

4.2.2 THE ELEMENT EARTH (PRITHIVI)

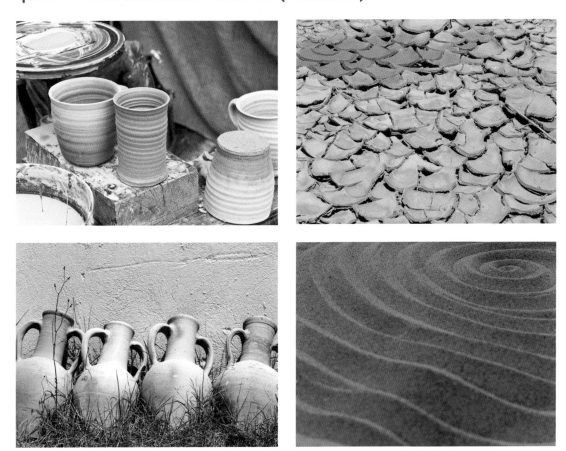

Earth is the most tangible of the five elements. The earth's qualities are described as heavy, solid, slow, inert, sturdy, steady, hard, rough, and dry. This is most apparent when imagining a large rock, a pebble, dry desert sand, a mountain, or a dried up riverbed. When adding water, earth becomes muddy, soft, and moist. Earth represents nourishment, matter, roots, steadfastness, sturdiness, and body. The equivalent to earth in the human body: bones, teeth, fingernails, hair, tendons, organs, and skin.

4.2.3 THE ELEMENT WATER (AP)

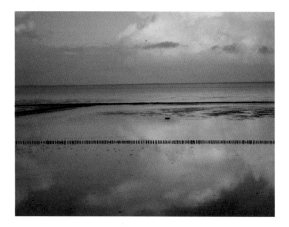
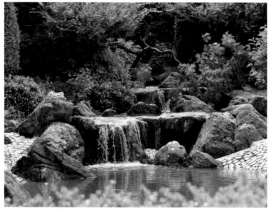
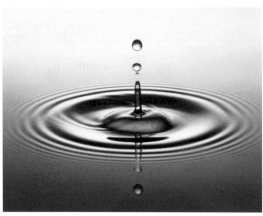
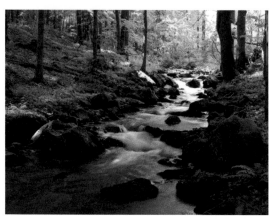

Water is fluid, fluctuating, lazy, slow, connective, soft, and cool. But water is no longer as tangible as the element earth. Water's structure is changeable. Think of an ocean whose waves surge or become calm depending on the wind. Or a thick layer of ice, icebergs, or snow. In the human body, water is the carrier of all fluids that flow inside us, like blood or lymphatic fluid. On a mental-emotional level, water corresponds to our feelings, which are in turn closely linked to our mental experiences, are constantly changing, and can greatly fluctuate.

4.2.4 THE ELEMENT FIRE (TEJAS)

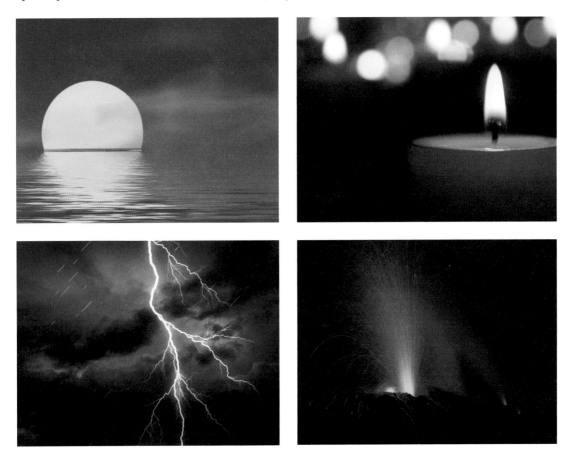

Fire is hot, warm, fast, light, sharp, and subtle. Fire brings us warmth and light but also possesses speed and sharpness. Think of lightning or an explosion. Inside our bodies, fire represents body temperature, which can be high (fever) or too low when we are cold. In yoga and Ayurveda, we refer to the digestive fire, which means the force of transformation of food into energy. On the mental/spiritual level, we talk about a fire when we are full of energy. But when we are too fiery we dry out, which can manifest itself in dry skin or chapped lips.

4.2.5 THE ELEMENT AIR (VAYU)

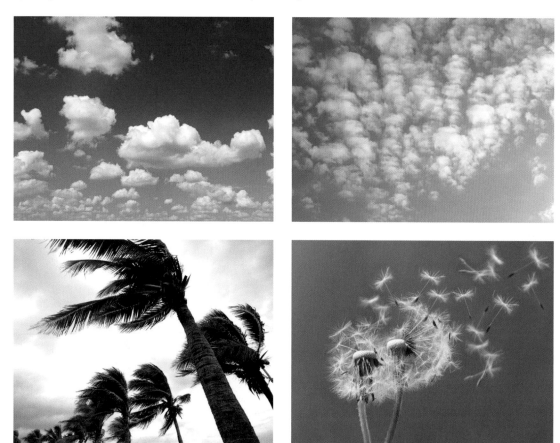

Air is light, clear, cool, delicate, and subtle. The term *Vayu* means *wind*. Wind has a drying effect; think wet laundry hung up to dry in the fresh air. Air is a very ethereal element. It cannot be seen but can be felt with our largest tactile organ, the skin. Think of a gentle summer breeze that caresses the skin, the hair. With respect to the body, air represents the breath, the air we breathe in and out. *Vayu* also stands for the five aspects of *Prana*, the subtle life force energy.

4.2.6 THE ELEMENT SPACE/ETHER (AKASHA)

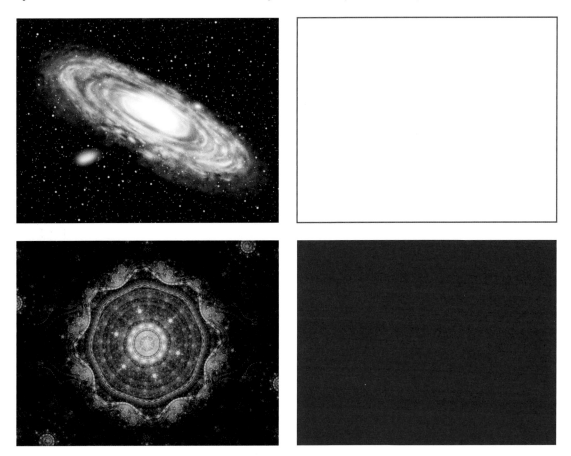

The attributes of the element space are light, delicate, subtle. Space stands for *vastness*, for *infinity*, and *freedom*. Space holds all of creation and is all-pervasive. We are generally only aware of space in terms of limits that can be distant or near. With respect to the body, in yoga we refer to breathing space, on the spiritual-mental level we refer to spaces of consciousness that can also be broad or limited. Humans long for great open spaces and freedom in spirit as in life. We instinctively reject anything tight, constricting, and restrictive if it limits our freedom. What makes the subject of space so interesting is that without external points of reference, we can quickly feel lost.

4.3   GUNAS – BASIC PROPERTIES OF NATURE

None of the five elements stands alone. All of them work with each other in different increments. The constant interaction between the five elements creates strong forces, the Gunas, which represent the basic properties of nature.

With respect to the yoga practice, the Gunas represent a mental-spiritual model that allows us to recognize trends of which forces are at work inside us. A deeper understanding of the effects of the Gunas can help us focus our yoga practice accordingly.

THE GUNAS

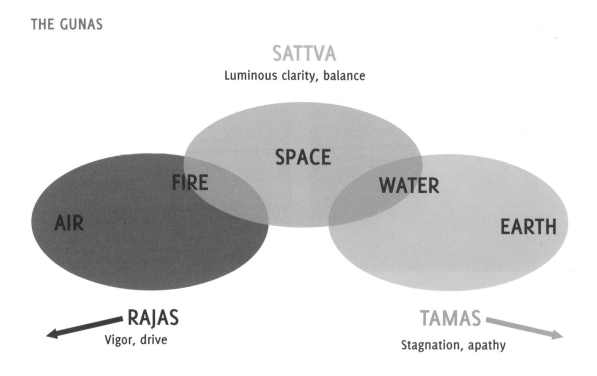

Fig. 6: All phenomena of life result from the interaction of the three fundamental forces: SATTVA, RAJAS, and TAMAS. [26]

---

26 Graphic illustration of the Gunas courtesy of Kriti Peter Michel.

4.3.1 RAJAS GUNA: FIRE, WATER, AIR

Rajas possesses primarily the properties of the elements fire and water and represents *drive, energy, vigor*. Rajas initiates movement. In nature, the energy of Rajas is particularly active in the spring, when plants sprout and all of nature practically explodes, grows, and renews itself.

The energy from Rajas gives us the ability to set things in motion. We need a good shot of Rajas for all our undertakings. Without Rajas we would not be able to "get off our ass". When fire and water work together they create steam. In the past, people used this knowledge to operate steam locomotives. When these two elements are active inside us, we are proverbially "under pressure." We are warmed up and full of creative power. This energy can help move mountains.

People under major Raja influence are very active and like to rush from one thing to the next. *Raja types* are ambitious and passionate. They have trouble staying still. They fan their inner fire with lots of activity and put pressure on themselves. They are spirited and can be very quick-tempered. They fight obstacles in their path with their fiery energy.

Extreme Raja types tend to be selfish. Their motivation is then characterized by greed and wish fulfillment. When Rajas become too dominant and take over, it results in extreme restlessness, edginess, jitteriness, and can ultimately lead to chaos. *Raja types* like to wear clothes that are flashy and expressive. They want to be seen and noticed.

The spirit that is dominated by greediness and passion is similar to a volcanic eruption or a raging storm.

Spicy, hot, stimulating foods, spices, and beverages, sugary foods, as well as coffee and alcohol have a major *Rajas effect*. *Rajas types* always eat in a hurry, devouring their food while simultaneously doing something else.

Bhagavadgita, chapter 17, verse 9: "Rajas types prefer foods that are bitter, sour, salty, too heavily seasoned, spicy, dry or stinging, and that cause pain, sorrow, and illness.[27]

4.3.2 TAMAS GUNA: EARTH, WATER

Tamas is primarily characterized by the energies of earth and water. Both elements are very tangible. In their interaction they represent matter, the dark, ignorance, inertia, laziness, lethargy, all the way to motionlessness. In nature we can experience the energy of Tamas in winter, when all growing and blooming comes to a rest. When the ground is covered with leaves that are slowly rotting, when the fields and meadows lie dormant under a blanket of snow. But the inhibiting force of Tamas is also represented by a pond full of stagnant, cloudy, stinking, brackish water.

---

27 Srimad & Swami Sivananda (1998). *Bhagavadgita* (pg. 345, chapter 17, verse 9). Lautersheim: Mangalam Publishing.

When the qualities of Tamas are dominant inside us, we are sluggish, feel dull and inactive. All of our actions are inhibited by lethargy. People under extreme Tamas influence can't get off the proverbial couch; they are unable to pick themselves up, and they feed their bodies with fast food and their minds with "trash". They are emotionally and mentally depressed; they are unable to pull themselves together, are lazy, and extraordinarily unmotivated.

Extreme Tamas can manifest itself in a lack of personal hygiene. The individual is dirty, slovenly, but is in a state of severe inhibition. Progress seems to be impossible. There is a lack of interest in material as well as spiritual goals.

On a mental-spiritual level, Tamas types have trouble expressing themselves, which can lead to rudeness or even violence. Extreme Tamas influence can lead to hatred, paranoia, and even megalomania.[28]

The spirit that is dominated by dullness, darkness, and lethargy is similar to a moldy pond.

All types of fast food, prepackaged foods containing preservatives with lots of chemicals such as, for instance, canned goods, foods that have been reheated multiple times, large amounts of meat and sausage and all types of stimulants have a severe Tamas effect on the body and the mind.

Baghavadgita, chapter 17, verse 10: "The stale, tasteless, rotten, leftover, and impure is the preferred sustenance of Tamas types."[29]

4.3.3   SATTVA GUNA: SPACE, AIR, FIRE (LIGHT)

Sattva represents the qualities of the element space/ether and stands for light, clarity, and purity. In nature we can experience the energy of Sattva when we think of a clear mountain lake, or when nature has brought forth its fruit in summer. The mango is considered a very *Sattva* fruit: juicy, naturally sweet, and fresh.

Sattva types are peaceful, focused, and even-tempered. They love tranquility and harmony. Their actions are characterized by love, selflessness, and creative joy. They prioritize the needs of others. They are not motivated by profit; their actions serve the common good. They are sensitive and are aware of their surroundings. They work for the sake of the matter, not out of greed or pressure, and they often complete even difficult tasks seemingly effortlessly.

Sattva types are focused on spiritual subjects; they enjoy meditation and therefore have a serene and pure presence. They are sincere, mentally stable, balanced. They are at peace with themselves and feel good about themselves.

Sattva types live in harmony with their environment. They exploit neither nature's resources, nor those of their fellow man. They have a clear intellect and are not interested in external things like looks, reputation or prestige. Their appearance is clean and pure. Their dress tends to be plain and inconspicuous.

---

28 Dr. Frawley, D. & Summerfield, K.S. (2003), Yoga for your Type: An Ayurvedic Approach to Your Asana Practice (pg. 41). Aitran. Windpferd Publishing Inc.
29 Srimad & Swami Sivananda (1998, pg. 345, chapter 17, verse 10).

The spirit that is characterized by clarity and freshness is similar to a crystal-clear mountain lake or the vast, clear sky.

Fresh foods like fruit and vegetables, spices, grains, sprouts, seeds, nuts, freshly pressed juices and herbal teas are considered *Sattva* and raise our awareness. Sattva foods are prepared with love and consumed with mindfulness.

Bhagavadgita, chapter 17, verse 8: "The Sattva (pure) person enjoys foods that increase life, purity, strength, joy and cheeriness (increase the good appetite), are tasty, fragrant and pleasant."[30]

4.4 TRIGUNA – INTERPLAY OF THE THREE GUNAS

The three Gunas do not exist independently of each other. They exist side by side and with each other. Their effect can be seen as a perpetual and continuous process in nature and inside of us. Although all three Gunas are active at all times, the effects of one are usually more prominent. One of the goals of a yoga practice is to strengthen the Sattva Guna and thereby establish the Sattva properties of clarity and light in us.

With respect to life and especially with respect to the yoga practice, the first step is recognizing which Guna characterizes our actions and experiences, i.e. figuring out under which mental type one generally tends to fall. But since this is also subject to fluctuation, possibly due to seasonal changes, the weather, the continent where one lives, physical age, professional or family situations, it is important to notice one's tendencies in everyday life:

» Are my actions shaped by greed and ambition?

» Do I rush from one thing to the next and have trouble being still?

» Or do I feel uninspired; are my thoughts and emotions destructive; do I tend to be lethargic and filled with resentment?

» Or are my actions and thoughts shaped by peace and compassion?

Most people initially want to balance the aspects of excessive Rajas or Tamas to create a foundation for the *Sattva* quality of life.

Of interest is that *Rajas* can actively work in two ways. On the one hand here in the West the effects of excessive *Rajas* are known as burnout. Too much fire ultimately burns precious matter, vital energy, and as a result can lead to the opposite state, *Tamas*. On the other hand, we need the *Rajas* energy to reduce *Tamas* and change the state of stagnation.

The *Sattva* state we seek is the balance between Tamas and Rajas. Sattva possesses its own properties that don't develop automatically if we can manage to balance the other two Gunas in a healthy way.

---

30 Srimad & Swami Sivananda (1998, pg. 345, chapter 17, verse 8).

4.5   THE GUNAS AND YOGA PRACTICE

With respect to yoga and the Asana practice, knowledge about the Gunas is a valuable tool with which we can influence and change our energy-related mental state. For yoga instructors, this knowledge is a valuable tool used to initially identify the current needs of participants, and to then direct the energy-related progression of the practice via appropriate content (perception, Asana, Pranayama, relaxation, meditation, the basic philosophical theme of the class).

At the beginning of a session, it is a good idea to allow the participants to settle down. By doing awareness exercises (body- and breath awareness, awareness of the mental content) the participants should have the opportunity to learn self-observation step-by-step.

Over the course of a yoga practice, it can be necessary to first reduce Rajas and Tamas by practicing flows/Karanas that are adapted to the group structure. On the one hand, you reduce restlessness and stress (Rajas) but also fuel energy and thus vitality (balancing Tamas). A deep, deliberate breath helps Rajas and Tamas to achieve energy balance.

Of interest here is that the different types of physical constitutions tend to want to intensify their energy-related dispositions on the yoga mat. *Rajas* types tend to want to intensify their restlessness, their activity and ambition on the mat via endless challenging flows and physically very demanding Asanas, whereby the state of inner calm and peace is frequently confused with exhaustion.

Here it would be beneficial to start out energized, but then incrementally transition to a calmer, meditative practice. On the one hand to teach what powerful calm feels like, but also to make the participants aware of their own tendencies in an appropriate manner. In a way, the "work" on the yoga mat is an incentive for self-observation, to become aware of those relevant and unhealthy tendencies in everyday life and change them.

People with a Tamas character generally don't like intense flows. They sometimes arrive to class, requesting to "practice only Shavasana today". *Tamas* types often like sustained and comfortable poses that accommodate their natural sluggishness and lack of energy. Here too, it is important to stimulate energy with a well-balanced practice and thus enter a state of clear, alert calm.

Too much Tamas impedes all types of relaxation and meditation that are meant to result in a state of clear, peaceful alertness. An excess of Tamas causes the participants to fall asleep during relaxation and get drowsy during meditation.

The manner in which we practice the Asanas gives us the opportunity to affect the Gunas:

Do I practice lots of Asanas in rapid succession and activate energy flow that way, or do I choose long, sustained Asanas that help one let go?

The types of Asanas also impact our energy-related experience: backbends have a stimulating effect, forward bends have a cooling, calming effect; twists provide balance, and inversions are clarifying and support the meditative experience.

Of course, the choice of Asanas and Pranayamas as well as their practice should be balanced. But as yoga instructors, we have leeway regarding intensity control and energy-related effects for which we should utilize our knowledge about the Gunas to reinforce the Sattva aspects.

Yoga is a process of constant self-observation and perception. Our knowledge about the elements and their interplay via the Gunas allows us to be self-reflective. It is also interesting to research which elements in us should be reinforced or reduced.

» Do I need more earth, meaning stability in myself and in my life?

» Or am I inflexible and rigid and have trouble accepting change?

» Is the aspect of water too dominant and do I constantly give my feelings free reign?

» Or am I too fiery and burn myself out?

» Am I an airy type, allowing myself to be blown away, having my head in the clouds, and losing myself in a thousand different ideas and needing more earth, e.g. via standing poses?

The closely related Ayurveda theory developed the three *Dosha systems* based on the elements. In his work *Yoga of the Five Elements*, the author and experienced yoga instructor Kirti Peter Michel explains these relationships from an Ayurveda point of view while also offering practice routines for each Dosha.[31]

With respect to the spiritual path, we must remember that the system of Gunas can help us get on the inner path, from the foliage back to the roots of the Ashwatta tree, through specific awareness and differentiation of Prakriti (matter).

The elements are also closely linked to the Chakra teachings, which can only be understood in depth when the knowledge about the elements has been internalized. All of the explanations here are intended to continuously show different approaches based on well-founded lesson plans that go far beyond the function of muscles during poses.

---

31 Michel & Wellmann, (2003).

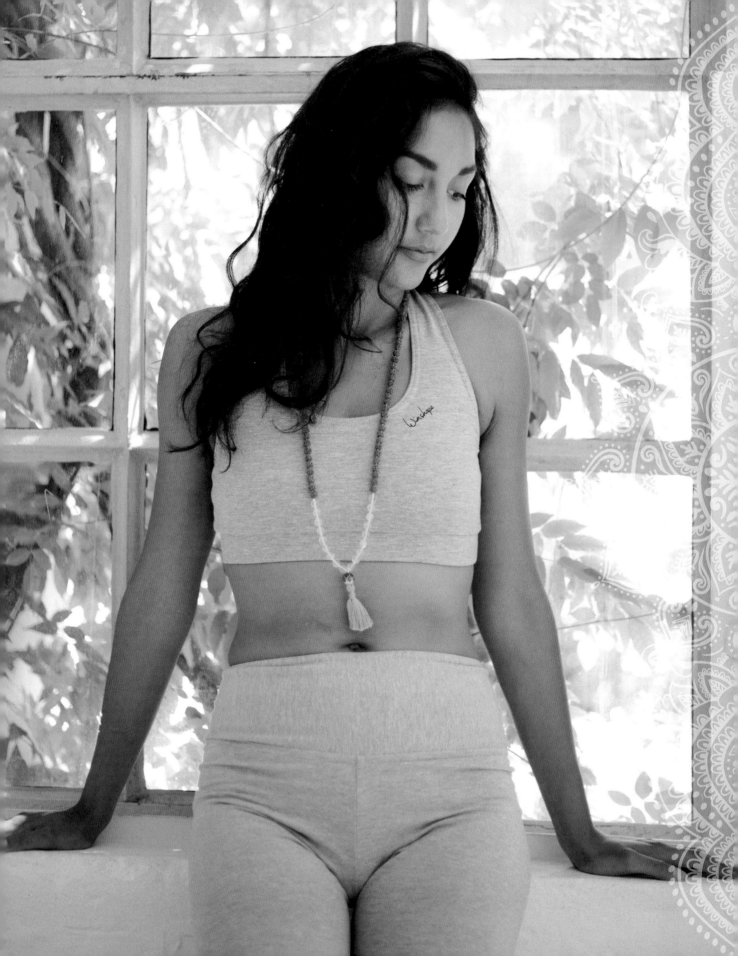

5 THE CHAKRA SYSTEM

5   THE CHAKRA SYSTEM

5.1   PANCHA KOSHA – THE FIVE SHEATHS

Pancha = five / Kosha = layer, sheaths

The energy system is the main focus and also one of the most interesting and exciting areas of Hatha Yoga. It is the theory of the energies that are active inside us, and their functions with respect to the body and the mental, emotional, energy-related, and spiritual experience.

When we talk about our body in everyday life, we generally mean our physical (tangible) body. By contrast, yoga philosophy does not just refer to a tangible body but four additional subtle layers or sheaths that permeate the physical body. These sheaths, the Koshas, are described in detail in the *Upanishads*.[32] These Koshas penetrate each other and interact with each other. One can imagine them as veils or shrouds that envelop the Self (the pure being).

"I recognize this Self, said the sage Shvetashvatara, as immortal and eternal. I know this Self, the Self of everything, he whom the wise men call the Eternal One."[33]

1.   ANNAMAYA KOSHA – THE NUTRITIONAL SHEATH (THE PHYSICAL BODY)

The visible and palpable tangible body consists of the five elements earth, water, fire, air, and space. The element earth stands for everything solid in the body, like bones, nails, hair, skin, muscle, and organs. Water stands for everything fluid inside us, like blood or lymphatic fluid. Fire is represented by body heat, and the element air is the air we breathe in and out. Space stands for the spaces our organs, limbs, in short the entire body occupies. The tangible body, the nutritional sheath, is everything we touch or feel on a tangible level and has many attributes based on the elements from which it is built. *Annamaya Kosha* is subject to the changes in life such as growth, age, disease, and death.

---

32 Easwaran, E. (2008, pg. 195-197, Taittiriya Upanishad).
33 Easwaran, E. (2008, Shvetashvatara-Upanishad, III, 21).

2. PRANAMAYA KOSHA – THE BREATH SHEATH, ENERGY SHEATH

This is also referred to as the vital or energy body and encompasses the Nadis (subtle energy pathways) and the *Chakras* (centers of energy). It is linked to the breath and the five aspects of Prana (Vayus). It controls vital processes like food intake, conversion of food into energy and elimination in the body.

3. MANOMAYA KOSHA – MENTAL SHEATH, THOUGHT SHEATH

This is where the intake and processing of sensory impressions takes place. *Manomaya Kosha* is the level of thoughts and emotions (wishes, fears, needs, feelings, memories), which largely move back and forth unfiltered between waking consciousness and subconscious. It is therefore also referred to as the outer "low" level of the intellect.

4. VIJNANAMAYA KOSHA – COGNITION SHEATH, WISDOM SHEATH

The intelligence sheath is inked to the ability to reflect and to differentiate. It is the sheath of higher knowledge and intuition. Decisions made on this level result in the release from attachments and more conscious living.

5. ANANDAMAYA KOSHA – THE SHEATH OF BLISS

The level of bliss that ensues when one is very close to the Self, the pure being. *Ananda* is the pure joy that we are beyond the duality.

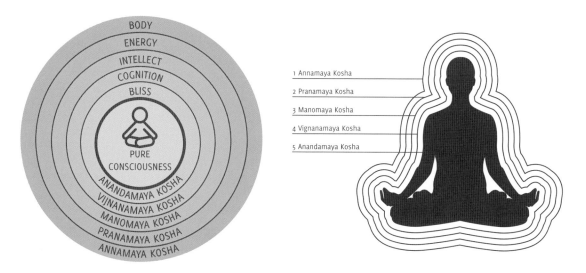

Fig. 7.a / b.: The Kosha model and the five sheaths.

5.2   PRANAMAYA KOSHA – THE ENERGY SHEATH

Nad = roar / Nadi = tube, canal, stream / Prana = subtle vital energy

In this chapter, we will focus primarily on the aspects of *Pranamaya Kosha*, which are extremely important to the Hatha Yoga practice, because this is where all vital processes take place.

From a Hatha Yoga point of view, our physical (tangible) body is permeated by an ethereal body. The same can be measured as an electromagnetic force field inside and around all living things. It contains a network of invisible energy pathways, the *Nadis*. *Nadi* means tube or *canal*, where *Prana*, the cosmic vital energy flows.

But we are (still) unable to detect the Nadis with modern scientific methods, for instance under a microscope. Yoga is an empirical science and with some practice the effects and functions of the Nadis can be quite perceptible. Experienced yogis, so-called *rishis* (sages), who have the gift of sensitive sight, have estimated the number of Nadis at 72,000 based on the *Hatha Yoga Pradipika*.[34] The reported number of Nadis can however fluctuate from one tradition to another.

Let anyone who requires concrete evidence to consider the existence of Nadis as real be reminded that in past centuries, much that was initially not visible to the naked eye was seen as utopian or simply crazy. For example, the discovery of X-rays, which initially seemed fanciful to generations at that time, or proof of viruses and bacteria that was long contested by the medical community of the past.

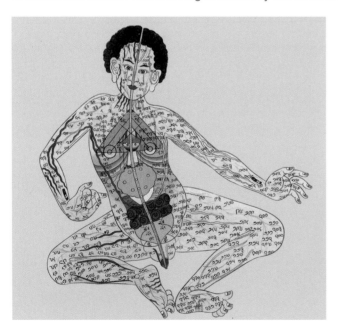

Fig. 8: The chakras and a portion of the Nadis.

34 Svatmarama, S. (2009, pg. 10).

Prana, the subtle life force and vital energy, streams and flows through the Nadis. Prana's function in turn is divided into the so-called five Vayus, the five winds that in various ways handle the intake and distribution of energy and the release of spent energy inside the human body.

» **Prana Vayu:** Its primary function is the intake of energy via the breath, the inflowing energy moves in the chest cavity.

» **Apana Vayu:** Regulates all elimination processes; the descending energy moves primarily in the lower pelvic area.

» **Samana Vayu:** Is in charge of the conversion of energy via the metabolism and moves primarily in the middle of the body.

» **Udana Vayu:** Controls the nervous and endocrine systems. As an ascending energy, Udana is responsible for speech, communication, and self-expression.

» **Vyana Vayu:** Controls the bloodstream and circulation at a higher level and distributes energy.

An energy body that is permeable and evenly perfused by Prana is one of the goals and simultaneously the effect of Hatha Yoga. We absorb Prana with our breath, but Prana should not be confused with the oxygen we inhale. Prana is an even subtler force and is also absorbed from food and through the skin. In the Far-Eastern perception the equivalent to Prana is *Chi = vital energy*.

When Prana's perfusion of the Nadi system is unimpeded and all aspects of vital energy function are well balanced, we are healthy, we feel even-tempered, and are in harmony with our surroundings and ourselves. But in daily life there are always circumstances and challenges that throw the sensitive energy system off balance. These include internal, emotional, and mental tensions, conflicts, and difficulties on an interpersonal level, or external influences such as weather, the seasons, all the way to natural disasters.

When energy doesn't flow in different areas of the body but is bogged down or blocked, on the tangible level we most likely perceive this at some point as some sort of malaise, tension, pain, all the way to disease. In fact, manifestation on a physical/tangible level is viewed as the final link in a chain of many reactions to an imbalance in the energy system. From the yoga perspective, everything originates in the etheric body.[35]

With the Hatha Yoga practice, we gently restore the flow of energy in the body by directing attention to the inner experience, through physical and breathing exercises, mindfulness, concentration, by directing energy, and meditation. In a way we free up constrained, frozen energy so it can begin to flow again. In fact, a tight muscle or a tense body uses much more energy than a relaxed muscular system. That is also the reason why we tend to not only feel pleasantly loose, but also full of vital energy after a yoga class. The energy flow we are referring to here acts on a tangible level as much as in the mental, emotional, and spiritual parts of the body.

---

35 See Aswhatta tree, pg. 47.

5.3 NADIS – THE ENERGY PATHWAYS

Within the system of Nadis there are three main Nadis that originate in the lower pelvic region, in the area of the pelvic floor, and the tailbone.

» *Susuhumna Nadi* (also called *Madhya Nadi*, the central canal) originates at the base of the spine in the lower pelvic region and stretches vertically along the axis and up to the crown of the head.

» *Ida* (the moon-like one) and *Pingala* (the sun-like one) Nadi also originate in the lower pelvic region and run upward along the vertical axis of the spine, crossing multiple times, and ending in the right (Pingala Nadi) and left nostril (Ida Nadi) respectively.

» *Ida Nadi* corresponds to the energy of the moon. When Ida Nadi is stimulated via appropriate breathing or Asana practice the effect is gently cooling, efferent, regenerative, and calming. Ida Nadi promotes relaxation and meditation and facilitates interiorization of the mind. Ida connects us to the feminine aspects, with the power of emotion, with intuition, imagination, with permeability, and softness. Ida Nadi is attributed to the right brain.

» *Pingala Nadi* corresponds to the energy of the sun and stands for joyful creative energy, for vigor and activity. When Pingala Nadi is stimulated, we connect with the power of the sun that supports all becoming and growing. Pingala stands for the masculine, strong-willed, mental and rational aspects in us. Pingala is attributed to the left half of the brain.

Please note: Labels like masculine and feminine should be viewed as relative since all of us, men as well as women, carry both polarities (sun-moon, male-female, active-passive) inside us to varying degrees.

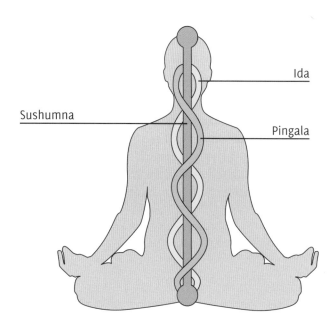

Fig. 9: The three main Nadis.

5.4   KUNDALINI SHAKTI

Kundala = ring, rolled up, wound

From the Hatha Yoga point of view, a strong, fiery force is located in the lower pelvic region, in the *Muladhara chakra* (root chakra), which is symbolically depicted as a triple-coiled serpent. It is referred to as *Kundalini Shakti* and is the primal creative energy. In most people, it rests peacefully coiled up in the root chakra. The serpent represents the latent spiritual energy inside us. When this energy awakens it moves in spirals inside our body. The snake stands for one of the aspects of the power of the absolute, the all-encompassing unity. It split off during the process of creation and as the Shakti force created the matter during its vigorous activity.[36] It now rests as a hidden force in our lower pelvic region. When it is awakened, it makes its way through *Sushumna Nadi* back to the upper crown chakra, and reunites with the primal cosmic energy.

Since *Kundalini Shakti* has an enormous force potential, the entire energy system, but particularly the *Sushuma Nadi*, must be cleared and cleaned out. The entire energy system must be free of impurities of any kind (physical, mental, emotional, spiritual). Massively forcing Kundalini energy is definitely not advisable as it can result in a premature awakening accompanied by very unpleasant experiences and consequences.

There are three blockages in *Sushumna Nadi*, the *Granthi*, which prevent the Kundalini Shakti from rising. *Granthi* means *knot*. According to *Hatha Yoga Pradipika*[37], *Brahma Granthi* is located at the heart level. *Vishnu Granthi* is in the throat area, and *Rudra Granthi* is located between the eyebrows. They stand for the marred or numbed aspects of our consciousness. When the energy inside the Sushumna gets backed up at one of the Granthi points or in one of the centers of energy, it can result in physical and mental suffering.

The *Kundalini Shakti* is the force of enlightenment. One way to let the Kundalini rise up through a blockage-free channel at a given time is to clear the chakras, the subtle centers of energy. When the vibrations in our bodies are synchronized via the chakras, the Kundalini flows quite naturally. This process can take years, an entire life, or many lifetimes. But time is relative, and excessive ambition often only leads us down painful detours, which is why patience, deep breaths, and mindfulness are the ideal companions on the yoga path.

---

36 See Ashwatta tree, pg. 47.
37 Svatmarama, S. (2009, pg. 21).

5.5   THE CHAKRAS

Chakra = Wheel, disk, whirl of energy

If one were to form an image of the Nadi system, a map comes to mind that consists of many small and large streets that crisscross the body.[38] Sushumna Nadi is a major traffic pathway flanked by Ida and Pingala Nadi. In addition, there are countless large, small, and tiny energy pathways. Wherever a particularly large number of energy pathways cross and are seemingly interwoven there are very strong centers of energy, the *chakras*.

With respect to their function *chakras* are subtle centers of energy and consciousness. They are both transmitters and receivers of energy. One can imagine the chakras as transformers that regulate the elemental cosmic energy on the human body's frequency. We absorb the cosmic life energy Prana through the chakras, and from there Prana is distributed throughout the body via the many large and small Nadis.

Moreover, constant communication with our environment takes place via the chakras, usually unconsciously. With every encounter, be it during a walk out in nature, or at a gathering with other people, chakra energy flows back and forth, and we communicate, in a manner of speaking, through our chakras. In most people this process takes place unconsciously. We often notice that we feel a fresh and clean energy after spending time out in nature, or feel energized after an inspirational encounter with other people. But sometimes we also feel completely weak and exhausted after some encounters, seemingly for no reason.

The reason is the chakras that are active without our conscious knowledge correspond with each other, receive energy and transmit it.

There are seven main chakras within the physical body and many secondary chakras. The seven main chakras ascend along the spine's axis from the lower pelvic region up to the crown of the head. They are round and funnel-shaped and they permeate our physical body at the front and back. All chakras are connected via the main energy pathway Sushumna Nadi and are in constant communication with each other.

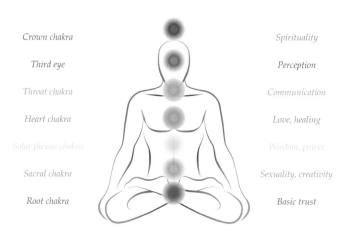

Crown chakra — Spirituality

Third eye — Perception

Throat chakra — Communication

Heart chakra — Love, healing

Solar plexus chakra — Wisdom, power

Sacral chakra — Sexuality, creativity

Root chakra — Basic trust

Fig. 10: The Chakras

---

38 See Fig. 2.

The chakras are the interfaces between physical, energy-related, mental, emotional, and spiritual experiences. They represent the link between the different planes inside us; they interact with each other and create interactions. Every chakra vibrates in its own frequency and at the same time is connected to a certain level of consciousness. It thereby represents certain qualities and controls areas of our experiences and actions.

The bottom three chakras stand for the existential aspects like food intake, our actions in the material world, emotions, sexuality, perseverance, energy balance, and mental strength. The top four chakras stand for feelings (love, compassion), relationships, communication, wisdom, sensitivity, intuition, and for the spiritual aspects of our development.

5.6 THE SEVEN MAIN CHAKRAS

1. The *Muladhara Chakra* (root chakra) is located in the lower pelvic region at the bottom of the spine. The dominant theme is survival.

2. The *Svadhisthana chakra* (sacral chakra) is located in the lower abdomen at a level with the internal sex organs. The dominant themes are emotions, sexuality, and pleasure.

3. The *Manipura chakra* (sun) is located at a level with the solar plexus. The dominant themes are power, will, self-esteem, and transformation.

4. The *Anahata chakra* (heart chakra) is located centrally behind the sternum. The dominant themes are love, compassion, sincerity, and balance.

5. The *Vishuddha chakra* (throat chakra) is located in the throat. The dominant themes are communication, sounds, and purification.

6. The *Ajna Chakra* (third eye chakra) is located between and slightly above the eyebrows. The dominant themes are intuition and clairvoyance.

7. The *Sahasrara chakra* (crown chakra) is located at the crown of the head. The dominant themes are higher knowledge and higher consciousness.

All of the individual chakras are linked via Sushumna Nadi. To get an even better visual of the individual levels of consciousness, one can imagine Sushumna Nadi as a cosmic elevator shaft that runs along the spine. The elevator itself moves from the bottom upward and connects apartments in the places where the chakras would be. The occupants of each floor represent the floor's themes.

» The *Muladharas* down on the first floor prefer earthy reddish hues and rustic furniture made of stone and wood. They are in close contact with nature. Their dominant theme is to have a decent meal on their plate and a warm roof over their head. Their pantry is always full. When they are in harmony, they practically brim over with basic trust. But when their harmony becomes shaky due to circumstances they feel they cannot control, they experience terrible existential fear. They worry a lot, especially about losing their home and worldly goods. They then see themselves as victims of their circumstances and complain and whine.

» The *Svadisthanas* live one floor above the Muladharas. Their apartment has an orange color scheme. Soft, orange fabric drapes on the ceiling and walls are reminiscent of a fairytale palace from Arabian Nights. There are small and large fountains with cascading water all over the apartment. The occupants are very in tune with their emotions and follow them. They are very sensual; they love the physical union and celebrate it like a ritual. But internally they are out of balance; their moods can change like the ocean in the wind. From calm and peaceful to being whipped up into a frenzy and feeling agitated, they are quite unpredictable. They then practice their sexuality to excess without an emotional connection, or they withdraw completely and become emotionally cold.

» The *Manipuras* on the third floor love anything that glitters and shines. They have chandeliers hanging from their ceilings whose crystals shimmer in the light of the many fireplaces. Everything glows in different bright yellow-tones, walls, furniture, curtains; there are candles and other light sources everywhere. They like warmth, love fire, and also like to play with fire in the figurative sense. They are full of self-confidence, creativity, and zest for life. When they get off balance, they become very power-conscious; they want to show everyone and focus all of their willpower on proving to others how strong, powerful, and valuable they are. Or they withdraw completely, mourn their perceived worthlessness, and lose all of their creativity.

» The *Anahatas* on the fourth floor love soft green and rose-colored hues. Everything in their home has gentle curves and exudes complete harmony. They are modest by nature; don't need much to feel comfortable. What little surrounds them is of excellent quality and was made with love. They radiate love and are full of compassion, especially whenever their fellow occupants go to the extreme again. They are always willing to listen and are not very focused on their own needs. They have a strong connection to their heart and follow it. When they are off balance, it can manifest itself on the one hand in an excessive willingness to help, all the way to self-sacrifice, or in a kind of cold-heartedness. Access to the inner self is then closed off, which can manifest itself in coldness.

» The *Vishuddhas* live on the fifth floor and love all shades of blue and turquoise. They also love music and always have the best tunes. They also like to communicate. They possess all of the technical equipment in the area of communications. They are the mediators in the building whenever there are disagreements between individual parties. When they are in harmony, they communicate from the heart and express themselves in a loving, explicit manner. They also know when to remain silent because not everything can be expressed through words. When they are off balance, they use all means of communication simultaneously, are in constant exchange with others, and talk nonstop. Or they stubbornly withdraw and block any kind of communication.

»   The *Ajnas* on the sixth floor are visionaries. Their walls and furnishings are different shades of purple. At the same time their home has an air of enlightenment. Spherical pictures and sculptures are skillfully arranged throughout the rooms. Anywhere the eye travels, one sees something new, viewed from different perspectives. The entire atmosphere exudes something barely perceptible. They are the artists in the building and always follow their intuition. The images they create with their art are created from the gift of their intuition. The other building occupants like to consult them because with their gift of clairvoyance, they often see and address things that are still hidden to others. When the Ajnas are off-balance, they complain of eye pain all the way to blindness. They then lose their gift of intuition and clairvoyance.

»   You never hear the *Sahasraras* on the seventh floor, and you rarely see them. Their apartment and the furniture are all shades of clear, warm whites, as are their clothes. They are the sages in the building and are usually meditating. They exude clarity, perfection, and bliss. When they are out of harmony, it can manifest itself in apathy, boredom, and confusion.

Of course this is just a rough transliteration meant to provide a first, highly simplified impression of the effects of the chakras.

In the yoga world, the lower chakras are sometimes viewed with some contempt as the purely worldly, material areas that must be escaped and forsaken based on the motto: "My car, my house, my boat", while the upper chakras are considered important to spiritual growth. In fact, all chakras are equally important to our development, our health and overall wellbeing. The themes of the lower chakras provide a vital, solid base for the higher chakras. In this respect it is useful to experience all of life's themes, to engage with them and integrate them in their entirety.

When we ignore the existential aspects, we run the risk of neglecting the material means of survival while focusing on spiritual highs. On the other hand, concentrating exclusively on the lower three chakras is also not desirable. This happens when people try to compensate for their feelings of meaninglessness – a result of a broken connection with the source – with material things or with validation and power; while this strategy may work briefly, in the long-term it results in burnout and depression.

Chakras are depicted as *wheels* or *disks*, which expresses their whirling and moving energy. They move clockwise when in action. A chakra can be open or closed. When we refer to closed chakras, it means that energy doesn't flow there, and the respective qualities are not being lived. If it is wide-open and also very strong, it is possible for the respective qualities to be expressed in excess.

When a chakra is weak and open only a little, it may be difficult for the chakra's qualities and attributes to unfold, and for this reason, we are cut off from important aspects of our being and our development. For instance, when the solar plexus chakra (Manipura chakra), which stands for the absorption of energy, metabolism, transformation, and willpower, shows little activity, it can result, on the one hand, in our having trouble processing things, and on the other hand we may lack the energy to get moving. We may have ideas and plans but don't lack the willpower to implement them. We give up weakly when met with the least resistance.

But when a chakra is hyperactive, individual functions or attributes are in overdrive. In the case of the throat chakra (Vishudda chakra), which stands for communication and expresses the connection between heart and mind but also carries the qualities of being silent and listening, hyperfunction can manifest itself in a continuous stream of speech. The person talks nonstop just to talk, usually about trivial things, repeating themselves frequently. But if the chakra is blocked, it can manifest itself in the individual not being able to make a sound, having a lump in the throat, or a stiff neck.

The *lotus flower*, which also stands for the opening center of energy, is a traditional symbol for a chakra. It can be viewed as an invitation to take a look at which chakras are too active or too inactive in which areas of our life, and to gently activate them through a targeted yoga practice such as physical exercises, breathing techniques, mental exercises, and inner focus on the respective theme, all the way to meditation on a specific theme.

Each of the lower five chakras is linked to one of the five elements (Mahabhutas), whose attributes are reflected in the function of the respective chakra. Every chakra is assigned a specific color according to the element. In practice this allows for many possible ways to get in tune with a chakra. In case of the root chakra (Muladhara chakra), one can internally attune to the qualities of grounding, stability, and trust, and internally attune to these qualities in the Asana practice. Another option would be to focus on the appropriate color red and to visualize it with its stimulating warmth in the own blood circulation.

On a physical level, the individual chakras are linked to the position and function of the nervous system and the endocrine glands (hormonal system). Chakra theory implies that everything happens in the ethereal sphere first before it manifests itself on the physical level. An imbalance in a chakra thus affects the corresponding part of the body.

In her comprehensive work *Wheels of Life*, Judith Anodea describes the link between the physical and energy-related plane:

"Body and spirit are inseparably linked. Each part controls and influences the other and can be accessed via the other. The seven main chakras also form an inseparable unit. When one chakra's function is blocked, it can affect the activity of chakras above or below. For instance, a blocked communication chakra (fifth chakra) may result in problems with inner strength (third chakra) and vice versa. But may be the problem actually lies with the heart (fourth chakra) and only manifests itself in the areas listed because it is so deeply buried. By engaging with the theoretical system in its entirety and applying it to your personal chakra system that is strictly your own, you learn to bring order to the subtleties and patterns and undergo positive change in accordance with your goals."[39]

---

39 Anodea, J. (2004). *Wheel's of Life: A User's Guide to the Chakra System*. (pg. 54/55). Goldmann Arkana Publishing.

By learning to see our reflection in the mirror of the chakras we can learn much about our consciousness, our behavior, our body, and our relationship with other people and our environment.

But before we know exactly what precisely we wish to heal or change and exactly where to start with our practice, it makes sense to take a closer look at the individual chakras in all their different facets and dimensions.

5.6.1   MULADHARA CHAKRA – ROOT CHAKRA

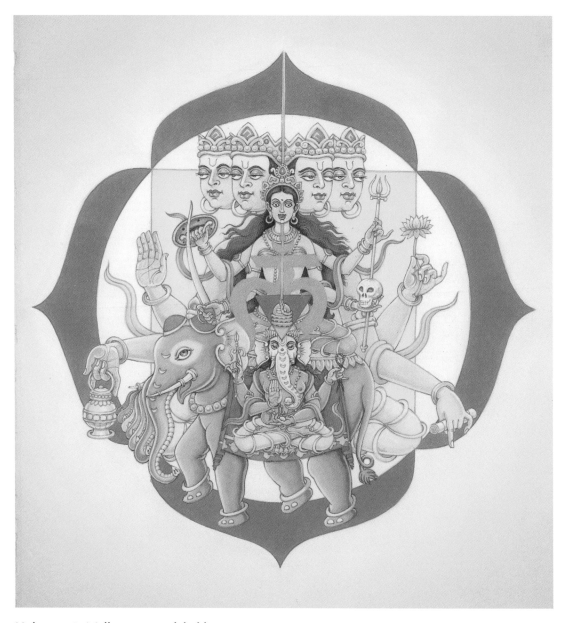

Mula = root / Adhara = vessel, holder, support

Muhladhara means root or support and forms the basis for all other chakras.

The *Muladhara chakra* is located in the lower pelvic region, in the area of the pelvic floor between the anus and the genitalia. The body parts assigned to this chakra are the lower pelvic region, anus, intestines, legs, feet, as well as bones, teeth, hair, and fingernails.

Element: earth

Color: red

Glands: adrenal glands

Neuroplexus: Plexus coccygeus (tailbone, coccyx)

Sensory organ: nose

Sensory function: smell

Bija-Mantra: LAM

Vayu: Apana (promotes elimination processes, e.g. stools, urinary excretion

Guna: Ganeesha (elephant god, son of Shiva and Shakti)

Function: survival, grounding, self-preservation

The lotus flower symbol shows four flower petals with a yellow square in the center, which symbolizes the four cardinal directions.[40] Depicted in the center is the single-syllable seed mantra (Bija Mantra) LAM. Above that is an arrow with its tip pointing downward. The shaft of the arrow symbolizes the main energy pathway Sushumna Nadi, accompanied by Ida and Pingala Nadi. The red downward pointing triangle stands for the Shakti force that developed into creation and lies hidden. In the center of the triangle is the snake coiled three times around a lingam, the Kundalini Shakti. The elephant with the seven trunks at which the triangle points represents the chakra's heavy, earthy, tangible quality. The elephant's seven trunks point to the seven chakras through which the Kundalini will move as it rises.

The elephant has an additional meaning. The Muladhara chakra's dominant deity is the elephant god Ganeesha who is considered a sign of good luck in Hindu mythology but also stands for wisdom. His long trunk reminds us of the importance of the breath and breath control, and the small eyes stand for alert observation. The giant ears remind us of taking on a receiving posture to cultivate the ability to lend an ear, to listen carefully, and thus absorb wisdom.

The Muladhara chakra represents the foundation of all earthly life. The Muladhara's main themes are grounding, stability, security, will-to-live, self-preservation, to be provided for on a material level, and basic trust. Solid and secure grounding is a requirement for all growth. A tree whose root system reaches deep into the ground will weather even strong storms and hurricanes. Just like everything that grows on the earth or is built on it by the hands of man requires a solid foundation, so, too, do we need a solid outer and inner foundation in our lives.

When we are constantly worried and insecure about our life situation, we lack the inner basis, the basic trust, and we trundle from one worry to the next, and from one insecurity to another like a leaf in the wind. Since in life the thing that manifests itself tends to be precisely that which resonates most with us internally, fears and worries unfortunately have a self-perpetuating effect.

---

40 Anodea, J. (2004, pg. 92).

Creating and cultivating a solid base of security for oneself is one of the Muladhara chakra's themes. If the Muladhara chakra is hyperactive, it can manifest itself in very rigid internal patterns that won't permit a second opinion or any mental flexibility. If the chakra is too weak, it can manifest itself in a "lack of groundedness". One floats with his head in the clouds, has many inspired plans but doesn't get anything done because there is no solid inner foundation.

In the Asana practice, perception-based, mobilizing, and strengthening exercises for feet, legs, and pelvis can provide a real sense of bodily grounding and stability. Strength and support poses can improve strength and stability in the entire body and create a sense for a secure "foundation". *Tadasana*, the Mountain, and Vrishasana, the Tree, are classic grounding exercises. Combined with visualizations like, for instance, letting vigorous roots from the pelvis, leg, and feet reach deep into the ground and being nurtured through them, can help reinforce faith in the process of life and one's own being.

5.6.2   SVADHISTHANA CHAKRA – SACRAL CHAKRA

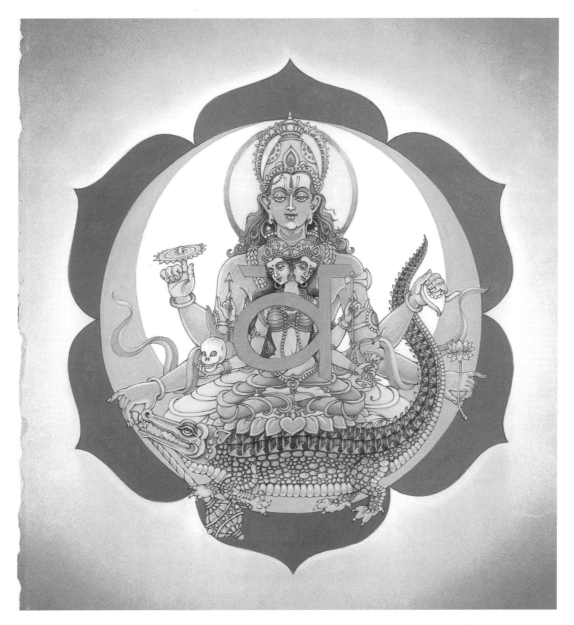

Sva = one's own, depending on the source also "Svad" the sweet, Adhisthana = dwelling, abode

Svadhisthana is the dwelling place of *sweetness*, *pleasure*, and *sexuality*.

The *Svadhistana chakra* is located in the sacral/bladder region at a level with the internal genitalia. The areas of the body associated with this chakra are the low back, genitalia, kidneys, bladder, as well as the cardiovascular system.

Element: water

Color: orange

Glands: gonads (ovaries, testes)

Neuroplexus: sacral plexus

Sensory organ: tongue

Sensory function: taste

Bija Mantra: VAM

Vayu: Apana (promotes elimination, e.g. ejaculation/menstrual blood)

Guna: Tamas (sluggishness) and Rajas (activity)

Deity: Narayana (great ocean of eternal time, embodiment of Vishnu)

Function: sexuality, procreation, creativity, emotional identity

The lotus flower symbol shows six orange petals that frame two additional lotus blossoms. A white crescent moon is located in the lower half of the lotus flower, which symbolizes water. In this context, one should think of the power of the moon with respect to the giant daily tidal movements of the oceans. On the crescent moon is the image of a crocodile (Makara). A crocodile can deploy enormous strength when it is hungry and on the hunt.

Since the Svadhisthana Chakra can be experienced by taste (tongue) as well as sexuality's pleasure center, the crocodile symbolizes inflamed passions. It can rest without moving for long periods of time, but once it has become active due to fierce desire, feral forces are unleashed. In this sense, the crocodile stands for unbridled passions and urges. Yoga masters have always recommended that their students should either practice asceticism (which can also become an impediment) or a moderate diet and sex life, to achieve enduring tranquility and peace.

The dominant element water stands for the aspects of movement, change, flexibility, and adaptability. On the physical plane water represents everything that flows within the body, such as blood, lymphatic fluid, digestive juices, sperm, and in the broadest (ethereal) sense also the flow of Prana along the energy pathways. On the emotional plane water expresses our constantly changing feelings. One moment one is engulfed in waves of excitement, and the very next moment the emotions stagnate again as though nothing ever happened. Like water, feelings are in constant motion.

When the Svadhisthana Chakra is hyperactive, it can manifest itself in hypersexuality as well as sex addiction or hedonism. Or one's emotions constantly run wild. A very weak Svadhisthana chakra can manifest itself in a lack of the ability to perceive or feel emotions, to express them, all the way to frigidity.

The Svadhisthana chakra is where the unconscious resides and the home of one's emotional identity. Anything we unconsciously hold on to, especially emotional issues that haven't been resolved, can manifest itself in vague muscular or organic tension. Unconsciously adhered to or suppressed emotions can consume a lot of the body's strength. The element of water and the associated quality of free flow represent another valuable aspect, letting go. Mindfulness and deliberate breathing allow the lower abdominal area to relax again. Many people are very tense in that part of the body without even noticing. Gently flowing pelvic movements like hip circles and pelvic tilt can release congealed emotions or energies in the stomach and pelvic region. Movements that gently get the body, the energy, to flow help stimulate the Svadhisthana chakra. Karanas/flows in time with the breath along with soft, relaxed movements enhance the feeling of flow. All variations of Markarasana (crocodile exercises) also gently stimulate energy flow.

Long, sustained stretches in the pelvic region like Baddha Konasana, so called *cooling exercises*, can calm revved up emotions and open the path to deeper perceptions and emotions. Focusing on the water element as a visualization exercise helps with embracing and letting go and promotes understanding for all of life's cycles.

5.6.3   MANIPURA CHAKRA – SOLAR PLEXUS CHAKRA

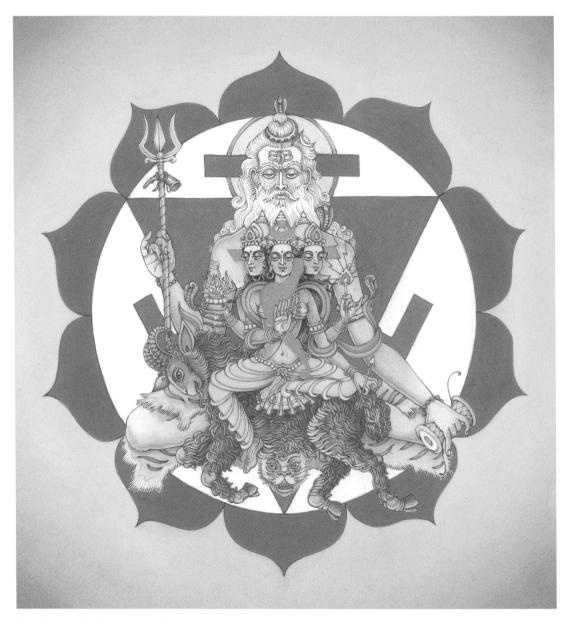

Mani = Jewel, Pura = city, place, center

The *Manipura chakra* is also referred to as *City of the Shining Jewel* and relates to the luminous power and brilliance of the sun's energy.

It is not located directly in the area of the navel but in the region between solar plexus (coeliac plexus) and navel. The associated areas of the body are the upper and middle abdominal region, digestive system, stomach, spleen, liver, gallbladder, and the vegetative nervous system.

Element: fire

Color: golden-yellow

Glands: pancreas, adrenal glands

Neuroplexus: solar plexus

Sensory organ: eyes

Sensory function: sight

Bija Mantra: RAM

Vayu: Samana (digestions: conversion of food to energy)

Guna: Rajas (activity)

Deity: Surya (sun)

Function: willpower, perseverance, power, discipline, self-esteem, transformation

The lotus flower symbol shows ten petals with a downward-pointing triangle in the center. The brilliant orange-yellow triangle stands for strength and the heat of fire, the downward-pointing tip of the triangle stands for the descending cosmic force. The three suggested vertical lines in the background represent the three main energy pathways Sushumna Nadi, flanked by Ida and Pingala Nadi, and remind us that all chakras are linked via Sushumna Nadi. The ram, the Manipura chakra's power animal, represents dynamic strength, heat, endurance, and willpower.

The Manipura Chakra is considered the place where the cosmic life force (Prana) is stored, which is depicted via the fire's radiant warmth/heat. On the mental-emotional level the power of the fire provides the necessary willpower, vital energy, and power to meet life's many challenges vigorously and with joyful enthusiasm. Without the force of the fire we would grow cold inside, withdraw, grow lethargic, and our development would ultimately stagnate.

But this chakra isn't about fulfilling the ego's many desires and wishes through power and willpower, thereby building up some perceived self-esteem.

The sensory function "sight" is associated with the Manipura chakra. Sight allows us to come into contact with things or products we want or think we need. The power of fire helps us develop discipline (Tapas) on the spiritual path. Tapas means *embers*, *inner heat*. This refers to establishing a joyful inner discipline, a regular practice (Asana, meditation, Pranayama, the study of spiritual texts). Fire means light. In terms of a spiritual practice, it is about distinguishing whether our motivation and actions facilitate inner growth in the sense of a higher light, or whether they are of a distressing nature.

Manipura chakra is closely linked to the digestive process. The activation of Manipura creates warmth in the body, which activates the metabolic processes all the way to cell metabolism. Digestion means transformation, conversion. On a physical plane food is transformed into energy, which is controlled by Samana

Vayu. But feelings are also transformed on the Manipura level. Some common expressions show roughly how this works: "My stomach is in knots", "I have to digest this or that experience", or "I have a queasy feeling about that".

Manipura chakra is activated by all forward bends and backbends. The Sun Salutation *Surya Namaskar* is a classic exercise to stimulate the sun's energy. On the one hand, the organs are alternately stretched and contracted by the successive forward bends and backbends, and on the other hand these whole-body movements, when executed at a fast pace, counteract sluggishness and lethargy because they build heat. All twists facilitate the process of transformation and purification. Strength and support exercises can help to also develop internal discipline, strength, and endurance. Visualization exercises that bring light to the body's center (e.g. a small sun) support a sense of warming inner strength and life force.

5.6.4   ANAHATA CHAKRA – HEART CHAKRA

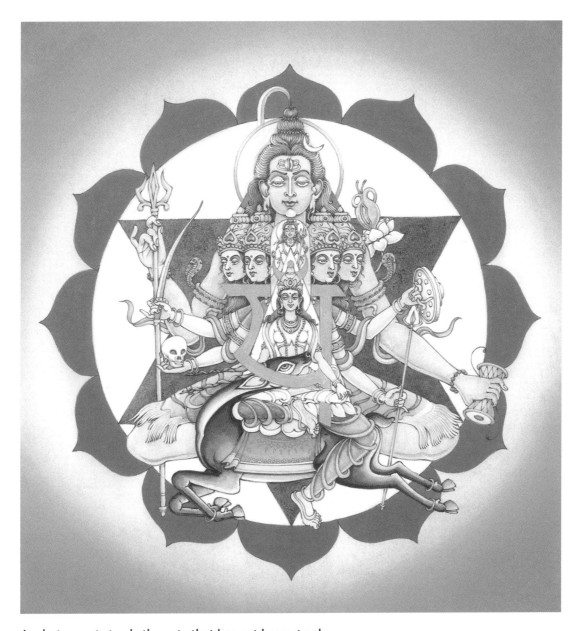

Anahata = not struck, the note that has not been struck

The term *Anahata* refers to the eternal, unstruck cosmic sound vibration in the heart of every living creature.

The heart chakra is located at a level with the physical heart, behind the sternum. The associated areas of the body are the ribcage, upper back, heart, lungs, arms, and hands.

Element: air

Color: green

Glands: thyroid

Neuroplexus: cardinal plexus (neuroplexus at the base of the heart)

Sensory organ: skin

Sensory function: touch, feel

Bija Mantra: YAM

Vayu: Prana Vayu (absorption of energy)

Guna: Sattva (clarity, purity) and Rajas (activity)

Deity: Vishnu and Lakshmi

Function: Universal love, tolerance, sincerity, balance, peace

The lotus flower symbol shows twelve petals. They frame a six-pointed star, which is formed by two triangles that penetrate each other. The light-blue triangles represent the endless expanse of the sky and the clarity in the space of the higher heart. The downward-pointing triangle stands for the cosmic Shiva force (highest consciousness force). The upward-pointing triangle stands for the Kundalini Shakti that rises from the lower pelvic region. Both penetrate each other in the Anahata chakra and thus express the union between Shiva and Shakti, or rather the oneness of Purusha and Prakriti (spirit/matter; consciousness/energy).

The flame in the center of the star represents the higher light, the higher self in the heart of every human being. The leaping antelope symbolizes the freedom and lightness of the heart quality.

"Hidden within the heart of every living creature lies the Self, more subtle than the subtlest, greater than the greatest[41]", according to the Katha Upanishad. The heart center is our spiritual center. It is also called our emotional center because that is where we get in touch with the aspects and polarities of our different feelings, such as passions and dislikes, love, disappointment, and pain.

The goal of the spiritual path is the transformation from damaging or (self-)destructive thoughts and feelings to inner peace and balance. "When you have peace in your heart, your shack becomes your palace" is a common expression. Deep inner peace lets conflicts melt away and breaks through the chain of the constantly revolving wish spiral.

Common expressions tell us that we can have a heavy heart, pierce someone to the heart, have a heart of stone or a heart of gold, have your heart in your boots, someone can have his heart in the right place, or wear his heart on his sleeve, or pour out his heart.

---

41 Easwaran, E. (2008, Katha Upanishad 2.20, pg. 125).

We often hear, "If only I had followed my heart". With the many assertions about the role of the heart it is surprising that everyone doesn't first consult their heart when it comes to important issues. In everyday life, the quiet voice of the heart is often drowned out by the more forceful activity of the mind.

And because often everyday life is also very fast-paced and sometimes requires quick decision-making, we usually don't get the necessary rest to place a hand over the heart and feel what the heart wants. The yoga practice provides participants with precisely that quiet time to relax and allow the voice of the heart to speak to us.

"When torn between the heart and the mind, follow the heart" (Vivekananda)[42]. From a physical standpoint, the heart is linked to the element of air and the breath. We gather energy by breathing. A conscious, deep and calm breath calms the mental-emotional level. Many people unconsciously try to protect their heart space by rounding their shoulders and upper back. If your job requires you to sit a lot, this posture can quickly become a habit, which means your breath can no longer flow freely.

42 https://www.aphorismen.de/zitat/19586

5.6.5 VISHUDDHA CHAKRA – THROAT CHAKRA

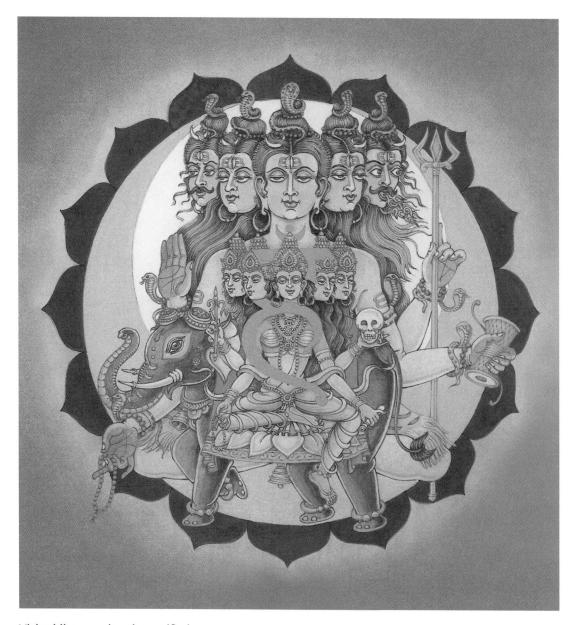

Vishuddha = purity, the purified

The *Vishuddha chakra*, also referred to as the throat or laryngeal chakra, is located in the center of the throat. The associated areas of the body are neck and nape, throat, vocal cords, vocal apparatus, thyroid, and esophagus.

Element: space (ether, Akasha)

Color: light-blue/turquoise

Glands: thyroid, parathyroid

Neuroplexus: plexus pharyngeus (plexus in the pharynx)

Sensory organ: ears, mouth

Sensory function: hearing, speech

Bija Mantra: HAM

Vayu: Udana (rising energy, controls speech, communication, self-expression)

Guna: Rajas (activity) and Sattva (calm, clarity)

Deity: Shiva and Ganga (purifying river goddess)

Function: communication, creativity, purification of the mind and vocal expression

The lotus flower symbol shows sixteen petals framing a downward-pointing triangle (descending cosmic force). Inside the triangle is a white circle that is reminiscent of the full moon. It stands for the element of space. In the center of the circle is the character for the Bija Mantra "Ham". In the Vishuddha lotus symbol, the elephant with the seven trunks (see definition of Muladhara chakra) is white. White symbolizes purification, the chakra's main theme.

The element *space*, which is assigned to the Vishuddha chakra, and is also called *ether* or *Akasha*, is the most ethereal of all elements. While the elements earth, water, and fire can be clearly described and experienced through their different qualities, the qualities of the elements air and space are extremely subtle. We can perceive air as the air we breathe or as wind on our skin, but we experience the qualities of space as vast, free, and clear. But when the capacity of external or internal space is markedly restricted, we feel constrained and oppressed; we lack the space to breathe or the space to form our own thoughts and impulses and to act on them.

Space is closely linked to vibration and sound since sounds and tones can only be transmitted through space. *Sound* means *language* and *voice* and is closely connected to *listening*, to *listening closely*. One of the overriding themes of the Vishuddha chakra is to get in tune internally with the subtler cosmic vibrations and to discern them.

The "OM" or "AUM" in the classical yoga texts is considered the primal cosmic sound. OM is the sound vibration from which all of creation originates and perpetually renews itself. In the book *Nada Yoga, Moving Towards the Inner Sound*, it is explained as follows: "The syllable 'OM' is the first level of manifestation, the sound vibration that is closest to the divine. Reciting this syllable allows us to connect to the divine origin."[43]

---

43 Irmer, B. & Mager, C. (2009). *Nada Yoga. Hinwendung zum inneren Klang.* (pg. 17). Bielefeld: Theseus Publishing.

Sound vibrations in the form of music, sounds, mantras, and words can evidently have a healing effect. But sound vibrations can also cause injury. In his book *The Message From Water*[44], the famous Japanese parascientist and alternative medicine practitioner Masaru Emoto describes and shows very vividly how the sound vibrations of different words affect water crystals. Words like love, gratitude, or wisdom show water crystal shapes of clear and brilliant beauty, while words like imbecile, war, or even aggressive, loud music full of expletives show vague, dark, and diffuse crystal shapes.

Compared to the rest of the body, the neck is rather thin and fragile and connects head and body. In a metaphorical sense, the neck center represents the connection between intellect and emotion. When these aspects are not in alignment the neck center is generally the target organ for inner, unresolved conflicts. There are many common expressions that describe this phenomenon: to breathe down someone's neck, someone's crest is rising, one has a lump in the throat, laughter sticks in one's throat, or one has a frog in the throat.

Most of these sayings imply that something cannot be said due to an emotional or physical blockage in the throat. But when someone has "a golden throat" it means a beautiful, clear voice. However, when someone has "eaten chalk" it is an attempt at sugarcoating something that isn't perceived that way. Muscular tension in the neck and nape can also express an unresolved, unclean Vishuddha chakra.

According to legend, to save the world the Hindu deity Shiva (god of the neck center) once took the deadly poison of the ocean, which threatened to destroy the entire universe. If he had swallowed it, it would have been the end of him. That is why he held it in his throat, which caused his neck to turn blue. The hidden message is that the throat as our speech center can both poison and heal, because words can have a salutary and clearing effect, too.

Gentle shoulder, neck, and nape mobility and stretching exercises, limbering exercises for the lower jaw, exercises that prolong exhalation, like humming or Ujjayi Pranayama, vowel sounding exercises, mantra recitations, kirtan singing, visualization exercises (e.g. visualizing the purifying color light-blue in the throat area or shifting the inner focus to the element space), consciously lending an ear (listening closely), gong meditation, periods of conscious silence (Mauna) are all exercises that help harmonize the Vishuddha chakra.

---

44 Emotu, M. (2001). *The Message from Water*, Vol. 1.

5.6.6   AJNA CHAKRA – THIRD EYE CHAKRA

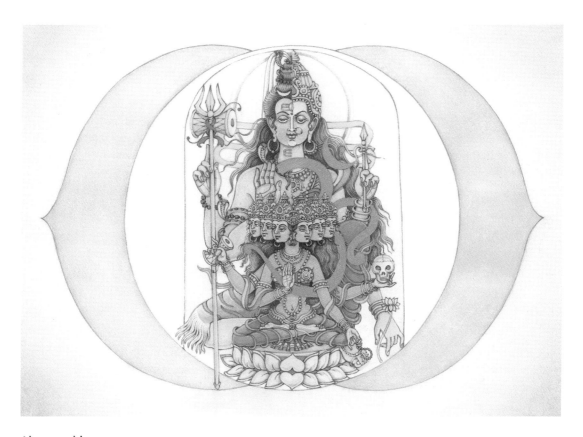

Ajna = guidance

Ajna means *perception*, but also *guidance*. *Directive*. This chakra is located in the center of the head, slightly above the eyes between the eyebrows, and can be perceived via *Bhrumadhya* (eyebrow center). It is therefore also referred to as the *third eye* or *eyebrow center*. The associated areas of the body are the forehead, ears, nose, sinuses, and nervous system.

Element: no allocation

Color: indigo blue

Glands: epiphysis (pineal gland)

Sensory organ: no allocation

Sensory function: no allocation

Bija Mantra: OM

Vayu: Prana, Vyana

Guna: Sattva (calm, purity)

Deity: Hakini Shakti, Shiva (pure power of consciousness), Sarasvati (goddess of wisdom)

Function: intuition, intellect, clairvoyance, visualization, receiving higher knowledge

The lotus flower symbol shows two white petals, one on each side of a circle. Inside the circle is a downward-pointing triangle. In the center of the triangle the Bija Mantra OM is pictured above a lingam, the symbol of the god Shiva. The flame symbolizes the higher light of consciousness but also represents vision.

Interesting here is the significance of the gland, the epiphysis (pineal gland) that is associated with the Ajna chakra. It is very light sensitive and controls the sleep-wake rhythm as well as other time-dependent rhythms in the body. The epiphysis is located in the brain just above the pituitary gland and is often associated with the seventh chakra. Judith Anodea bases the association of the epiphysis (pineal gland) with the sixth chakra on the one hand on the superior function of the pituitary gland, and on the other hand on the light sensitivity of the epiphysis and the resulting control of the sleep-wake rhythm.[45]

Correspondingly the three main energy pathways Sushumna, Ida, and Pingala Nadi merge on the energy plane in the Ajna chakra. That is why this chakra is also viewed as the control center for all vital processes. Ida Nadi represents the lunar aspects (regeneration, calm, intuition, emotional experiences) and Pingala Nadi represents the solar aspects (light, fire, activity, intellect). From there Ida and Pingala Nadi run along the right (Pingala) and left (Ida) side of the nose. The polar qualities can be stimulated and experienced via Pranayamas like Surya- or Chandra Bhedan, among others, Ajna Chakra also controls the lower five chakras.

The Ajna chakra represents higher knowledge, intuition, and clairvoyance. We get in touch with our inner wisdom via the Ajna chakra. Just like we carefully tune a radio channel for better reception we can also tune into and focus on the Ajna chakra to boost intuition. All of us are much more intuitive than we think, and focusing on the Ajna chakra provides the link to increased sensitivity. When the mind's loud voices calm down or grow quieter, we can enter the field of refined awareness. This connects us to our inner guru and opens us up to inner guidance.

When we cannot see the forest for the trees, have lost sight of what matters, our vision has grown foggy, we lose perspective, or have a thorn in our eye, we can see this as a definite hint to close our eyes and return to experiencing life slightly more with our inner eyes.

Ajna chakra allows us to receive or develop visions and inner images that support us on our inner or spiritual path. All meditative visualization exercises (focusing on a flame, inner light, vastness or clarity) strengthen the Ajna chakra. The Ajna chakra can be strengthened via eye exercises (blinking, etc., working on practicing with eyes closed), focusing on Bhrumaddhya (the third eye), reciting the OM mantra, concentration exercises, and all twists (allow us to feel the polar qualities), and by focusing on the inner center (Madhya).

---

45 Anodea, J. (2004, pg. 338).

5.6.7 SAHASRARA CHAKRA – CROWN CHAKRA

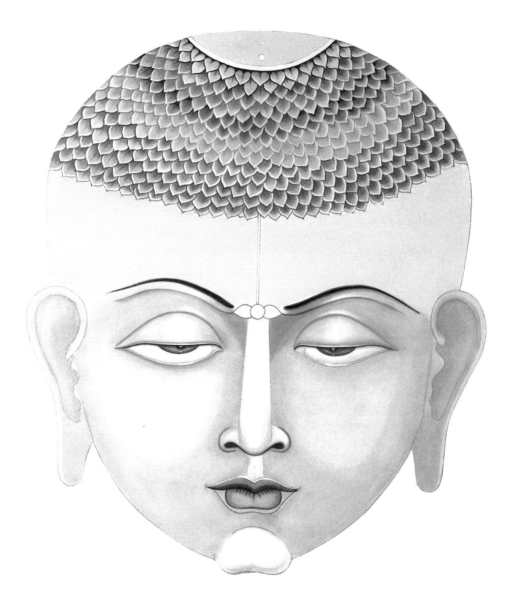

The *Sahasrara Chakra* is located centrally on the highest point of the head, which is why it is also called the vertex chakra. The associated areas of the body are the skullcap, fontanel, and cerebral cortex.

Element: no allocation

Color: white, colorless, transparent

Glands: pituitary gland (controls the function of all other glands)

Neuroplexus: no allocation

Sensory organ: no allocation

Sensory function: no allocation

Bija Mantra: no allocation

Vayu: no allocation

Guna: Sattva (clarity, purity)

Deity: Parashiva (absolute consciousness)

Function: consciousness of oneness, transcendence, wisdom, deliverance, meditation

Sahasra means *1000*, *Ara* means *spoke* (of a *wheel*). This refers to the number of petals of the lotus flower symbol, which is said to be 1000 and is the symbol for infinity. Other interpretations are that 1000 refers to the chakra's thousand-fold power. But it could also refer to the many energy pathways (Nadis) that radiate from the crown chakra, since the chakra is located at the upper end of Sushumna Nadi, the central main energy pathway.

Each petal bears one of the 50 letters from the Sanskrit alphabet. The lotus flower symbol is often depicted in color; all of the colors of the lower six chakras are represented. They merge in the crown chakra and ultimately become white or colorless because all qualities have transcended. This is expressed with the brilliantly white moon in the center of the lotus symbol (Chandra Mandala).

The crown chakra is also called the "gateway to infinity". Another term is *Brahmarandhra*, the home of Brahman. In Hindu philosophy, *Brahman* is the eternal source of all being, the unchanging, transcendent, immanent reality. That is why *Brahmarandhra* is also called the *cosmic hole* through which consciousness can ascend to higher planes in the course of spiritual development and with the help of yoga practices.

Sahasrara reveals itself through the cleaning of the chakras and the associated inner development. It is also the gateway to higher consciousness:

"So what is 'higher consciousness'? Higher consciousness is the knowledge of a higher or lower -a comprehensive-order. Higher consciousness is sometimes also called cosmic consciousness. This refers to the knowledge surrounding a cosmic or celestial order. The lower chakras contain endless information about the material world and its cycles of cause and effect. By contrast cosmic consciousness reaches far into the galaxies and beyond. It opens us up to knowledge about the truths that unite us. It is the awareness of the Meta patterns, the comprehensive organizational principles of our cosmic classification system."[46]

---

46 Anodea, J. (2004, pg. 381).

During the Asana practice, awareness of the Sahasrara chakra can be activated via the king of Asanas, the headstand. Tadasana or standing forward bend can also facilitate focus on the vertex. There are many visualization techniques that focus on the Sahasrara chakra. Some also include focusing on the lower six chakras.

The more overly intellectual we are, the faster the carousel of our mind spins, or the more we are at the mercy of our emotions, and the farther away we get from the lucid quality of the crown chakra.

Quiet meditation with an inner focus on deliverance, calm, and vastness of spirit is consistent with the crown chakra, which can be prepared via purifying or balancing Pranayama/breathing exercise.

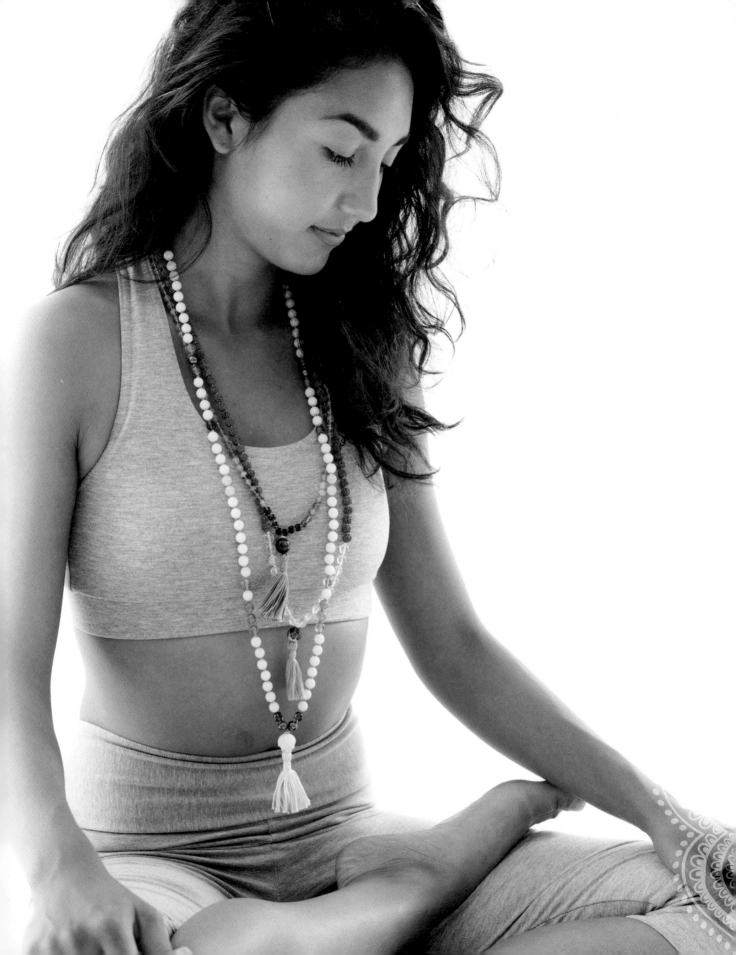

6 SIGNIFICANCE AND PRACTICE OF ASANA

6 SIGNIFICANCE AND PRACTICE OF ASANA

6.1 SIGNIFICANCE

ASANA

As = seat

The Sanskrit name *Asana* is derived from the root word as, which means seat. There were references to yoga poses in the writings[47] long before the Hatha Yoga practice system developed: the seated pose. This refers to the *seated meditation pose*. While the headstand is generally considered the king of the Asanas and the shoulder stand the queen, the seated meditation pose in its different variations can be considered the mother or father of the Asanas.

Information varies with respect to the number of Asanas. The *Hatha Yoga Pradipika*[48] refers to 8,400 yoga poses, of which – according to legend – Shiva, the patron god of yogis chose and taught 84 Asanas for preservation of good health and development of self-reflection. Of these, four poses (Siddhasana, Padmasana, Simhasana, Bhadrasana) were considered the essential ones, all of which describe variations of the seated meditation pose.

As easy as this seated pose may look at first glance, as demanding does it become in practice. When looking at the classic meditation seat strictly from a physical point of view, it requires flexible, nimble hips and inner thigh muscles. In addition the spine must be held upright and relaxed along its natural curvature for an extended period of time.

People who are used to sitting every day primarily with a rounded back and possibly even have tension in the shoulders and nape, will hardly be able to sit relaxed and upright for an extended period of time with inflexible hips and a rounded spine. This being the case, the Asanas with their many different effects are a perfect system with a wide bandwidth to systematically prepare the body for meditation or the seated posture.

---

47 Skuban, R. Patanjali's Yoga Sutra, pg. 146 / Bäumer, B. & Deshpande, N.Y.: Patanjali: Die Wurzeln des Yogas, pg. 121 / Autobindo, S. Bhagavadgita, chapter 6, verse 11-13, pg. 43 and 44
48 Swami Svatmarama. *Hatha Yoga Pradipika, The Yoga of Light.* pg. 25.

When we talk about Asana today, we refer to *yoga* poses. A popular point of view is that ultimately the primary goal of all Asanas is to prepare the body and mind for the seated meditation pose. This perspective is convincing particularly in view of the Yoga Sutra according to Patanjali, because first the physical preconditions (Asana) are created to then create a basis for the subtler aspects (breath control, pulling back the senses, concentration), which in turn is the foundation for meditation.

The emergence and development of Asanas can be seen as a dynamic process. Some Asanas are still relatively recent, meaning they were only created in in the past 100 years. This includes most of the standing poses. Others, as verified by archeological discoveries in the Indus valley (today's Northwestern India), show yogic seals, symbols, and poses whose origins are estimated to date back to approx. 5000 BCE.

Since the names of many of the Asanas were taken from nature (tree, mountain) or creatures (cobra, locust, camel), it can be assumed that individual poses were created by observing and imitating nature, or at least were heavily influenced by it. By assuming and experimenting with physical poses, people found out that certain poses have purifying, health-maintaining, and invigorating effects.

Asanas and practices derived from the Tantric line of development grew from the wealth of experience regarding the subtle energy system (chakras, Nadis). They were developed by yogis with a deep inner vision, which resulted in knowledge about the effects of and links between physical poses and Prana. Other orientations that prioritized the aspect of asceticism placed more emphasis on overcoming the physical body and its deliverance through Asanas, self-discipline, and concentration.

Over time, very different ideas and orientations developed from the many approaches to the practice of Asanas. There was never an overriding, mutual consensus and there still isn't today. The bandwidth of the Asana practice includes orientations whose poses are acrobatic and challenging in nature. There are versions that prioritize the physical aspect (practice Asanas with abandon and the rest will just happen on its own). In some traditions, Asanas are practiced in specific sequences or series with varying degrees of difficulty, while others prioritize effects or spiritual themes that provide the framework for the Asana practice. Some schools teach primarily static practices while others teach primarily dynamic ones. And these days many schools and instructors combine different methods.

6.2 BASIC POSES

As previously explained, the practice of Asanas is an organic system that over time evolved in different ways and along different lines of tradition. Even today, new Asanas and variations on Asanas are still being added. The number of Asanas commonly used today is approx. 30-40 poses.

But the following twelve basic poses are generally viewed as most essential.

1. Headstand – Shirsana

2. Shoulder stand – Sarvangasana

3. Plow – Halasana

4. Fish – Matsyasana

5. Extended leg seated forward bend – Paschimottanasana

6. Cobra – Bhujangasana

7. Locust – Shalabhasana

8. Bow – Dhanurasana

9. Seated twist – Ardha Matsyendrasana

10. Crow – Kakasana

11. Standing forward bend – Uttanasana

12. Triangle – Trikonasana

There are many variations, amplifications, and modifications of these twelve poses. They can be categorized in different ways to provide an overview of the entire system, regardless of the number of Asanas.

6.3 DIRECTIONS OF SPINAL MOVEMENT

6.3.1 BASED ON THEIR FORM AND ORIENTATION IN SPACE

STANDING POSES

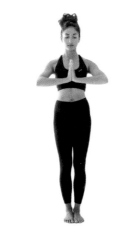

Tadasana (mountain pose)

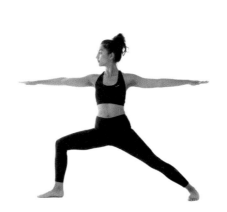

Virabhadrasana 2 (warrior 2)

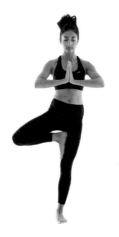

Vrikshasana (tree)

SEATED POSES

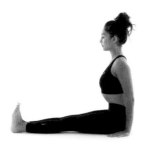

Dandasana
(staff pose)

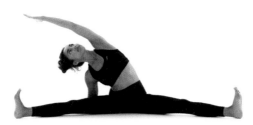

Upavista Konasana
(open angle pose)

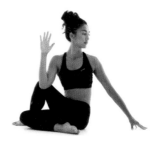

Ardha Matsyendrasana
(seated twist)

RECUMBENT POSES

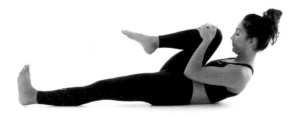

Eka Padana Apanasana

Setu Bandha (shoulder bridge)

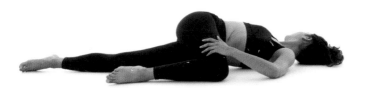

Makarasana variation (crocodile pose)

6.3.2 BASED ON THEIR FUNCTION

STRENGTH AND SUPPORT POSES

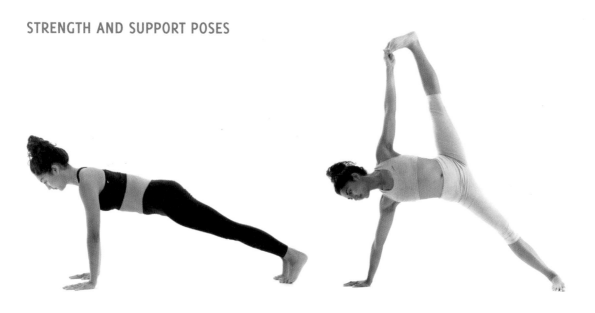

Phalakasana (plank)

Vasisthasana (bound side plank)

BALANCE POSES

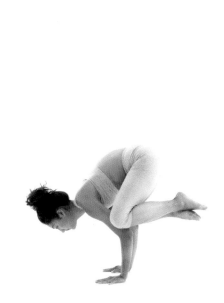

Kakasana (crow)

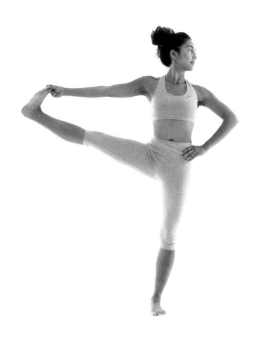

Hasta Padangusthasana (standing hand-to-foot pose)

INVERSIONS

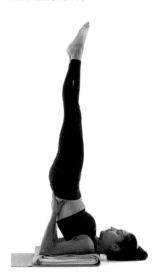

Salamba Sarvangasana
(shoulder stand)

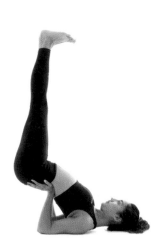

Viparita Karani
(half shoulder stand)

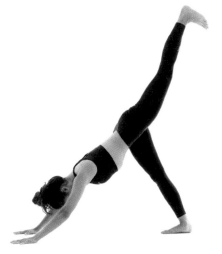

Adho Mukha Svanasana Eka Pada
(downward facing dog with leg split)

RELAXATION POSES

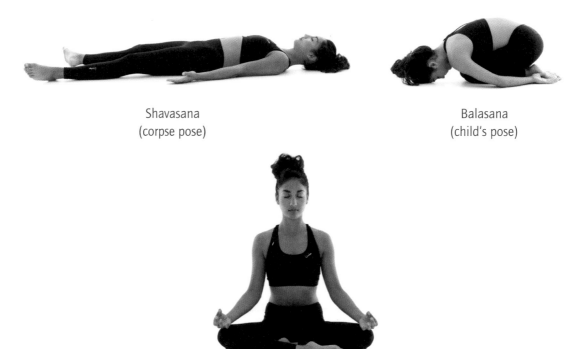

Shavasana
(corpse pose)

Balasana
(child's pose)

Sukhasana (upright-seated pose)

6.3.3 BASED ON THE SPINE'S DIRECTION OF MOVEMENT

Arranging Asanas based on the spine's directional movement is a differentiated arrangement that includes simple as well as more complex Asanas and provides a more comprehensive overview. To capture and understand the structure of a pose, one must first look at the spine's direction of movement before putting the pose in one of the following categories.

a) "Meru Danda" the axis of the world – the spine and its directions of movement

Meru[49] is a mythological mountain in the center of the universe that stretches over hundreds of thousands of kilometers and is the meeting place of the gods. It is said that the source of the Ganges (Sushumna Nadi) is on its summit and the seven low worlds (the chakras) are below it.

In yoga and in the Tantric view, *Meru Danda* represents the human spine. It forms the vertical axis for physical movements and also the pathway for the nervous system and energy-related processes.

---

49 Source: Huchzermeyer, W. (2015, pg. 115).

From a yoga perspective, anything that affects the spine affects the entire system. Thus the spine is always at the center of the practice. All Asanas affect the spine without exception.

From an anatomical point of view, there are six directions of movement of the spine: flexion, extension, lateral flexion (right-left), rotation (right-left).

b)   The eight basic spinal movements in yoga

1.   Axial extension
Tadasana (mountain pose)

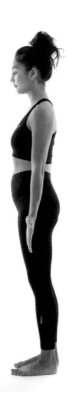

This is the erection of the spine along its vertical axis. The spine is consciously lengthened beyond its neutral position (double-S curve). The axial extension is an important basis and prerequisite for every additional movement. All active poses always begin with the axial extension. Creating length is both a requirement for energy flow as well as injury prevention.

2.   Compression

The opposite of "axial extension" is the spine's collapse along the vertical axis. This generally happens because of too much sitting or an awkward body position for an extended period of time. This movement in particular will be counterbalanced by the yoga practice, so the natural posture is closer to the axial extension.

3. **Forward bend (Flexion)**

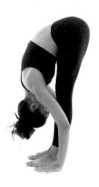

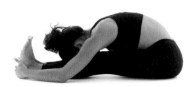

Uttanasana (standing forward bend)   Paschimottanasana (seated head to knee posture)

4. **Backbend (Extension)**

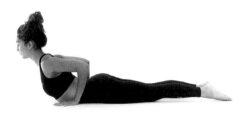

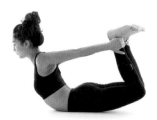

Bhujangasana (cobra)   Dhanurasana (bow)

5. **Side bend right (lateral flexion)**
6. **Side bend left (lateral flexion)**

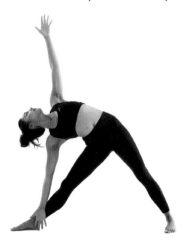

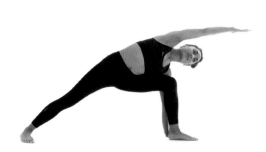

Trikonasana (triangle)   Utthita Parsvakonasana (extended side angle)

7. Twist right (rotation)
8. Twist left (rotation)

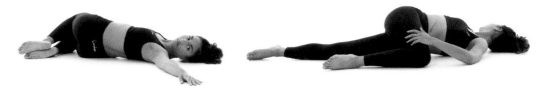

Makarasana variations (crocodile pose)

6.4   GENERAL EFFECTS OF ASANAS

"No amount of praise is too much when we talk about the almost supernatural effects of physical poses on the human organism and their role in preserving vitality and promoting health."[50]

Asanas work on a physical, energy-related, mental, emotional, and spiritual level. But the Asanas' effects depend more specifically on how they are practiced, both in terms of the type of practice and the inner attitude and focus. Traditionally an Asanas is a static pose, but many dynamic approaches have been established over time. From a muscular standpoint, the practice of Asanas can be very intense or more accessible. The method of choice always affects the overall experience.

The following effects can be observed with respect to the different physical systems:

Locomotor system

» Improves bone structure,

» Strengthens the core muscles (deep trunk-erecting muscles),

» Erects and stabilizes the spine,

» Corrects muscular imbalances and thus improves posture,

» Strengthens and stretches the skeletal muscles,

» Improves motor skills (mobility, coordination, balance).

Cardiovascular system

» Improves blood circulation and perfusion of internal organs,

» Regulates blood pressure.

---

50 Yesudian, S. & Haich, E. (1984, pg. 140).

Digestive system

» Massages internal organs and thereby improves organ health,

» Stimulates metabolism,

» Stimulates digestive fire and elimination process.

Respiratory system

» Improves breath awareness,

» Opens airways,

» Deepens breaths and improves breath volume,

» Deacidification of the body via deeper exhalation,

» Increased oxygen uptake.

Nervous system

» Calms the nervous system,

» Facilitates relaxation ability,

» Improves conductivity of nerve pathways (sensory and motor signals are processed more quickly).

Endocrine system

» Release of endorphins (act as a kind of analgesic body-purifying opiate and can trigger a sense of wellbeing),

» A direct effect of Asanas on the endocrine system such as is often mentioned in yoga literature with respect to head and shoulder stands, is now considered debatable.[51]

Mental and emotional effects

» Improved concentration ability,

» Improved cognition,

» Improved body awareness.

Intellectual-emotional effects

» In a way the Asana practice is a mirror for us. By focusing our awareness on what happens inside of us and with us during the practice, we can reflect on our behavior and make incremental internal adjustments. At the start of the yoga path, the Asanas are generally practiced the same way we operate in our lives. For instance, someone who always functions full throttle in everyday life and is very performance-oriented, initially tends to also live that out in the Asana practice: The behavior that actually requires a correction continues to be fueled by the same performance-standard pattern on the yoga mat.

---

51 Viveka, Hefte für Yoga: http://www.viveka.de/pdf/viveka_22_Asanas_und_Druesen.pdf

» But when awareness-oriented and meditative elements are incrementally integrated into the practice, the experience of balance, mindfulness, and reflection can help bring more inner calm and deep strength to the way we function in everyday life.

» By contrast, someone who tends to be physically and mentally rather more unstable can learn how to consciously build up strength and tension with a physically more intense practice, and apply that experience in everyday life. Someone who tends to give up when faced with the smallest difficulty can learn through the practice to build up patience and stability. When we develop and learn "witnessing awareness" within the practice, reflect our behavior, it gives us the opportunity to recognize habitual patterns that are harmful to us and break new ground. Hence the practice on the mat is the ideal practice ground for everyday life. And in our daily lives we can then remember which experiences on the mat helped us gain more energy, stability, and inner calm.

Spiritual effects

» The spiritual effects of the Asana practice are very individual and should always be viewed in combination with the practicing individual's inner attitude and level of development. For instance, the extent to which a chakra's qualities express themselves over the course of the practice depends on different factors. The spiritual effects gradually appear very individually in the course of the practice.

» The possible spiritual effects on the yoga path are described in detail in Patanjali's Yoga Sutra, chapter 3 (Vibhuti Pada: Disengagement) and chapter 4 (Kaivalya Pada: Deliverance).

6.5   STRUCTURES AND EFFECTS OF ASANAS

6.5.1   STRUCTURE AND EFFECTS OF THE FORWARD BEND

A *forward bend* involves flexion of the hip joint and depending on the type of forward bend, flexion of the spine. There are different kinds of forward bends like, for instance, the forward bend with a straight spine (e.g. Utkatasana/chair pose, Ardha Uttanasana/half forward bend) and forward bends with a rounded spine (e.g. Marjarie Asana/cat pose; Balasana/child's pose). There are standing, seated, and supine forward bends.

From an anatomical standpoint forward bends are deep stretches of the body's entire backside, especially the muscle chains at the back of the legs and low back. The back muscles are stretched, depending on the type of forward bend, as well as the structures of the lumbar spine and sacrum, and the deep erector spinae muscles and ligaments within the spine. In the case of a forward bend with an extended spine, the trunk-erecting muscles of the back are strengthened, while the posterior lower pelvic region and the back of the legs are deeply stretched.

♦ HATHA YOGA

In the course of a yoga class, the forward bends are usually practiced first from a standing position as transitional Asana in the form of Sun Salutations or as part of a flow. Further into the practice the holding phases get longer based on how warmed up the practicing individual is, how flexible he is, and his ability.

Most of the forward bends are done in closed poses that don't permit outside "entertainment". This can occasionally cause internal friction. Opposing physical, mental, and emotional aspects can be experienced very intensely during the holding phase of a forward bend when, for instance, areas of the back of the body are very much shortened and one is confronted with limitations and "stretching pain". One might grow impatient with this and want to give up on a particular exercise or pose.

The challenge of the pose isn't in taking it higher, deeper, farther. In situations where muscles are tight and we can get no farther, we can learn to develop permeability, to meet stiffness with softness, patience, and leniency.

Pausing, accepting, and breathing through it. Developing serenity. In this manner, we can learn to accept strains and observe them during the Asana practice, which in turn is a valuable exercise for everyday life and also a way to prepare for meditation.

From an energy anatomy standpoint, hardening, tightness, or shortening of the muscles is energy that has solidified on a material level. It is energy that no longer flows. One of the goals of the Asana practice is to dissolve this energy and allow it to flow so it no longer blocks the body, but is once again available as vital energy.

Tight muscles demand a lot of energy; they take up a lot of the body's strength. By being mindful in feeling the muscles and breathing into them (or via appropriate preparatory exercises) these structures can over time loosen up, and the energy begins to flow again and is once again available to the system. That is also a reason, among other things, why often feel not only relaxed but also energized after a practice.

Forward bends are also called devotional and submissive poses. The pose's symbolism says: We bow deeply; we bow our head before that which is higher and greater than our thinking and planning mind. We thereby relinquish control with the forward bend, which can be quite a challenge. We lose sight of what is going on around us, expose our unprotected necks, we are vulnerable, violable in terms of the archaic experience. At the same time we delve into ourselves. Linked to this is the invitation and also the great opportunity to release ourselves from controlling thoughts and to open the external and internal organs of perception to delve deeper inside ourselves, into the powerful calm of the heart.

During the forward bend, particularly while standing or seated, the internal organs are vigorously massaged due to the compression in the abdomen. This massage effect is aided by long deep belly breaths, whereby the diaphragm puts gentle pressure on the internal organs during inhalation.

From an energy standpoint, forward bends activate Apana Vayu, meaning the aspect of Prana that is responsible for all elimination processes. Depending on how vigorously the individual poses are taken and practiced, forward bends, when they are held for an extended period of time, always have a cooling, calming effect on the mind and on the energy system. Forward bends at the end of a practice allow the mind to quiet down. The Rajas Guna retreats in favor of a clear, Sattva quality.

6.5.2 STRUCTURE AND EFFECTS OF BACKBENDS

A *backbend* is a stretch, or more accurately, a hyperextension of the spine, often combined with a hip extension. The backbend is ideally initiated from an axial extension.

Depending on the degree and intensity of the backbend, it is performed standing (e.g. Natarajasana/Shiva's dance pose), kneeling (e.g. Ustrasana/camel), on the floor in supine position (e.g. Setu Bandha/Shoulder Bridge), seated (e.g. Eka Pada Raja Kapotasana/pigeon), and in a prone position (e.g. Bhujangasna/cobra).

The primary function of backbends is to stretch the front of the body, particularly the ribcage, the front of the shoulder girdle, the abdominal muscles, the hip flexors, and the front of the thighs. Depending on the type and execution of the back bend, the back of the body is strengthened, and the erector spinae muscles in particularly are play an important role. All backbends support the erection of the spine with their structure, which can result in the correction of kyphosis (rounded back). Blockages or imbalances resulting from excessive sitting in daily life can be corrected with backbends.

There are suggested backbends and very deep backbends, which affect different areas of the spine depending on the intensity. Suggested backbends, like *upward-facing dog* or *crescent lunge*, are performed during a class to prepare for deeper backbends like *cobra*, *camel*, *locust*, or *bow*. Karanas/flows like, for instance, sun-salutation variations that include backbends can help prepare for more intense backbends.

Backbends can have a dynamic buildup, can be held for extended periods of time, and deepened via arm or leg resistance. In contrast to forward bends, where the idea is to let go, most backbends require active strength and muscle engagement. To provide backbends with a solid foundation it is important to remember which parts of the body form the base for the respective pose to sufficiently stabilize it. Since backbends require more strength, the holding phases aren't as long as those for forward bends. Passive backbends that are practiced with aids such as bolsters or blocks are the exception.

Backbends have a stimulating effect on the energy system and generate heat; they deepen respiration and open the chest. This stimulates Prana, the aspect of Prana that is responsible for energy intake. They create a sense of openness in the heart space and affect the space of the higher heart, the Anahata chakra, which stands for themes like love, self-love, and empathy.

On an emotional level, backbends help to develop a strong back, the ability to sit or stand up straight. The upright body position supports the internal experience and helps us move through life tall and confident.

6.5.3   STRUCTURE AND EFFECTS OF SIDE BENDS

Side bends, *lateral flexion* tilt the trunk to the left or right. The ability to perform side bends involves the entire spine fairly equally, but is most pronounced in the cervical spine. Side bends are initiated from the axial extension of the spine.

Side bends are performed primarily in a standing (e.g. Trikonasana/triangle; Parsvakonasana/extended side angle) and seated position (e.g. Parighasana/gate pose). Moreover, side bends are often performed as a continuing combination of an Asana.

Since side bends are always practiced in both directions, they compress and stretch the deep back muscles around the spine. The entire trunk musculature, especially the flanks and chest (intercostal muscles), is alternately vigorously stretched and strengthened. The compression stimulates the internal organs such as lungs, kidneys, liver, intestinal tract, and diaphragm. Side bends can correct imbalances and asymmetries of the spine and trunk and thereby support a healthy posture.

Side bends require a solid base from which one can bend to the side. They promote stability as well as supple lightness. The quality of the side bend is like a bamboo stalk that moves pliably in the breeze yet is solid and sturdy enough to withstand severe storms.

Due to the opposing directions of movement, side bends are able to shift awareness to the inner axis, to the in-between space, and thus deepen awareness of the inner center.

From an energy standpoint side bends stimulate Samana Vayu, the aspect of Prana that is responsible for the conversion of energy.

6.5.4   STRUCTURE AND EFFECTS OF TWISTS

During *rotation poses*, more commonly referred to as *twists*, the spine rotates in both directions around the longitudinal axis via the individual vertebrae. The spine's ability to rotate is limited in the lumbar spine and is greatest in the thoracic and cervical spine. In a healthy spine, the rotating ability is about 120°. The lumbar spine can rotate up to 5°, and has a primarily stabilizing function. The rotating ability of the thoracic spine is between 35-40°; the cervical spine (C7-C2) can rotate up to 40°, and the atlanto-occipital joint (C1-C2) can also rotate up to 40°.

The most common twist is the *seated twist*, *Ardha Matsyendrasana*. There are many variations of supine twists, which are referred to as *crocodile poses/Makarasa*. Twists can also be combined with almost any standing Asana. There are very intense and gentle twists depending on the starting position. One can rotate the pelvis towards the fixed shoulder or away from it. Twists can be static as well as gently dynamic.

The foundation for a twist is the extended, vertical axis of the spine (axial extension). Since the body loses much of its rotating ability in the course of a lifetime, it is important to regularly practice twists. They promote and maintain flexibility of the intervertebral discs and ligaments and equally strengthen and stretch the deep as well as the superficial trunk muscles. Thus twists also correct posture, imbalances, and asymmetries between the left and right side of the body can be balanced.

Twists are purification exercises that help the body to purge on every plane. The alternating compression and stretching of the entire trunk deepens respiration and vigorously massages the internal organs, which stimulates the metabolism. Compression of the intestinal tract also stimulates digestion, which in turn has a cleansing effect. Yoga and Ayurveda theory tells us that a sound intestinal tract is the foremost requirement for good health.

On an energy level, twists support *Samana Vayu*, the aspect of Prana that supports digestion and is responsible for the conversion of food into energy. Samana Vayu is closely linked to Agni, the digestive fire.

Active dynamic twists have a stimulating effect, but when the twists are held for some time, they have a cooling, discharging, loosening effect. Here respiration plays an important role. Because during trunk twists, there sometimes is a tendency to allow the breath to get shallow. Deep, slow breaths during the twist greatly intensify the effect on an organ level.

A sense of the polar experience in terms of sun/moon – active/passive can also be experienced. The right side of the body is associated with our active, energetic, fiery, rational, and intellectual side, while the left side is associated with our intuitive, emotional, cooling, soft, and yielding aspects. Like all asymmetric poses, the twists promote a sense of the inner center, the fusion of all opposites.

6.5.5 STRUCTURE AND EFFECTS OF INVERSIONS

Inversions are Asanas during which the heart is above the head. The most common inversions are the head- (*Salamba Sirshasana*) and shoulder stand (*Salamba Sarvangasana*). There are also a number of half inversions like downward-facing dog/*Adho Mukkha Savasana* or standing forward bend/*Uttanasa*. During half inversions the feet maintain contact with the floor. They ultimately prepare the body and organism for full inversions.

Inversions such as head- or shoulder stands are demanding Asanas that should be practiced only after the necessary strength, flexibility, coordination, and awareness have been developed through previous practice. This can be done via many suitable preparatory and introductory exercises. The neck, nape, and shoulder areas are very vulnerable in humans as well as the spine should first be sufficiently flexible and strong.

During an inversion, our perspective changes. That requires a sure sense for possible deviations in the body to be able to quickly make the appropriate compensatory response. The main risk of injury in these poses occurs while moving into and out of the pose. If one relies on momentum because they lack strength or coordination, one unnecessarily exposes oneself to risk of injury. The poses should have a good foundation and should always be performed in a way that does not compress, nor put a lot of weight on neck, nape, and shoulders.

Inversions improve strength and flexibility both in the deep but also superficial musculature. Since inversions are also balance poses they improve both intra- (inside the muscle) and intermuscular coordination (synergy of muscles and muscle groups), which improves intrinsic balance.

They have a revitalizing effect on the entire system of organs because during an inversion, gravity causes the organs to sink into the dome of the diaphragm. Deep, slow belly breaths allow the diaphragm to push the organs back in the direction of the pelvis, which has a massaging and stimulating effect on digestion and metabolism. Inversions promote venous return and return of lymphatic fluid from the legs, which is particularly beneficial in cases of varicose veins and heavy, swollen legs.

Inversions are meditative Asanas that are static in nature and held for longer periods of time because the mind is supposed to quiet down. They have both a calming and refreshing effect on the mind. The deeper meaning of inversions is intended as a pause that invites one to take a look at and experience oneself and life's themes from a different, opposite perspective.

6.6　THE PRACTICE OF ASANAS (ALIGNMENT CRITERIA)

Every Asana consists of:

»　**Body alignment: the position of joints relative to each other**
This knowledge is the basis for every Asana, because the position of the joints gives an Asana its shape. The orientation criteria for each Asana are based on the joints' position relative to each other. This creates a solid foundation. Hyperflexion of the knee joints, hyperextended, compressed necks, or twists with a rounded back present a high risk of injury, impede energy flow, and create muscle tension.

»　**Muscle contraction**
To assume a pose, to lend the pose stability, or to determine the center of gravity of a pose, one must first ascertain which muscles/muscle groups are primarily active (agonists) and which play a supporting role (synergists). This knowledge is essential to the composition and introduction of an Asana. Asanas like strength, support, or balance poses can then be built up systematically over weeks or months when one chooses exercises and poses that incrementally build up the respective muscles.

>> **Stretching**

Since Asanas have a multi-joint structure, it is necessary to determine the muscles that are contracted as well as the muscle groups that are being stretched. Certain parts of the body have a tendency to shorten like, for instance, the back of the legs. These areas should be prepared with appropriate pre-stretches to facilitate the aspect of Sukha (light, free, permeable) during Asana. Once sufficiently familiar with the poses, one can use advanced techniques, like *assisted stretching*[52] (brief contraction   of the stretched muscle) or *reciprocal inhibition*[53] (briefly contracting the antagonist), to deepen the stretch within an Asana,

>> **Breathing**

Every yoga pose is based on the breath. We absorb energy through the breath and eliminate waste matter. A long exhale deacidifies the body. Most of the poses affect the internal organs. Without even, deep, and calm breaths, the poses lose their function and effect. Moreover, respiration is the key to body awareness. When the breath is held or doesn't flow freely, it is a sign that the pose is either too intense or the alignment is incorrect (also see chapter 9, *Yogic breathing*).

>> **Body awareness**

One of the main goals and effects of the yoga practice is improved awareness. For many people, the demands of our everyday working life and lifestyle have caused awareness to take a backseat while our mental processes are very active. Body awareness means actively directing your attention to the internal processes. Developing body awareness is generally the first step on the path to the inner self, from head back to body, from the tangible to the ethereal. Imbalances and tensions can only be discerned through body awareness. It is also the basis for alignment and any processes that pertain to body alignment.

>> **Directing energy and consciousness**

On the basis of body awareness, during the Asana practice the focus is shifted to the energy-related experience. This includes observing the energy-related processes in the body as well as purposefully directing our awareness to specific areas of the body. Directing energy takes place within the breathing rhythm. For instance, as you inhale you direct your attention downward along the spine to the lower pelvic area, and as you exhale you direct it from the pelvis to the crown of the head. The combination of concentration, imagination, body awareness, and breathing causes Prana, the vital energy, to noticeably flow and greatly intensifies an Asana's effect.

"The ancient muscle-building gymnastic exercises of the Dandalos and Bhaskis differ from Western gymnastic exercises primarily in that they don't consist of soulless repetitions, but of "holding exercises" that are performed with great mental focus. Just as the mind, and not just the muscles, participates in interesting work or an exciting game, so does the yogi perform his exercises with great interest, and while engaging his willpower observes the currently moving limbs and mentally showers them with Prana."[54]

---

52 Long, R. (2015). *3-D Yoga Anatomy, volume 1-4*. Munich: Riva Publishing.
53 Ebenda.
54 Yesudian, S. & Haich, E. (1984, 29th edition). *Sport + Yoga*. pg. 246. Munich, Drei Eichen Publishing.

6.7   THE QUALITY OF ASANAS

In Patanjalis' Yoga Sutra the qualities of the seated pose are described as follows:

Chapter 2.46 sthira-sukhma-asanam: The seated pose should be firm and comfortable.[55]

» *Sthira* is translated as *firm* but also *still* and *immovable*. Sthira means that every pose needs a solid and firm foundation so it can be held for an extended period of time.

» *Sukha* means *comfortable*, but is also translated as *happy*, *light*, and *free*. This refers to a certain permeability and lightness of the posture. When our posture is too rigid, too firm, we usually cannot breathe, cannot perceive and feel.

Although Patanjali's *Yoga Sutra* focuses exclusively on the description of the meditative pose, the upright-seated pose, the *Sutra* does offer valuable advice on the practice of the Asanas. Regardless of whether we practice standing, seated, or lying on the floor, every pose first requires a solid foundation that provides grounding and stability. This foundation is initially created via body alignment and stability of the respective muscles. Muscle imbalances prevent a solid foundation, which is why it is necessary to determine where in the body an imbalance might interfere with a solid foundation.

This foundation is the basis for the lightness and freedom required to remain in a pose for an extended period of time and be able to breathe calmly and consciously. Sthira and Sukha can be seen as opposites that are supposed to find balance in every pose in order to merge into a powerful unit.

All human beings vary in their nature. Some need more stability, others more flexibility. Often both are needed in different areas. And the poses also differ a lot in their structure. With each pose we must therefore figure out anew the appropriate degree of firmness (Sthira) and permeability (Sukha) for that moment.

6.8   STATIC AND DYNAMIC ASANA PRACTICE

The traditional classical Asana practice is primarily static. But *static* doesn't mean rigid, but rather *focused, calm, steady*. More motionless on the outside but not inanimate. One assumes an Asana according to the alignment criteria and holds it for a certain amount of time. The advantage of a static practice is that one can concentrate completely on the Asana and the moment since no external movement diverts attention from the internal processes. Here breathing, body awareness, and energy and consciousness control have particular significance in the holding phase.

Along with the static form of practice, there are also active forms of practice. They can be called *dynamic* or *active*. The term *dynamic* is easily misunderstood.

---

55 Bäumer, B. & Deshpande, P. Y. (1990). *Patanjali. Die Wurzeln des Yoga*. Bern, Scherz Publishing.

Dynamic does not imply fast, sweeping, or particularly powerful movement in the sense of athletic momentum. With respect to the yoga practice, the dynamic practice is best described as *gentle movement*.

A dynamic practice can include circling motions for joint mobility, gentle, active pre-stretches of certain muscle groups, or targeted strengthening or stabilization of certain areas of the body in time with the breath. When two poses are linked through movement and the breath, or when various arm and leg variations are practiced in time with the breath, it is also a dynamic practice.

Most of the time a dynamic practice is combined with a static practice. Gentle forms of dynamic practice are very helpful when introducing an Asana because the active movement warms up the body and prepares it for the Asana. These practice forms are also used in yoga therapy.

6.9   TO BUILD UP AN ASANA (FROM DYNAMIC TO STATIC PRACTICE)

1. **Preparation**

   During the preparation phase, the areas of the body that are relevant to the pose are loosened up, pre-stretched, and stabilized. For instance, for a pose like *downward-facing dog*, the back of the legs, the low back, and the chest are pre-stretched, the spine, shoulder girdle, and wrists are loosened up, and the trunk muscles are stabilized.

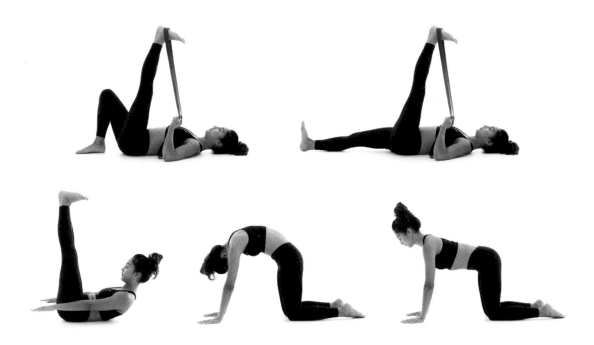

2. Introduction

Introducing a pose is generally done via a form of dynamic practice, meaning one moves into the pose multiple times before holding it. But dynamic does not imply the use of momentum or speed. It means that one moves slowly in time with the breath. Examples of dynamic practice are pedaling the feet during *downward-facing dog (walking dog)*,or linking an all-fours position and *downward-facing dog*.

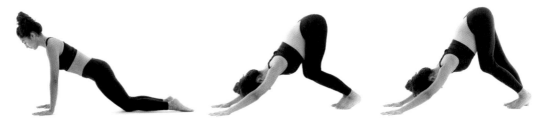

3. Holding phase

You have arrived in the Asana, the outside of your body is quieting down, and you are focusing on the breath and lend the pose the quality of "sthira-shukam". This is also called "working in Asana". It means that one melts into the pose in accordance with the principles of alignment of the respective Asana; consciousness spreads across the entire body. This also includes modifying the pose appropriately when strength and flexibility are not yet sufficient. For instance, during *Downward-facing dog* one can bend the knees so that the back of the legs is shortened to maintain the length of the spine. The holding phase is a constant sensing and feeling inside the body.

Once the physical body is in proper alignment, the focus on the energy-related experience begins. Where does the energy flow, where is it backed up? How can we direct or intensify the energy flow through breath control? The more familiar one is with the Asana practice on a physical level, the more the subtler aspects of energy control and inner alignment can unfold. It is an incremental process that develops over the course of regular practice.

There is a rule of thumb that one should practice Asanas at only about 80% of possible intensity because too much exertion inhibits the subtler perception. The exception to this rule is strength and support poses. But in general it is important to make sure that a healthy amount of intensity and feeling is maintained during the holding phase.

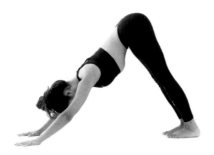

4. **Exiting the pose**

You exit the pose as carefully as you entered it. This is also done step-by-step in time with the breath. Particularly in complex poses, exiting the pose step-by-step protects the body from injury. Ending a pose slowly also sets an example for everyday life. Over the course of a day, we sometimes rush from one thing to the next. Before we have even completed one activity, our mind has already moved on to the next step or the one after that. Exiting a pose helps us remember that we must first complete something before tackling the next thing.

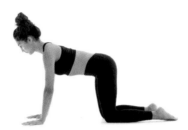

5. **Rest and reflection**

The rest and reflection phase is the pause after exiting an Asana. It is also a moment of composure, relaxation, and turning inward before entering the next Asana. Here we can assess what has changed after the Asana. The brain can form a new image of the body. That is the actual purpose of the rest and reflection phase.

It is also about turning inward to align yourself with your inner self, the intention of the practice, or the higher power. The rest and reflection pose depends on whether one practiced standing, seated, or lying on the floor. When completing a series of standing Asanas it would make little sense to lie on the floor to reflect after each one. It would inhibit the flow of the practice and the energy flow. After a standing practice one can reflect in Tadasana; a relaxing seated or supine pose would be appropriate after a seated or reclined practice.

When practicing multiple poses from one category (e.g. backbends) as a series, it is possible that an extended reflection phase could have an adverse effect on the energy flow. Over the course of the practice, one generally develops a feeling for when and how long a reflection phase is appropriate.

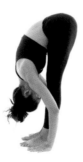

6.10 IMPORTANCE OF PREPARATORY AND INTRODUCTORY EXERCISES

Preparatory and introductory exercises prepare the practitioner for the specific requirements of an Asana. They help the body to incrementally prepare for an Asana or a group of Asanas. They help to safely enter the Asana while simultaneously avoiding the risk of injury. Before practicing or teaching an Asana one should look at the structure of the pose and determine which areas to activate, where a pre-stretch might support the practice of the Asana, and which areas might benefit from strengthening and stabilizing.

Preparatory exercises activate the joints and stretch and strengthen the relevant muscles for an Asana.

» *Activating* the joints helps produce synovial fluid, a gel-like substance that nourishes the joint cartilage. The cartilage envelops the joint surfaces and protects them by keeping the contact between the individual joints soft and smooth. This production of synovial fluid via activating movements increases cartilage elasticity and thereby protects the joint surfaces.

Examples: For any poses that require arm support, like *Downward-facing dog / Adho Mukha Svanasana* or *Plank / Chaturanga Dandasana*, it is recommended to warm up the shoulder joints and wrists beforehand, e.g. with circular movements. Also activating the hip joints supports joint suppleness for any hip-opening Asanas. Ankle joints are activated before standing poses, neck and nape are warmed up prior to inversions, and the entire length of the spine is activated before every practice.

» *Pre-stretching* certain muscle groups makes it easier to enter and achieve an Asana.

Examples: The back of the legs is pre-stretched for *Adho Mukkha Svanasana / Downward-facing dog* because many people have severely shortened muscles in that area, particularly the ischiocrural muscles in the hollow of the knees and the calves. Extended-angle poses are prepared by pre-stretching the inside of the legs (adductors). Backbends are prepared by pre-stretching the chest and shoulders. Twists are prepared by pre-stretching the gluteal muscles.

» Preparatory *stabilization / strengthening* prepares for any Asanas that include strength and support elements. It protects the joints from overloading, and one learns in small increments how and which muscles are being activated.

Example: To prepare for a plank both the trunk muscles as well as shoulders and arms are stabilized in preparation. This can be done with dynamic or static exercises.

Introductory poses means the positions from which one can move into an Asana. There are usually multiple options. Introductory exercises and a dynamic practice can be easily combined. Possible introductory exercises for *Cat / Marjryasana* can be *Child's pose / Balasana* and the *neutral all-fours position*.

Preparatory and introductory exercises should not be more demanding than the ultimate Asana. Within a sequence the final Asana is always the culmination. All of the preceding poses should incrementally prepare participants for the Asana.

Example: Preparatory and introductory exercises for Anjaneyasana/Deep lunge

Preparatory exercises:

» Warm up shoulder girdle, hip flexors, and hips.
» Prestretch primarily the hip flexors (m. iliopsoas) and the quadriceps.
» Stabilize the trunk muscles.

Introductory exercises:

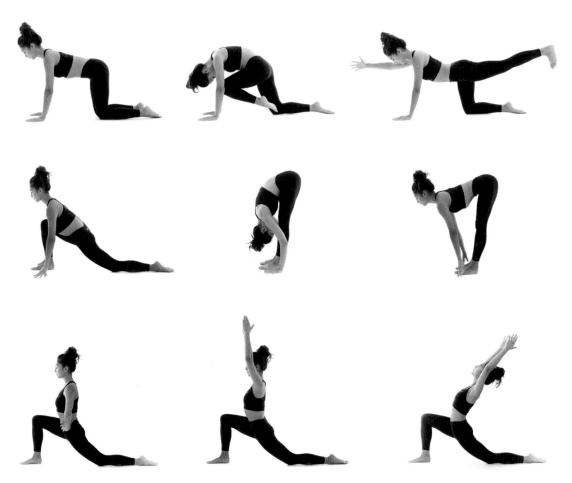

Photo series 6.10 a-i

Exit and reflect:

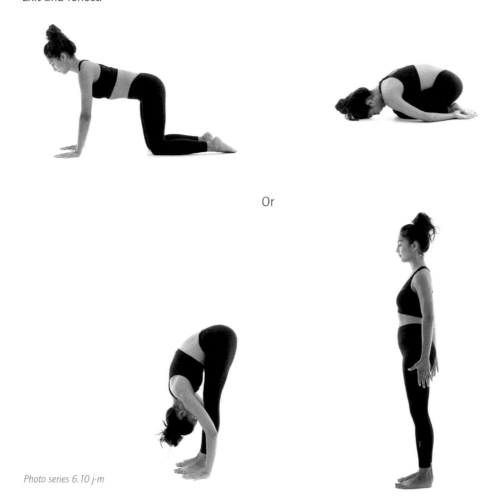

Or

Photo series 6.10 j-m

» From an all-fours position (PS 6.10 j) (you can insert a back warm-up PS 6.10 b + c), move one leg forward into a lunge and stretch the hip flexors (PS 6.10 d). This can be done gently and dynamically.
» To switch sides, move into Uttanasana and practice the dynamic combination of Uttanasana (PH 6.10 e) and Ardha Uttanasana (PS 6.10 f) several times (stabilizing the erector spinae muscles).
» Step into a lunge with the other leg and pre-stretch the hip flexors (PS 6.10 d).
» Straighten the back and lift and lower the arms in time with your breath (PS 6.10 g + h).
» Finally hold your arms in the raised position and deepen the backbend (PS 6.10 i).
» Exit the posture (PS 6.10 a) or (PS 6.10 e).
» Rest and reflect (PS 6.10 l) or (PS 6.10 m).

6.11   KARANA – MOVEMENT SEQUENCES

Karana = cause(doing, making, affecting)

When three or more Asanas are linked, creating a sequence that is repeated without interrupting the breathing rhythm, it is called a *Karana* or *Vinyasa Flow*. In the Hatha Yoga practice system this refers to a movement sequence consisting of several Asanas (also see chapter 8/Surya Namaskar).

6.12   THE THREE BANDHAS – THE BODY LOCKS

Bandha = bond, connection (join, hold)

Bandha means *bond*. The term is also translated as *join*, *tie*, *bind*, or *hold*. On a physical plane the Bandhas are deliberate, specific muscle contractions in the area of the pelvic floor (Mula Bandha), the diaphragm (Uddiyana Bandha), and the throat (Jalandhara Bandha).

Chapter III of the *Hatha Yoga Pradipika* offers a detailed description of the Bandhas. In advanced Pranayama techniques like, for instance Kumbhakas (holding of the breath) they are absolutely essential to directing the released energy in certain directions and to absorbing any pressure in the body created by holding the breath. The Bandhas are also called the *holy seal of Hatha Yoga* because they have such a profound effect on the energy system.

The Bandhas are also used in the Asana practice. But for beginning yoga practitioners the focus is initially on the Bandhas' physical aspect. First they must learn to isolate the respective parts of the body and muscles and contract them before adding the aspect of energy control.

There are three Bandhas in classical Hatha Yoga.

6.12.1   MULA BANDHA – ROOT LOCK

Mula means *root*. As the name suggests, the *Mula Bandha* is located in the area of the Muladhara Chakra in the lower pelvic region. Contracting the pelvic floor muscles activates the Mula Bandha.

The pelvic floor consists of three layers. It is a complex network of muscle fibers and connective tissue layered on top of each other about the size and thickness of the palm of the hand. While the diaphragm closes off the abdomen at the top, the pelvic floor delimits the trunk at the bottom and also forms the support base for the internal organs. The muscle fibers within the individual layers run in different directions, giving the pelvic floor a sturdy, reticular structure. It extends from the pubis to the tailbone, and laterally to the ischial tuberosity. It has a passage for the sex organs, the urethra, and the rectum, and plays an important role during urination, defecation, and sexual intercourse. Its main functions are:

» Contraction (you can hold stools and urine and have elimination control).
» Relaxation (it relaxes during the elimination processes as well as sexual intercourse). During an orgasm, a woman's pelvic floor begins to pulsate (quick contracting and relaxing).
» Resistance reflex (when there is increased pressure in the abdomen such as while laughing, sneezing, coughing, jumping, or while carrying heavy loads).

Furthermore, the pelvic floor can be purposefully contracted. Doing so is recommended in cases of pelvic floor weakness, which results in pelvic organ prolapse and usually also incontinence. The individual pelvic floor layers can be activated with purposeful subtle contractions. Since we can feel the pelvic floor but cannot see it, it helps to target it via cognitive and visualization exercises to then learn to place the contractions.

During the yoga practice the pelvic floor supports all trunk-erecting exercises and Asanas. It can also be triggered and activated particularly when a high degree of stability is required. This prepares the body and the practitioner for the subtler aspects of energy control, which become important in the Pranayama practice.

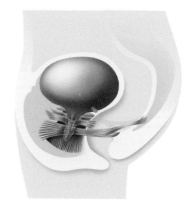

Fig. 11: The pelvic floor – side view

Exercises for contracting the pelvic floor

In yoga contracting the pelvic floor is referred to as engaging the *Mula Bandha*. There are a number of more or less flowery descriptions of contracting the pelvic floor or to practice engaging the Mula Bandha:

» Interrupting the stream while urinating.
» Imagining avoiding passing gas by locking the anal sphincter.
» Pulling the sit-bones (ischial tuberosity) towards each other without contracting the gluteal muscles.
» Pulling the vagina and anus (or scrotum and anus) inward into the abdomen.
» Pulling tailbone and pubis towards each other.
» Since it is more difficult to target the central area than the muscles surrounding the organs of elimination, the following are imagination aids for women: slowly pulling a marble upward along the vagina or pulling grass with the labia. Imagination aids for men: pulling the scrotum (the scrotal sack) upward.

Anything one deliberately contracts should also be relaxed again, including the pelvic floor. It is unnecessary, nor advisable to engage the Mula Bandha during the entire yoga class, as that can result in painful tension when the pelvic floor becomes rigid due to too much tonus.

Breathing and the pelvic floor

When breathing naturally, the pelvic floor is the antagonist to the diaphragm. When the diaphragm contracts during inhalation, it arches into the abdomen. Due to compression of the organs, this results in some slight pressure on the pelvic floor, which relaxes and drops slightly. When the diaphragm relaxes again during exhalation the pelvic floor also slightly lifts again. That is also why in the Asana practice, engaging the *Mula Bandha* is initially practiced while exhaling.

But when breath awareness has been practiced and one is familiar with engaging the "Mula Bandha", there are many exercises and variations in the Asana practice and particularly in Pranayama (while engaging the Kumbhakas) during which the Mula Bandha is initiated and held while inhaling.

6.12.2 UDDIYANA BANDHA – ABDOMINAL LOCK/ UPWARD LOCK

Uddiyana means *flying upward*, *flying open*. It is a major contraction of the lower and central abdominal muscles (the oblique and transverse abdominals work synergistically), whereby the navel area is pulled inward and up. At the same time the ribcage is lifted and the diaphragm is practically sucked into the chest (it flies upward). The upper abdomen remains relaxed, the ribcage widens, and the intercostal muscles are stretched. A kind of vacuum is created in the abdomen. In addition, holding the breath can simulate an inhalation. This exercise should only be practiced on an empty stomach.

During Pranayama, Uddiyana Bandha is primarily initiated after exhalation and suggested after inhalation. Uddiyana Bandha stimulates metabolism and the digestive fire, directs energy upward, and creates quiet mental clarity. The classical form of Uddiyana Bandha is practiced exclusively in combination with Pranayama/Kumbhaka.

The Asana practice uses a modified variation of Uddiyana Bandha. One contracts the external and internal obliques along with the rectus abdominus and transverse obliques. In doing so, one pulls the flexible lower ribs inward and back and pulls the navel in. This modified version of Uddiyana Bandha is often practiced in combination with Mula Bandha. It supports all balance, strength and support exercises as well as all trunk-erecting poses.

6.12.3 JALANDHARA BANDHA – THROAT LOCK

Jala = net

The neck, throat, or chin lock consists of stretching the neck followed by lowering the head to tuck the chin into the depression between the collarbones. The ribcage and shoulder girdle are raised slightly to prevent overstretching of the neck. Jalandhara Bandha is practiced exclusively in advanced Pranayama/ Kumbhakas.

On an energy plane, the pressure of the chin is supposed to prevent the rise of energy.

Bandha Codex

The name Bandha Codex as a synonym for the supporting, stabilizing contracting of muscles and muscle groups in the entire body is an integral part of the Yoga Anatomy by Ray Long (2015). It combines modern scientific findings with the Asana practice and expands the same by several key principles. *"Bandhas or 'locks' can be set in the entire body by co-activating muscle groups. They represent the physical and mental focus areas of a pose. Bandhas stabilize the joints, stimulate the sensory nerves, and intensify the imprint of a pose on the brain."*[56]

6.13　INJURY RISKS/CONTRAINDICATIONS

Due to its many beneficial effects on the body and the mind, Hatha Yoga is so popular that today around three million Germans practice yoga regularly. But as with any other form of exercise, there are risks of injury in the Asana practice as well.

In January 2012, there was a huge outcry from the yoga community after an article by the journalist William J. Broad was published in New York Times Magazine with the title *"How yoga can wreck your body"*[57]. In the article he describes, in some cases hair-raising injuries, yoga practitioners have suffered as well as their causes.

Although yoga is praised for its health benefits, the focus on its injury risks made yoga the focus of previously unknown criticism. What once had been a taboo topic in the world of yoga was now openly debated. The American yoga scene and the European/German yoga culture are not identical, but for the past three decades, the yoga movement in Europe is also clearly being shaped by American influences.

Also in 2012, the book *"The Science of Yoga"* was published by the same author and became a global bestseller. In chapter 4, "Injury risk"[58] W.J. Broad examines the reasons and causes for typical yoga injuries. It is surprising that this topic was not addressed much sooner. With everything humans do in terms of physical activity, there is always a certain risk of getting hurt. The more intense, complex, or faster the activity is, the higher the risk of injury.

When we try to force the body into poses that are not appropriate for the practitioners because they don't meet certain requirements, the consequences are obvious. People who have gotten little or no exercise throughout their lives should not be surprised when the body responds to demanding and seemingly acrobatic poses with injuries. Someone who has spent his free time as a couch potato surely would not begin exercising by running a marathon but rather start by taking a brisk walk around the block.

56 Long, R. (2015, pg. 30).
57 http://www.nytimes.com/2012/01/08/magazine/how-yoga-can-wreck-your-body.html?mcubz=3
58 Broad, W. J. (2013). *The science of yoga.* (pg. 161-204). Freiburg im Breisgau: Herder Publishing.

And that is precisely the case with the Asana practice. Classical head and shoulder stands or extreme backbends or forward bends are not suitable for beginners. These poses should be systematically built up over an appropriate period of time and/or heavily modified.

It is primarily the instructors who must see and decide which poses and practices are appropriate for their participants. They are the ones who must protect their students and participants from damaging overloading during a yoga class

In summary, one can say that the biggest injury risks are people attempting poses that are not appropriate for them, excessive ambition, and ambitious practicing.

In principle, there are no wrong or damaging Asanas. All poses, without exception, have their benefits and effects. But with respect to the practitioner, it has to be determined whether the risk of a pose outweighs the benefits.

This means that the type of practice must be adapted to the practitioner. To his background, his age, his lifestyle habits, and most of all his physical qualifications. The old saying: "No pain, no gain" with respect to the Asana practice does not mean that one has to suffer pain to grow. On the contrary, one is asked to be aware of pain signals and heed them.

In sports there are terms like *warning pain* and *good pain*. Good pain is the sensation we get when muscles are working, being strengthened or stretched. It can be a slight "burning" that results from dynamic strength training. Or a pulling sensation in the muscles when the muscle is being stretched. All of that is normal when one works with the body. Even slight to moderate muscle soreness is considered good pain.

In contrast, *warning pain* usually occurs in the form of an unpleasant straining or stinging sensation in the muscles, the spine, or the joints. Feeling nauseous, seeing black or feeling dizzy, organ pain or headaches all are warning signs that something is wrong. In such an event the activity should be reduced or interrupted and the potential causes examined.

In this case, a well-trained yoga instructor should be able to communicate with the practitioner and make suggestions as to any possible causes. Sometimes the solution is simple (forgot to breathe, did not eat or hydrate enough, weather sensitivity, etc.). In other cases, the intensity was not appropriate, or the body alignment needs work. Yoga instructors are not physical therapists, which is why when in doubt, a trip to the doctor is recommended.

Along with breath awareness, body awareness is a critical element in performing a properly crafted Asana practice from the very beginning. It allows the practitioner to build a sense of his own body, become aware of loading limits, and recognize warning signals early on.

Creating lessons plans with small steps also makes it easier to ensure correct joint alignment in participants, and to guard against possible injury.

Asana practice is not recommended with certain disorders or symptoms and should be abstained from. These include:

» Severe colds,
» Influenza and flu-like illnesses,
» Gastro-intestinal infections,
» Acute inflammation of joints or abdomen,
» Acute herniated discs,
» Acute sprains,
» Acute low back pain,
» Acute muscle injuries, sprained ligaments, tendonitis, as well as
» Severe heart or lung disease.

After severe illnesses, surgeries, or in cases of major degenerative problems of the joints a doctor should be consulted to determine if, when, and in what form physical exercise/Asana practice is possible, as well as any possible exclusion criteria (things that should not be practiced).

Areas of the body with an increased risk of injury during the Asana practice include neck, shoulders, lumbar spine, and knee joints.

6.13.1 NECK

While the thoracic and lumbar spine is built primarily for stability and strength, the cervical spine is built primarily for mobility. This flexibility also makes it susceptible to injury.

The nape, in particular, is a target for all sorts of afflictions. Many participants come to yoga class with tight muscles in the neck and nape. Hours of sitting at a desk and working on a computer, pushing a computer mouse back and forth, or the one-sided carrying of babies and young children can easily cause posture problems and result in painful muscle tension in the nape (cervical spine issues).

This is amplified by chronic stress and too little physical activity. When adding emotional pressure, the muscles increasingly shorten and grow more rigid.

Moreover, the likelihood of degenerative changes in the cervical spine increases with age, including cervical spine disorders resulting from wear such as herniated discs, arthritis, or rheumatic diseases.

Exposing a nape that is already pre-stressed to lots of pressure or tensile strain as happens in some classical Asanas, increases the risk of injury.

Yoga poses that are potentially risky for the neck/nape:

» **All exercises that require extreme neck hyperextension**
   This includes *Cobra* (*Bhujangasana*), *Fish* (*Matsyasana*), and *Camel* (*Ushtrasana*). The reason for this extreme hyperextension of the neck is that it deeply stretches and widens the larynx area, which is supposed to stimulate and open Vishuddha Chakra, the throat center. This is not a problem for healthy bodies.

In cases of cervical spine issues or other neck problems, performing these poses can easily be modified by tilting the head back with maximum axial extension of the cervical spine, only so far that no wrinkles form in the nape. The head should be a natural extension of the thoracic and cervical spine.

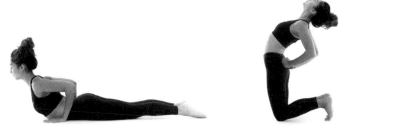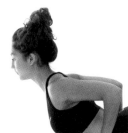

» **All exercises that include hyperflexion of the cervix**
This includes the classical *shoulder stand* (*Salamba Sarvanasana*) and *plow* (*Halasana*). An easy remedy here is placing a folded blanket under the shoulders to take weight off the back of the neck.

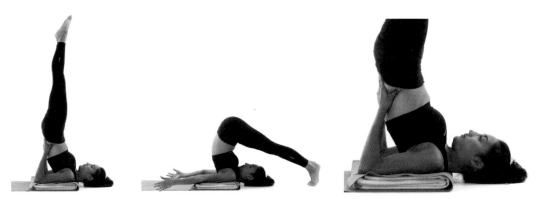

» **All exercises that put pressure on the neck**
The *headstand* (*Sirshasana*) has a broad action spectrum. But when the neck and shoulder muscles (as well as the core muscles) are not strong enough, it can easily lead to compression and injuries of the neck/cervix. Inversions present the greatest potential for injury of the cervical spine, specifically while entering and exiting the pose.

» **All exercises that require extreme neck rotation**
During twists like the *seated twist* (*Ardha Matsyendrasana*) participants are frequently instructed to turn the head as far possible in the respective direction of rotation. But during rotation emphasis should be on the area of the thoracic spine. Excessive rotation of neck and cervix should also be avoided in *Triangle* (*Trikonasana*) or *Extended Triangle* (*Urdhva Parsvakonasana*).

6.13.2 SHOULDERS

Due to its complex joint structure, the shoulder is the most movable part of the human locomotor system. It is capable of carrying heavy loads, but compared to the hip joint, it is quite unstable. The reason is that unlike the hip joint the shoulder is not stabilized by bones but primarily muscles and ligaments (rotator cuff). The rotator cuff provides the necessary joint stability by centering the humeral head in the socket. The complex structure of the shoulder makes it prone to injury.

Yoga poses that are potentially risky for the shoulder area are:

» **Strength and support poses**
   Strength and support poses can easily result in overloading and incorrect loading when the alignment of the pose is incorrect and the necessary strength for the pose has not been developed. The participant then "hangs in his joints", which can result in irritations, bursitis, and tears in muscles or tendons.

   Poses like *Chaturanga Dandasana* or *Adho Mukkha Svanasana* should be appropriately prepared beforehand (see preparatory and introductory exercises). Instructors should offer modifications, particularly for movement sequences like Surya Namaskar (Sun Salutation).

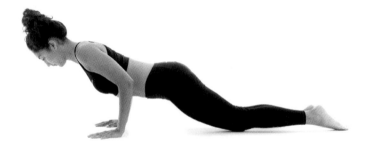

Modified Chaturanga Dandasana on knees

» Exercises in which the arms are held overhead for a long period of time are also risky for tight shoulders.

6.13.3 LUMBAR SPINE

Problems in the lumbar spine are very common. About 80% of people have had an issue there at least once in their life. Muscle tightness (acute low back pain in the lumbar spine with muscular imbalances) is considered the main cause. It is usually preceded by unfamiliar lifting or carrying of heavy loads 2-3 days prior.[59]

Many beginning yoga students have a shortening of the muscles in the back of the legs (ischiocrural muscles). Here extreme forward bends can easily aggravate the lumbar spine.

---

59 http://www.leading-medicine-guide.de/Medizinische-Fachartikel/Schmerzen-der-unteren-Lendenwirbelsaeule
   Author: Dr. Joachim Schuchert

Yoga poses that are potentially risky for the lumbar spine are:

» **Deep forward bends**
Very deep forward bends (standing or seated) should always be performed with extreme caution, particularly in cases of back problems. These include seated forward bends (Paschimottanasana) and an exercise during which one balances on one leg and moves into a forward bend (Utthita Padangusthasana). If the muscles in the back of the legs are shortened this poses a high risk of injury to the intervertebral discs.

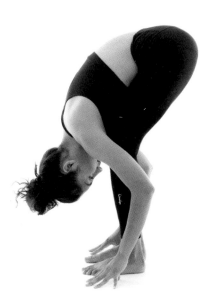

In cases of lumbar spine problems the knees should be slightly bent in these poses.

» **Long levers with forward bends during a flow**
The Asana practice includes some poses with very long levers. For instance, moving from *Urdhva Hastasana* into a forward bend Uttanasana with extended arms and back again during a *Sun Salutation* placesenormous tensile forces on the lumbar spine.

This deep forward bend is potentially dangerous for a novice participant with weak back muscles and shortened hamstring and low-back muscles. Until the necessary stability and flexibility required for this motion sequence has been built up, the practitioner should for safety reasons practice with short levers (the arms are lowered to the sides and the knees are slightly bent.

» **Sloppy practice during backbends**
During backbends it is important to avoid compression of the lumbar spine.

6.13.4   KNEES

The knee joint is the largest joint in the body. It is a hinge joint and facilitates flexion and extension of the leg as well as minor internal and external rotation. The knee is stabilized by a complex set of ligaments. Knee problems can be due to incorrect weightbearing and wear.

Yoga poses that are potentially risky for the knees are:

» Incorrect weight-bearing of the knee joints. During all standing poses with bent knees, it is important to make sure that the knees are lined up with the ankles, creating a right angle between calf and thigh and preventing the knee from veering to the right or left.

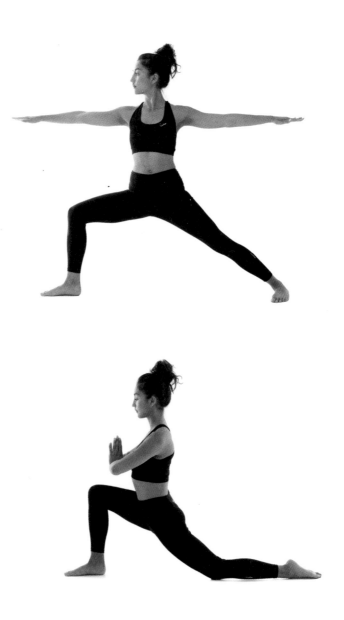

» Often knee problems are also associated with imbalances in the hip joints or the lumbar spine. This can make cross-legged seated positions problematic if the hips aren't flexible enough and one tries to force the knees into a cross-legged position. Poses like *King Pigeon* (*Kapotasana*) or *Hero* (*Virosana*, *Supta Virasana*) can also be problematic if the execution is sloppy.

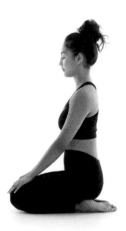

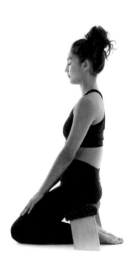

In cases of knee problems or a lack of flexibility, Virasana can be performed on a meditation bench.

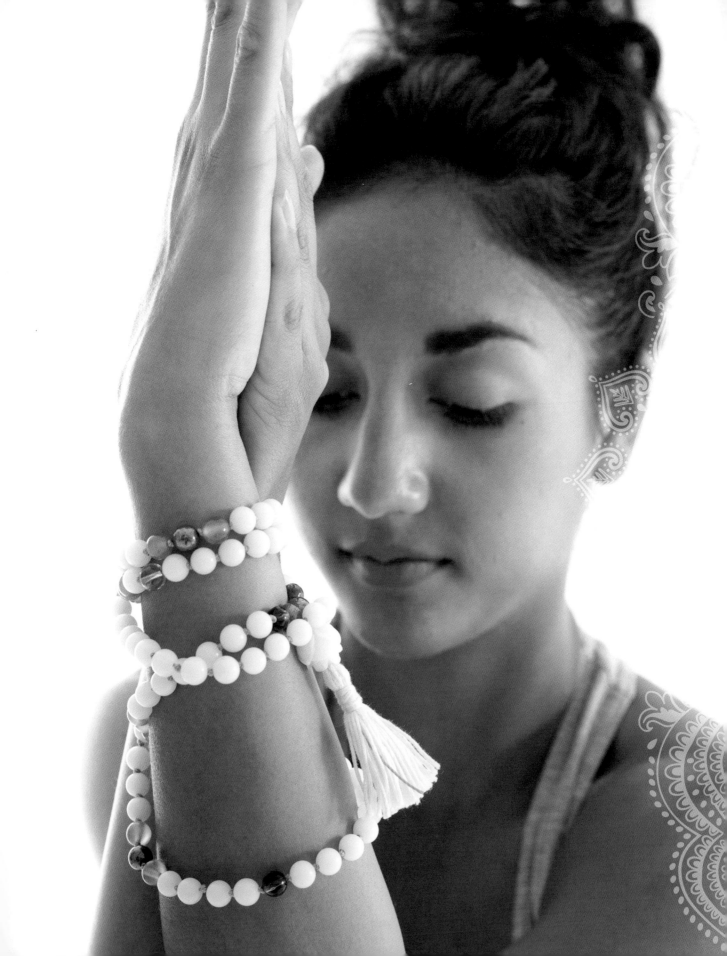

7 THE ASANAS

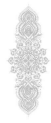

7 THE ASANAS

7.1 ASANA PRACTICE AND PROPS

We deliberately excluded typical yoga props like blocks and straps from the descriptions of the practice, effect, and function of the following 34 Asanas. While they doubtlessly are very helpful during the practice, not every place where yoga is practiced or taught has these aids available.

One reason one might forgo the use of props is that Asanas can be practiced without aids with zero limitations. For instance, if there aren't any blocks available during standing forward bends and the arms are just hanging in the air, it helps to bend the knees so the hands can touch the floor. There is a variation for nearly every exercise that can serve as a substitute for aids. It teaches us to be independent of external circumstances so we can practice yoga anytime.

Another argument against the use of aids in beginning classes is the practicing of body awareness. Every "implement" we use in the practice has the tendency to shift the focus away from the body and the inner processes, especially when the physical practice or concentration ability has not been practiced very much.

The Asanas presented here apply to the DTB course instructor modules 1-4, which means the first 100 hours of the 200 hours total comprehensive training. In the advanced courses 1-3 of the DTB yoga instructor training, we dedicate an entire module to the use and application of typical yoga aids such as blocks, straps, blankets, headstand stools, back-bending benches, etc.

7.2 ABOUT ASANA DESCRIPTIONS

First we will explain the impact and symbolism of the following Asanas. Even just the Sanskrit names of the Asanas offer information about their background. Along with the physical aspects of the poses (what type is it?) we will offer information on their energy-related, emotional, and in some cases psychological impact.

The pose structure gives a brief breakdown of how to enter the Asana. The section "Working in the pose" offers suggestions on how to deepen a pose.

The variations provide ways to introduce and modify a pose when the target Asana is too difficult. The introductions and modifications in particular are key topics of the DTB yoga course instructor modules 1-4. The anatomical explanations that accompany each Asana are best learned with the use of one or more anatomy books and muscle charts. There currently is a great selection of excellent yoga anatomy literature as well as animated websites that are listed in the book's appendix.

With everything that is described here, there is still one thing that matters above all: personal experience, the experience that comes with engaging in the practice. Books and descriptions offer information, but your body provides the answers.

7.3   INDIVIDUAL ASANAS

7.3.1   ADHO MUKHA SVANASANA – DOWNWARD-FACING DOG

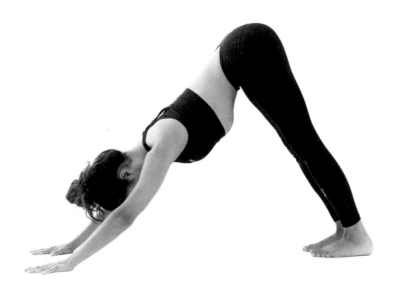

SYMBOLISM/IMPACT

Adho = down, Mukha = face, Svan = dog, Asana = pose

Adho Mukha Svanasana is reminiscent of a dog stretching languorously. This Asana is one the most common and most popular poses. It combines a forward bend with an inversion and is one of the arm-supported poses.

The effect of this Asana is varied: The entire back of the body is extended and stretched, and the entire spine is in a straight line. The energy-related effect is stimulating while it also allows the mind to rest in this pose due to the deep breathing. A.M.S. is a grounding pose during which both hands and feet have contact with the ground. Depending on the intensity of the execution, the chest, the heart space, is being stretched and opened in this position.

In the beginning, A.M.S. is often considered strenuous, which is usually due to the fact that many people have shortened muscles at the back of the legs and therefore shift their weight too far forward to their arms and hands.

POSE STRUCTURE

» Enter the pose either from a *forward bend/Uttanasana* via a lunge, or from a wide *all-fours pose*.

» Hands are about shoulder-width apart; knees and feet are hip-width apart.

» You will find the appropriate distance between feet and hands by getting into a brief *Plank* position. The distance is ideal when the shoulders are over the wrists.

» From here push the hips far back and up until the pose, when looked at from the side, looks like an inverted V.

» Fingers are fanned and wrists and arms are extended.

» It is important to avoid over-extending or locking the elbows.

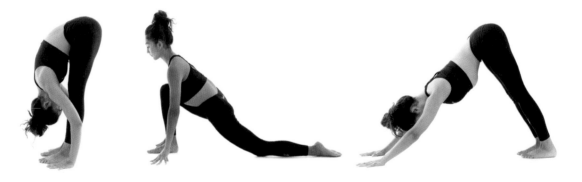

Forward bend/Uttanasana   Lunge   Inverted V

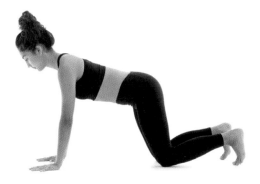 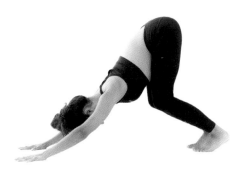

Wide all-fours position

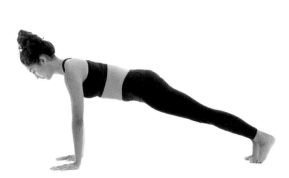 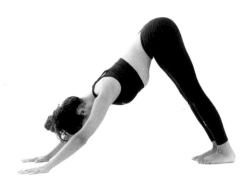

Plank

WORKING IN THE POSE

» Press your thumbs and the fleshy part of the index fingers into the mat. The muscles of the forearms are rotated slightly inward.

» The extension begins with the arms. With respect to shoulder alignment, imagine your armpits (the area where hair grows) facing each other or moving towards each other.

» The head either sinks towards the floor or is an extension of the spine (ears between upper arms).

» Let the sternum sink towards the floor (in case of a hyperextended spine it is advisable to stabilize the back with the core muscles by pulling the lower ribs inward).

» Tailbone and sit bones reach diagonally upward. There is a slight suggestion of a backbend in the lumbar spine.

» The heels sink towards the mat. The outside edges of the feet are parallel to the edges of the mat.

» Enter the pose with knees slightly bent to deepen extension of the spine. Then slowly straighten the legs. If the muscles at the back of the legs are severely shortened, begin by keeping the knees bent as the extension of the spine takes priority.

» **Energy control:** As you inhale, absorb energy through the hands and feet and direct it to the heart. As you exhale, spread the energy across the entire body.

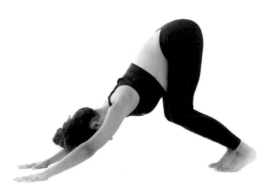

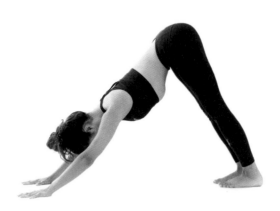

VARIATIONS

» **Walking Dog:** Alternate pedaling the feet without lifting the balls of the feet (preparation).

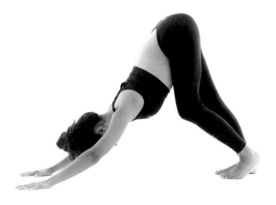

» **Eka Pada Adho Mukha Svanasana (with leg split):** Lift one leg into an extension of the spine.

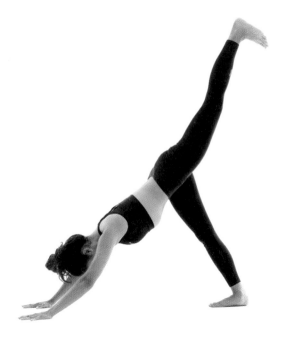

ACTIVE AND STABILIZING MUSCLES

Trunk

» The quadriceps femoris muscle straightens the leg.

» The muscles along the shin and calf (tibialis anterior and peronaeus longus) flex the foot.

Trunk

» The transverse abdominal muscles stabilize.

» The erector spinae muscles straighten the spine.

» The serratus anterior muscles stabilize the shoulder blades.

» The trapezius muscles, lower and middle section, pull the shoulder blades down.

» The rhomboids pull the shoulder blades together, stabilize.

» The small chest muscles (pectoralis minor) pull the shoulder blades forward, lower the shoulder girdle.

Shoulders/arms

» The deltoids lift the arms.

» The triceps straighten the arms.

STRETCHED MUSCLES

Legs

» Back of the thighs (ischiocrural muscles).

» Calf muscles (gastrocnemius and soleus)

Trunk

» Large gluteal muscles (gluteus maximus).

» Straight abdominal muscle (rectus abdominis)

» Large back muscles (latissimus dorsi)

» Large and small chest muscles (perctoralis major and minor).

PREPARATORY EXERCISES

Stretch the muscles at the back of the legs, the gluteals, low back, and flanks. Loosen up the spine, hips, shoulders, hands and fingers.

COUNTERPOSES

Tadasana, Backbends, Balasana (rest and reflection).

7.3.2   ALANASANA – HIGH LUNGE

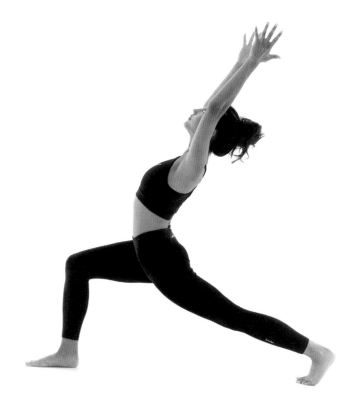

SYMBOLISM/IMPACT

Alanasana means *high lunge with backbend* and is actually not one of the classical Asanas. It is a variation on *Anjaney Asana* (*Deep Lunge*) and is also used as preparation for and introduction to *Virabhadrasana 1* (*Warrior 1*). The difference to *Virabhadrasana 1* is the position of the back leg. In *Virabhadrasana 1* the heel of the back foot is rotated in about 30°, which stabilizes the pose, but requires lots of flexibility in the back leg/hip. By contrast, in *Alanasana* hip, knee, and foot are parallel, which makes it easier to execute the pose. Alanasana is often practiced as a transitional pose in flows.

POSE STRUCTURE

See *Anjaney Asana*, except that the back leg is straight.

WORKING IN THE POSE

See *Anjaney Asana*. The extended back leg remains active, and it is important that hip, knee, and foot are parallel.

ACTIVE AND STABILIZING MUSCLES

See *Anjaney Asana*, except here the quadriceps muscle is active.

STRETCHED MUSCLES

See *Anjaney Asana*, except here the quadriceps muscle is active.

PREPARATORY EXERCISES

See *Anjaney Asana*.

COUNTERPOSE

See *Anjaney Asana*.

7.3.3   ANJANEY ASANA – LOW LUNGE

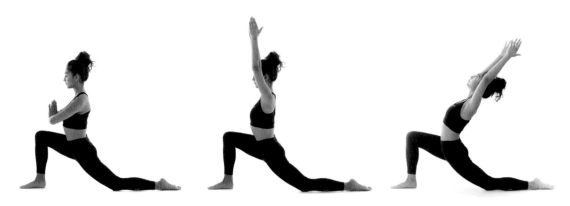

Photo series 7.3.3 a-c

SYMBOLISM/IMPACT

Anjaneya = crescent moon, one of the names of Hanuman (Monkey God)

Anjaneya is one of the names of the monkey god Hanuman who is known for his giant leaps. This Asana consists of a wide lunge, in which the back knee rests on the ground while the arms are extended upward in extension of the shoulders.

In some traditions, this Asana is also called *crescent moon* if a backbend is added.

Anjaney Asana can be practiced by itself or as part of a Karana. Due to its deep stretch of the hip flexors with simultaneous extension and backbend of the trunk, it is a good preparation for *Alanasana* (*High Lunge*), *Virabhadrasana 1* (*Warrior 1*) and all backbends.

POSE STRUCTURE

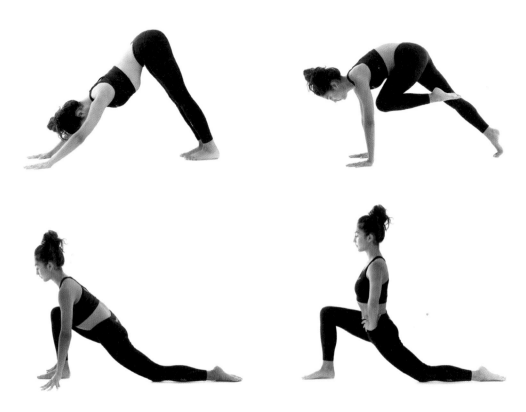

Photo series 7.3.3 d-g

Either take a big step forward from *Adho Svanasana* (PS 7.3.3 d) as you exhale, or a big step back from Uttansana (Standing Forward Bend) as you exhale. The forward knee forms a right angle and the calf is in a vertical position. Knee and ankle form a vertical line. The back knee is positioned far behind the hip. Place a folded blanket under a tender knee. Once the hips are parallel, the trunk is lifted during inhalation. The arms are raised as an extension of the back and shoulders; the hands are open shoulder-width apart.

If you are unable to move the foot far enough forward between the hands from Adho Mukha Svanasana, modify the pose by doing it on all fours or on your knees.

WORKING IN THE POSE

» In a lunge, pull the hip of the forward leg forward slightly so the hips are parallel. (Hips often shift when stepping backwards into a lunge).

» To give the pose more stability, pull both legs towards each other with an isometric contraction (tightening of leg muscles without visible change in length). This also corrects hip alignment.

» Support the trunk extension by activating the pelvic floor muscles.

» Pull the shoulder blades back and down while the sternum reaches upward.

VARIATIONS

» **Low Lunge:** Lunge with hands on the floor (pose from *Rishikesh Sun Salutation*).

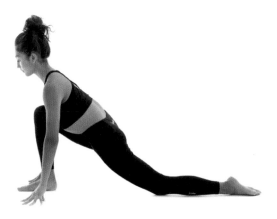

» **Crescent moon:** Here the palms come together overhead, moving into a deep backbend.

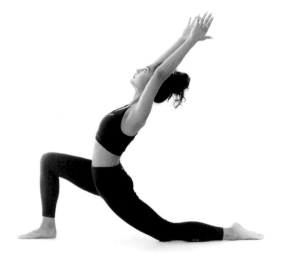

ACTIVE AND STABILIZING MUSCLES

Front leg/pelvis

» The hip flexor flexes the hip.

» The quadriceps muscle stabilizes the leg.

» The ischiocrural muscles flex the knee.

Trunk

» The erector spinae muscles extend the spine.

» The transverse abdominals stabilize the trunk.

» The lower section of the trapezius muscles pull the shoulder blades down and stabilize.

» The external and internal obliques stabilize the trunk.

Shoulders/arms

» The deltoids raise the arms.

» The triceps straighten the arms.

STRETCHED MUSCLES

Back of leg/pelvis

» Quadriceps femoris

» Hip flexors

» Adductors

Trunk

» Rectus abdominis

» Pectoralis major

» Serratus anterior

» Latissimus dorsi

PREPARATORY EXERCISES

Stretch the hip flexors and quadriceps; loosen up the spine and the shoulders.

COUNTERPOSE

Forward bends like Uttansana (relaxed form), Balasana.

7.3.4 APANASANA – KNEE-TO-CHEST POSE

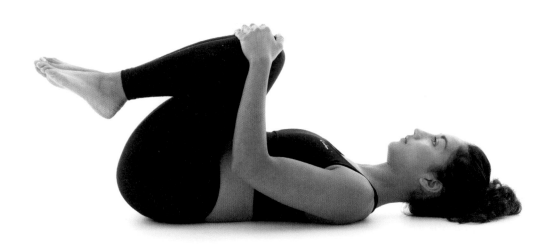

SYMBOLISM/IMPACT

Apana = descending energy (breath, air)

Apanasana activates *Apana Vayu* (the aspect of Prana responsible for all excretion processes). Lie on your back and pull your knees and thighs into your chest with your hands. Pulling the legs into the chest moves the diaphragm upward, which stimulates and deepens exhalation. *Apanasana* is considered a purification exercise, as it can also release excess gas (flatulence) in the abdomen. Also lift head and shoulders to facilitate a massaging effect on the internal organs. The low back stretch can loosen tight muscles in the lumbar spine.

POSE STRUCTURE

» Lie on your back and grip your bent knees with your hands.

» Shoulders and head rest on the floor.

» Knees and feet remain in a parallel position; ankles and knees form a straight line.

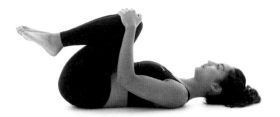

WORKING IN THE POSE

» As you exhale, pull your thighs towards your belly; as you inhale, push the knees away from your belly until the arms are extended.

» To intensify the pose, you can lift head and shoulders while you exhale.

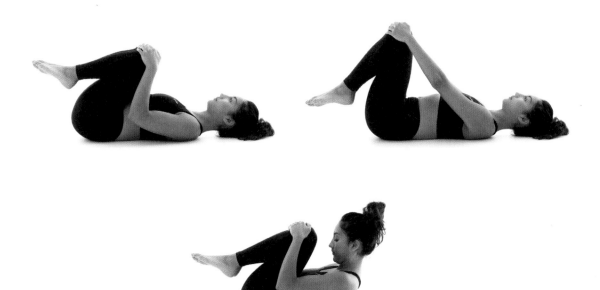

ACTIVE AND STABILIZING MUSCLES

If head and shoulders are also lifted during the exercise:

Trunk

» Rectus abdominis – trunk flexion.

» Transverse abdominals – stabilize.

» Internal and external obliques – stabilize.

» Sternocleidomastoid muscles – stabilize and turn the head.

Arms

» Biceps – bend the arms while pulling in the legs.

STRETCHED MUSCLES

Legs

» Back of the thighs (ischiocrural muscles/hamstring).

Trunk

» Gluteus maximus

» Quadratus lumborum

» Erector spinae muscles (lower section)

VARIATIONS AND COUNTERPOSES

Apanasana can be used as a preparatory exercise as well as a counterpose, for example after backbends.

7.3.5 EKA PADA APANA ASANA – (SINGLE) KNEE-TO-CHEST POSE

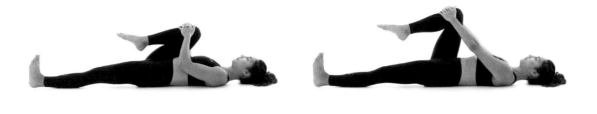

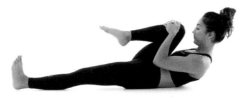

Photo series 7.3.5 a-c

SYMBOLISM/IMPACT

Eka = one / Pada = foot, step/ Apanasana = wind-relieving pose

Like *Apanasana*, *Eka Pada Apana Asana* is considered a wind-relieving pose. This form of execution intensifies the effect. In some traditions, it is also referred to as *Pawanmuktasana* (Pawan = air / Mukhta = liberation). The compression this movement creates in the abdomen massages and stimulates the internal organs, which is said to stimulate metabolism. This exercise also has a positive effect on the tonus of the internal organs, which can get tight just like muscles and are gently relaxed by this movement. The exercise is also an ideal introduction to and preparation for stretches of the back of the legs as in *Supta Padangusthasana* 1, 2, and 3.

POSE STRUCTURE

» Lie on your back, grip the bent knee with both hands and pull it close to the chest. (PS 7.3.5 a).

» Head and shoulders rest on the floor.

» Extend the "floor leg" and create close contact with the mat/floor.

WORKING IN THE POSE

» Pull the "working leg" close to the chest several times as you exhale and release as you inhale, while keeping the other leg extended on the floor. (PS 7.3.5 a-b). If you have trouble keeping the extended leg on the floor it is a sign that your hip flexors are shortened.

VARIATIONS

This exercise can be performed in different variations:

» Pull the bent knee into the chest several times as you exhale (PS 7.3.5 a), then hold it close to the chest for several breaths, and release. Rest and reflect (PS 7.3.5 e) and repeat on the other side.

Photo series 7.3.5 d-e

» Alternate pulling your legs into the chest several times, and extend the body completely as you inhale (PS 7.3.5 f); arms extend overhead.

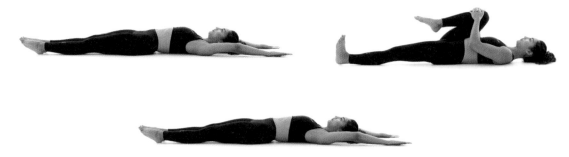

Photo series 7.3.5 f-h

» Also lift head and shoulders as you exhale (PS 7.3.5 k). It is recommended that you begin by alternately pulling the knees into the chest before performing the more intense variation with the upper-body lift.

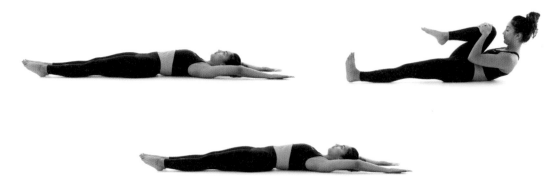

Photo series 7.3.5 i-k

ACTIVE AND STABILIZING MUSCLES

When head and shoulders are also lifted during the exercise:

Trunk

» Rectus abdominis

» Transverse obliques

» External and internal obliques

» Sternocleidomastoid muscles

Arms

» Biceps – while pulling in the leg.

PRIMARILY STRETCHED

Legs

» Back of thighs (ischiocrural muscles/hamstring

Trunk

» Gluteus maximus

» Quadratus lumborum

» Erector spinae muscles (lower section). When the trunk is also lifted the entire length of the erector spinae muscles is stretched.

» Hip flexors on the side of the extended leg (but only if the leg rests on the floor).

PREPARATORY EXERCISES

Apanasana, loosen up hips.

COUNTERPOSE

Shoulder Bridge, Shavasana.

7.3.6 ARDHA MATSYENDRASANA – HALF LORD OF THE FISHES POSE

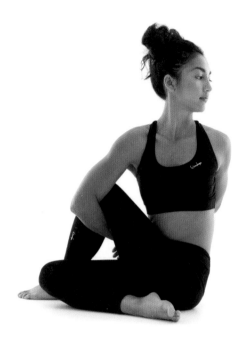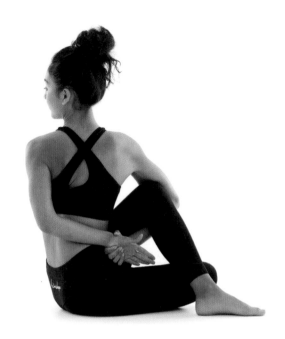

Photo series 7.3.6 a-b

SYMBOLISM/IMPACT

Ardha = half, Matsyendra = name of the yoga master who founded Hatha Yoga

The *Seated Twist* is one of the asymmetrical poses. It has a particular effect on the internal organs as the deep twist combined with long, deep breaths puts gentle pressure on the organs (the diaphragm pushes into the abdomen during the inhale), which has a massaging and stimulating effect. This in turn stimulates metabolism and benefits digestion, which is why twists are also considered purifying poses. If the twist is first performed to the right and then to the left, it also supports vermicular movement in the intestinal tract.

Ardha Matsyendrasana is a twisting of the trunk in a seated position. Prerequisite to the rotation is a stable seat from which the vertical spine twists in the respective direction. The spine's rotational ability is about 120° in a healthy spine. The lumbar spine can rotate about 5°, and has a primarily stabilizing function. The rotating ability of the thoracic spine is 35-40°, the cervical spine (C7-C2) can rotate about 40°, and the atlanto occipital joint (C1-C2) can also rotate 40°.

From an energy standpoint, the *Seated Twist* stimulates *Samana Vayu*. It is the aspect of Prana that is responsible for converting food into energy.

The *Seated Twist* is always performed in both directions. From an energy- anatomy standpoint, the twist stimulates both Ida and Pingala Nadi.

When we twist to the right, we internally connect with our active, joyful, and fiery aspects. When twisting to the left, we get in touch with our cooling, intuitive, and emotional aspects. The pose thus triggers a balance between the lunar and solar forces inside us.

Symbolically this pose represents inner flexibility. Not only does it eliminate physical stiffness, but it also facilitates the release of very rigid inner mental or emotional patterns. The seated twist always begins and ends with a stable center. In this sense, it equally promotes the experience of opposites and reinforces a sense of the inner center.

POSE STRUCTURE

» Sitting with your legs extended on the floor (*Dandasana*), line up hips and pelvis, and move the spine into axial extension. When twisting to the right, the right foot is planted to the outside of the left knee.

» The left leg is bent and slides under the propped up right leg; the left foot rests next to the right hip.

» The left arm wraps around the right leg; the crook of the left arm is wrapped around the right knee.

» The right arm is propped behind the body. Lift the spine one more time, initiate rotation, and look back over the right shoulder. Move the right bottom ribs farther to the right; the left lower ribs move closer to the right thigh. During this pose the entire back is in an upright position, the shoulders move down and to the outside.

WORKING IN THE POSE

In this pose, take long, even breaths into the belly and ribcage. The structure of the pose facilitates deep exhalation. Make sure to also inhale again because during deep twists the breaths can easily become too shallow. The spine is in an upright position for the duration of the holding phase. Hyperextension of the lumbar spine should be avoided as it blocks the thoracic spine. The propped-up arm can be used as a lever to deepen rotation; build up isometric tension by pushing the hand into the floor and away from the body. The gaze over the back shoulder is relaxed; excessive rotation of the cervical spine should be avoided.

VARIATIONS

Depending on flexibility, there are different arm positions for the seated twist:

» *Marichyasana*: the lower leg can also be extended if hip mobility is limited. In addition, a double-folded blanket can be placed under the sit bones, which aids an upright spinal position. The back hand can also be propped on a block to make it easier to straighten the spine. Extension always precedes rotation.

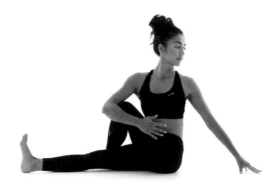

Photo series 7.3.6 c

» In a classic *Seated Twist*, the front arm either reaches past the propped up leg towards the outside edge of the front foot, or moves into a bind (*see PS 7.3.6 a*).

» But the front arm can also act as a lever against the inside of the propped up leg to deepen the stretch, which would be considered a modification.

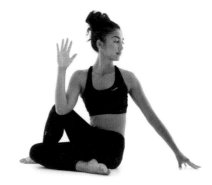

Photo Series 7.3.6 d

ACTIVE AND STABILIZING MUSCLES

Trunk

» All erector spinae muscles - help move the spine into an upright position.

» Short and long rotators (rotatores thorax longus and internus) – rotation of the spine.

» External and internal obliques – rotation of the spine.

» Hip flexors – on the side of the propped up leg.

Shoulder girdle and neck

» Rhomboid major (stabilizes shoulder blades) – head rotation.

» Sternocleidomastoid – head rotation

» Splenius muscle of the head – head rotation.

» Upper section of the trapezius muscles – head rotation.

Propped up leg

» Gracilis muscle – flexes and adducts the leg.

» Pectineus muscle – flexes and adducts the leg.

» Adductor magnus – adducts the leg.

Bottom leg

» Biceps femoris – bends the leg in the knee joint.

STRETCHED MUSCLES

All active muscles participating in the rotation (see above) are also being stretched on the opposite side.

Hips/legs

» Large, medium, and small gluteal muscles.

» Piriformis muscle.

» Superior and inferior gemellus muscle.

» Obturator internus and externus.

» Quadratus femoris muscle.

PREPARATORY EXERCISES

Crocodile poses (*Makarasana*), gluteal stretches, activation of erector spinae muscles, lateral movements that facilitate trunk extension.

Introductory Asanas: *Dandasana* (*Staff pose*), *Janu Shirasana* (*Head-to-knee pose*), *Parivritta Janu Shirasana* (*revolved Head-to-knee pose*), *Parsva Sukhasana* (*Seated Twist with bent knees*), *Marichyasana III* (*Seated Twist variation with extended leg*; the propped up leg is placed against the inside of the extended leg).

COUNTERPOSE

Forward bend, Shoulder Bridge.

7.3.7 BALASANA – CHILD'S POSE/UTTHITA BALASANA

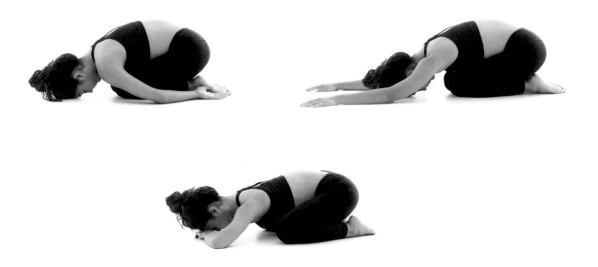

Photo series 7.3.7 a-c

SYMBOLISM/IMPACT

Bala = child, Asana = pose / Utthita Balasana = extended child's pose

Balasana means *pose of the child*. It is one of the forward bends, and its primary bending of the spine is reminiscent of an unborn child in the womb, gently drawn together and protected. As with all forward bends, Balasana has a calming effect on the nervous system.

When *Balasana* is performed by itself, it stimulates Apana Vayu, the aspect of Prana that represents letting go. *Balasana* is an ideal pose for rest and reflection and is often done after backbends as a counterpose. *Utthita Balasana*, extended child's pose, is often performed as a starting or transitional pose.

POSE STRUCTURE

»   From an all-fours position (PS 7.3.7 d) push your bottom back over your feet (PS 7.3.7 e).

»   Place a folded blanket under your knees if you have tender knees. To remain in the pose for an extended period of time or in case of stiff joints, a folded blanket can also be placed between calves and buttocks (slide the blanket into the hollows of the knees).

»   Rest your forehead on the floor (PS 7.3.7 f), on the back of the hands (PS 7.3.7 c), or on your stacked fists.

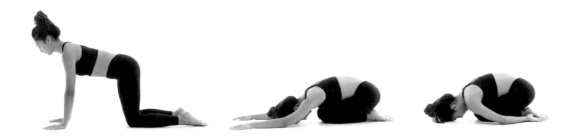

Photo Series 7.3.7 d-f

WORKING IN THE POSE

» Allow the lower back to open up and relax your buttocks.

» Breathe evenly.

» The contracted structure of the pose limits breath movement in the belly and ribcage, requiring more movement in the back, particularly in the area of the ribcage and waist.

VARIATIONS

Variation 1: As a starting position for a flow or an All-fours pose: place feet and knees shoulder-width apart; the back is long; lift the sternum; the nape is long, the forehead faces the floor, arms are extended forward shoulder-width apart, the humeral heads pull into the shoulder joints, the elbows are turned up (slight external rotation of the upper arms), elbows do not touch the floor, hands are fanned, the middle finger points forward (PS 7.3.7 g).

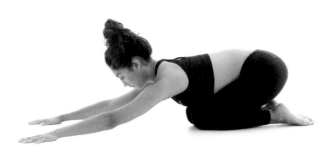

Photo series 7.3.7 g

Variation 2: As a rest and reflection pose: The buttocks rest on the heels, the back is loosely rounded, the forehead rests on the floor, and the arms rest alongside the body.

Variation 3: For pregnant women or people with lots of soft abdominal tissue: Knees are open wide so the stomach has room (PS 7.3.7 h). The straddle position of the legs allows the spine to achieve a near neutral position.

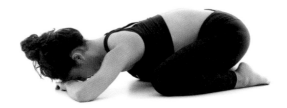

Photo series 7.3.7 h

ACTIVE AND STABILIZING MUSCLES

In a resting or reflecting pose, Balasana is a relaxation pose. All of the muscles can be relaxed.

As a starting position with an active spine and arms extended forward:

Trunk

» The erector spinae muscles − extend the spine.

» The lower trapezius muscles − pull the shoulder blades down.

» The posterior deltoids − lift the arms.

Arms

» Triceps (medial head) − extend the arms.

Primary muscles being stretched in a resting pose:

Trunk

» Erector spinae

» Quadratus lumborum

» Gluteus maximus

Legs

» Quadriceps femoris

» Tibialis anterior

PREPARATORY EXERCISES

Apanasana, *Eka Pada Apanasana*, *Marjaryasana*, *Hero*, stretches the muscles at the front of the shin.

COUNTERPOSE

Savasana

7.3.8   BADDHA KONASANA – BOUND ANGLE POSE AND UPAVISTHA KONASANA – WIDE-ANGLE SEATED FORWARD BEND

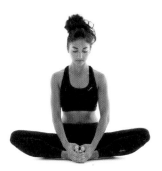 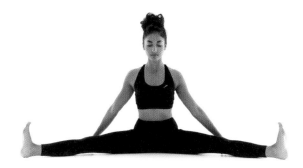

Photo series 7.3.8 a-b

SYMBOLISM/IMPACT

Baddha = bound, closed, Kona = angle, Upavishtha = open

Baddha Konasana (45) is also known as *Cobblers*. It is a symmetrical pose in which the groin and inner thigh muscles are deeply stretched while simultaneously placing the spine in an upright extended position. This pose is in the hip-opener category and is used to prepare for seated poses such as *Sukhasana* (*Basic Cross-legged pose*), *Svastikasana* (*Half Lotus*), and *Padmasana* (*Full Lotus*). A relaxed and upright-seated posture is the basis for Pranayama and meditation. Practicing *Baddha Konasana* is therefore particularly beneficial for inflexible and stiff hips and legs.

POSE STRUCTURE

» In *Dandasana* (*Staff pose*) bend first one leg and pull it in with your hands, then pull the heel as close to the groin as possible (based on flexibility). Then repeat with the other leg. The soles of the feet touch.

» The outside edges of the feet rest on the floor. Grip the outside edges of the feet with your hands. Let the knees drop while simultaneously fully extending the spine upward. If the pelvis tends to tilt backward (pubis points towards the chin) due to a lack of flexibility in the hips, it is not possible to move the spine into an upright position. In this case place a folded blanket under the sit bones, which will help to move the pelvis and spine into an upright position.

WORKING IN THE POSE

» Take calm and even breaths. The gaze is horizontal.

» Press the sit bones into the floor, while allowing knees and thighs to sink towards the floor.

» As the spine stretches upward, the outside of the shoulders pull slightly out and down.

» Make your neck long by slightly tucking the chin and moving the back of the head back until the earlobes are in line with the shoulders.

» Lift the sternum, but make sure the lumbar spine maintains its natural curve.

» The pelvic floor muscles can be activated (pull them in and up) while exhaling to help move the spine into an upright position.

VARIATIONS

» Baddha Konasana is often combined with a forward bend with simultaneously supinated feet (soles of feet point upward with the outside edges touching).

» Supta Baddha Konasana / Reclined Cobblers. (PS 7.3.8 c-d)

» Upavishtha Konasana / Open Cobblers, seated straddle. (PS 7.3.8 e-f)

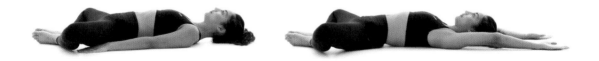

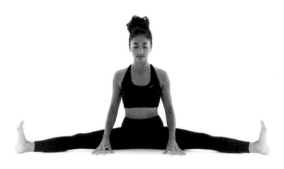 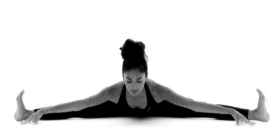

Photo series 7.3.8 c-f

ACTIVE AND STABILIZING MUSCLES

Trunk

» Erector spinae muscles − extend the spine.

» Multifidi muscles − extend the spine

» Serratus anterior muscle and rhomboids must both work to stabilize the shoulder blades at the ribcage.

Arms

» The biceps bend the elbows (especially when combining *Baddha Konasana* with a forward bend).

Pelvis/legs

» Piriformis muscle − external rotation.

» Superior and inferior gemellus muscle − external rotation.

» Obturator internus − external rotation.

» Quadratus femoris − external rotation.

» Hip flexor: iliopsoas muscle − flexes the hip.

» Rectus femoris − flexes the hip.

» Sartorius muscle − flexes the hip.

» (But if these three are extremely shortened they pull the knees upward and inhibit the ability to sit tall in the posture.)

» Biceps femoris − flexes the knee.

STRETCHED MUSCLES

Pelvis/legs

» All three adductors (adductor longus, magnus, brevis).

» Gracilis muscle

» Pectineus muscle

» Gluteus medius and minimus

» Tensor fasciae latae

PREPARATORY EXERCISES

Shoulder Bridge, Balasana, Apanasana

7.3.9 BHUJANGASANA – COBRA

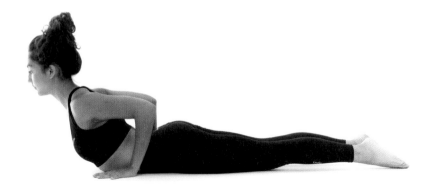

Photo series 7.3.9 a

SYMBOLISM/IMPACT

Bhujanga = serpent, cobra / Asana = pose

In India, the *serpent* is considered a symbol of wisdom. In Hatha Yoga the serpent has a special meaning. It represents the coiled up Kundalini Shakti at the base of the spine. *Bhujangasana*, also called *Cobra pose*, is a prone backbend. It is one of the basic poses. Cobra is performed by itself, usually in preparation for a number of other, more complex backbends. It is also part of the classic *Sun Salutation* of the Rishikesh series. And is practiced in many Vinyasa flows.

There are different ways to perform the Cobra pose depending on the tradition. In this pose, it is important that feet, legs, and pelvis touch the floor during the backbend. Due to its structure, the Cobra pose helps to lift the spine into an erect position, which can correct extreme kyphosis, especially if it is a result of poor posture, e.g. rachitic humpback. In *Cobra*, the legs and pelvis have a stabilizing effect. The backbend is concentrated primarily in the thoracic spine area.

During the backbend, the front of the body is stretched and opened, especially the chest, which allows for deeper breaths. This stimulates the Prana Vayu, the aspect of Prana that is responsible for energy absorption. *Cobra* is a good preparatory pose for Pranayama exercises because it works on breath awareness and increases breath volume.

With respect to energy, it affects the higher heart space, the *Anahata chakra*, which represents themes like love, self-love, and empathy.

POSE STRUCTURE

» In a prone position, first extend the legs and feet from the hips and position them hip-width apart.

» The trunk is on the floor as an extension of the body, the forehead faces the floor. (PS 7.3.9 b)

» Hands are planted on the floor below shoulders and next to the lower ribs. The elbows are bent at right angles and are held close to the trunk. Shoulders pulled back and down.

» To initiate the pose, activate the leg muscles: press the tops of the feet into the floor and pull the sit bones down slightly. The pubic bone pulls down towards the floor. The gluteal muscles are engaged without "squeezing".

» From this base position the upper body lifts into Cobra: lift the sternum and push it forward and up.

» The arms can gently aid this process, but it is important that the back muscles and not the arms facilitate the backbend. Don't let the elbows splay out to the sides.

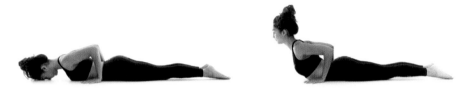

Photo series 7.3.9 b-c

» Traditionally in this pose, the head is moved far back to stretch the front of the neck (opens up the *Vishuddha chakra / throat chakra*), whereby the gaze is upward. But since many people have neck and cervix problems, yoga novices should avoid tilting the head back very far in this pose, meaning the head should tilt back only far enough to avoid wrinkles at the back of the neck. Experienced practitioners can decide how much to integrate the head into the backbend.

WORKING IN THE POSE

» Before entering the pose, make sure the spine is in axial extension, and then steadily build the backbend from the bottom up.

» Enter the pose as you inhale, and breathe evenly and calmly into the chest.

» The thoracic spine benefits most from the backbend. To deepen and support the backbend in the thoracic spine, pull the shoulder blades back and down.

» The pose is stabilized by actively pulling the lower abdominal muscles inward and up and by contracting the pelvic floor muscles.

» Visualization aid: imagine a small light at the center of the sternum that first shines its beam of light forward and during the course of the exercise moves gradually upward.

» How deep the backbend is depends entirely on flexibility. Many people can just barely lift the upper body while others are able to lift the upper body and arms nearly vertically. What matters is that the extension is spread out over the entire spine without compressing an area.

VARIATIONS

» Lift the arms and extend them alongside the trunk, hands reach towards feet, shoulder blades squeeze together (PS 7.3.9 d).

» To deepen the backbend in the chest area cross the hands behind the back (bound pose) and actively squeeze the shoulder blades together (PS 3.7.9 e).

» *Sphinx*: Plant the elbows below the shoulders; forearms are parallel (PS 3.7.9 f).

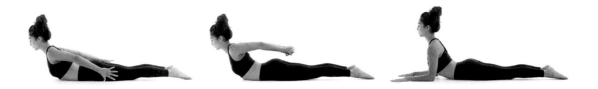

Photo series 7.3.9 d-f

ACTIVE AND STABILIZING MUSCLES

Trunk

» Erector spinae muscle – extends the spine.

» Quadratus lumborum – extends the spine.

» Gluteus maximus – extends the spine.

» Pelvic floor muscles (pubococcygeus muscles) – help the trunk move into an erect position.

» Rectus abdominis and transverse abdominals – act eccentric for stability.

Legs

» The ischiocrural muscles at the back of the thigh – extend the hip.

Shoulder girdle/arms

» The middle and lower trapezius muscles – pull the shoulder blade down.

» Infraspinatus muscle – stabilizes the shoulder blade.

» Serratus anterior muscles – stabilizes the shoulder blade.

» Teres minor – stabilizes the shoulder blade.

» Posterior deltoids – extend the arm backward.

» Triceps – arm extension.

STRETCHED MUSCLES

Trunk

» Rectus abdominis

» External and internal obliques

» Intercostal muscles

Shoulders/arms

» Lattisimus dorsi, upper section (Large back muscle)

» Pectoralis major and minor

» Teres major

Legs

» Rectus femoris

» Iliopsoas muscle

» Tensor fasciae latae

PREPARATORY EXERCISES

Loosen up the entire length of the spine, stretch the hip flexors and the front of the thighs, loosen up the shoulder girdle and chest, stretch the front of the shoulders, extend the spine.

COUNTERPOSE

Marjaryasana, Balasana, Apanasana

7.3.10 CHATURANGA DANDASANA – PLANK (PHALAKASANA)

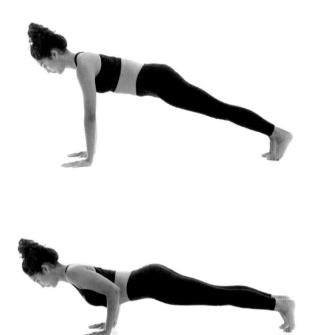

Photo series 7.3.10 a-b

SYMBOLISM/IMPACT

Chatur = four, Anga = link, Danda = stick/staff, Asana = pose (PS 7.3.10 a)

Phalakasana – the Planke / Phalaka = plank (PS 7.3.10 b)

Chaturanga Dandasana is the *Four-link Staff* pose and falls in the category of strength and support poses. The weight rests on hands and feet, and the elbows are bent at right angles. The entire body is straight and solid like a stick or a plank, which is why the exercise is also called *Plank pose*. *Chaturanga Dandasana* is often practiced as part of a Vinyasa flow. The pose requires a lot of physical strength and stability, especially in the shoulders and arms along with the core. There are a number of modifications to build up the required strength.

From an energy standpoint, *Chaturanga Dandasana* unites the qualities of *Muladhara chakra* (stability, strength, faith, grounding) and the fire of *Manipura chakra*. The power and the will to move something, to apply strength, and in doing so, leave one's comfort zone. For the overall yoga path, it is not just necessary to be permeable, to be able to feel and perceive. Occasionally the path also requires a certain inner discipline and perseverance, such as when we must leave behind habitual patterns or habits that would impede our long-term inner growth.

Here the practice of *Chaturange Dandasana* can be of mental, emotional, and physical help. Anyone who has mastered this demanding Asana is also able to muster the necessary strength in other situations and not collapse under the load of burdensome events.

Moreover, *Chaturanga* is an excellent basis for all arm-balance poses.

POSE STRUCTURE

» From *Downward-facing Dog* (*Adho Mukha Svanasana*, PS 7.3.10 c) lower the body into *Plank* (*Phalakasana*, PS 7.3.10 d); shoulders are stacked over wrists.

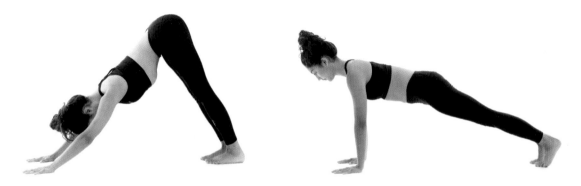

Photo series 7.3.10 c-d

» Another way to enter this pose is from all fours, and then extending first one and then the other leg.

» Next push the shoulders forward and bend the elbows at right angles in *Chaturanga Dandasana*. The body remains straight as a plank (PS 7.3.10 e).

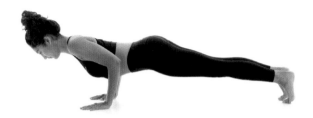

Photo series 7.3.10 e

WORKING IN THE POSE

» Pull the stomach in and up so the pelvis doesn't sag and the pose is stable.

» For stability, also pull the bottom ribs, the "floating ribs" in.

» Push the body away from the floor with fingers fanned. Both shoulders pull back.

» The entire back is wide and stable. Make sure you don't "sprout wings" on the upper back due to unstable shoulder blades. Pull the shoulder blades together and down.

» The gluteal muscles are engaged, legs are actively extended; pull the kneecaps up.

» As soon as body tension has been established, shift your bodyweight farther forward and bend the elbows at right angles. The body stays in plank position, shoulders are at a level with the elbows.

» In the pose, press your toes into the mat and back while pushing the hands forward on the mat. This isometric tension lends the pose additional stability.

» During the pose, allow the breath to flow calmly into the ribcage.

VARIATIONS

» If there is not yet enough strength in shoulders and arms, make the lever smaller and rest the knees on the mat (PS 7.3.10 g).

» This pose can also be dynamic by alternately bending and straightening the arms (PS 7.3.10 g).

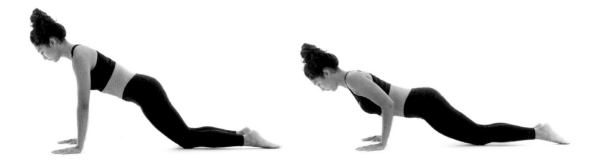

Photo series 7.3.10 f-g

» Bending and straightening the arms as well as building stable body alignment can also be practiced against a wall, standing upright.

» The pose can also be built from the floor. Place hands next to bottom ribs, tuck the toes, build up whole-body tension, and begin by lifting the upper body into a slight backbend, then lift the pelvis and stabilize the entire body.

ACTIVE AND STABILIZING MUSCLES

Trunk

» Rectus abdominis – stabilizes.

» Transverse abdominals – stabilize.

» External obliques – stabilize.

» Pectoralis major – pulls the arm forward.

» Erector spinae – extends the spine.

» Quadratus lumborum – stabilizes.

» Gluteus maximus and minimus – stabilize.

» Pelvic floor muscles/pubococcygeus – stabilize.

» Iliopsoas muscle – stabilizes.

Shoulder girdle

» Anterior deltoids – raise the arm.

» Serratus anterior – stabilizes.

» Rhomboids – stabilize the shoulder blade.

» Middle and lower trapezius muscles – pull the shoulder blade down.

Arms

» Triceps – extend the arm.

» Biceps – flex the arm.

» Brachialis muscles – bend the arm/elbow.

Legs

» Quadriceps femoris – extends the knee, stabilizes.

» Tensor fasciae latae – stabilizes.

» Ischiocrural muscles (back of the thigh) – stabilize.

» Gastrocnemius (large calf muscle) – stabilizes.

» Tibialis anterior (front of shin) – flexes the foot (dorsal flexion).

PREPARATORY EXERCISES

Loosen up the hand and shoulder joints; strengthen core, shoulder, and arm muscles.

COUNTERPOSE

Child's pose (Balasana), Cat (Marjaryasana)

7.3.11 DANDASANA – STAFF POSE

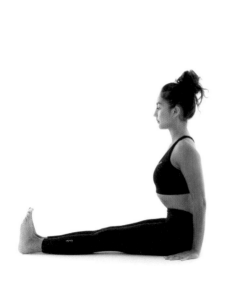 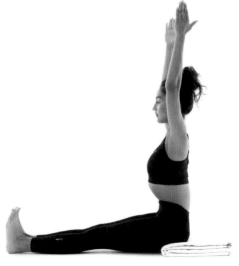

Photo series 7.3.11 a-b

SYMBOLISM/IMPACT

Danda = stick, staff / Asana = pose

In *Dandasana, Staff pose*, the spine is in an upright position and as stable as a stick, whereby the axially extended spine maintains its neutral curve. This pose is a basic pose and falls in the category of seated poses. It can be practiced by itself, but is generally used to prepare for more advanced Asanas such as forward bends, twists, or even support poses (e.g. *Purvottanasana / Upward Plank*).

POSE STRUCTURE

» Sit on the floor with legs extended forward and use your hands to gently spread your buttocks to expose the sit bones, creating a solid base in the pelvis.

» The insides of the legs touch, kneecaps point up.

» Feet are flexed, toes point up. The outside edges of the feet pull towards the outside of the hips, the inside edges of the feet push away from the body. The middle of the heel touches the mat.

» The back is in an upright position while maintaining the spine's natural curve. If the muscles at the back of the legs are severely shortened or the back muscles are tight, making it impossible to straighten the spine while seated with legs extended forward, it helps to place a folded blanket under the buttocks/sit bones.

» Hands rest next to hips on the floor with fingertips pointing forward. If the arms are too long or too short relative to the length of the trunk, they can either be extended via a block (if too short) or must remain bent during the pose (if too long).

» Arms are extended and shoulders pull back and down.

» The head is a neutral extension of the spine.

WORKING IN THE POSE

» Breathe naturally. Energy control: let the breath travel along the spine, lengthening its axial extension.

» The pelvic floor can be engaged to lend support to the pose.

» Pull the abdomen in slightly for stability.

» Lift the sternum without allowing the bottom ribs ("floating ribs") to drive forward.

» Engage the muscles at the front of the thighs, pull the kneecaps up to activate the quadriceps, press the muscles at the back of the thighs into the floor.

VARIATIONS

» In the pose, laterally raise the arms overhead and lower them in time with the breath to support the upright posture (PS 7.3.11 c).

» Lateral flexion to the right and the left to lengthen the sides of the trunk (PS 7.3.11 d).

» Maintain contact between buttocks (sit bones) and floor.

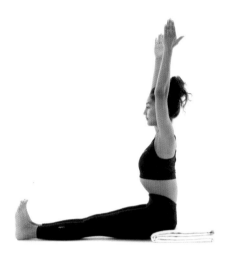 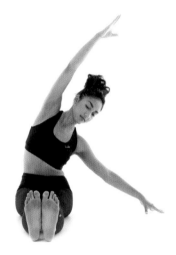

Photo series 7.3.11 c-d

ACTIVE AND STABILIZING MUSCLES

Trunk

» All erector spinae muscles help to put the spine in an upright position.

» Ilipsoas muscle for hip flexion.

» Transverse abdominals for stability.

» Serratus anterior muscles to stabilize shoulder blades.

Legs

» Large adductors and pectineus muscles for adduction and internal rotation of legs.

» Quadriceps to extend the knees.

» Muscles at front of the shins (tibialis anterior) flex the feet (dorsal flexion).

STRETCHED MUSCLES

Legs/hips

» Ischiocrural muscles (back of thighs)

» Gluteus maximus

» Piriformis

» Gemelli muscles

» Obturator internus

» Gastrocnemius (calf)

» Popliteus (back of knee)

PREPARATORY EXERCISES

Pre-stretching the back of the legs: *Eka Pada Apanasana*, *Reclining Hand-to-big-toe pose* (*Supta Padangusthasana A*), straightening and activating the spine, pre-stretching the flanks.

COUNTERPOSE

Shoulder Bridge (Dwi Pada Pitham), relaxed supine position (Shavasana)

7.3.12   DHANURASANA – BOW POSE

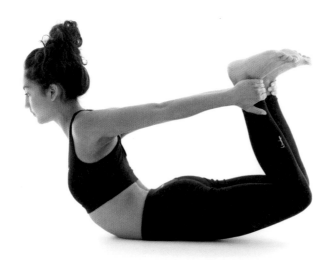

Photo series 7.3.12 a

SYMBOLISM/IMPACT

Dhanur = bow / Asana = pose

Bow pose is one of the backbends. It connects the upper with the lower extremities. The pose is reminiscent of a bow: Arms and legs form the bowstring, the trunk forms the bow. The mind directs the arrow of inner alignment.

This pose stretches and opens the entire front of the body. The pose is a combination of *Cobra* (*Bhujangasana*) and *Locust* (*Shalabhasana*), but the binding of arms and legs takes it a step further. The structure of the pose deepens the breath. The opening of the breathing apparatus, especially in the chest area, stimulates Prana Vayu, the aspect of Prana that is responsible for energy absorption.

When breathing deeply and evenly in this pose, the pressure created in the solar plexus by the deep backbend also strengthens the respiratory system and respiratory muscles, particularly the diaphragm. With respect to energy, this pose affects the *Manipura chakra*, which represents the absorption and transformation of vital energy/Prana and is linked to the willpower and power themes. The increasing pressure on the abdomen in this pose also has a stimulating effect on the digestive system and vermicular movement of the intestinal tract, particularly when rocking back and forth in this pose.

POSE STRUCTURE

» Lie on your stomach, bend the knees and grip your ankles with your hands. To stabilize your grip, pull the tops of the feet towards the shins (PS 7.3.12 b).

» To form the bow, pull with ankles against hands while simultaneously pulling with hands against ankles. This draws the bow and moves the body into a backbend.

» The head remains an extension of the spine (PS 7.3.12 c-d).

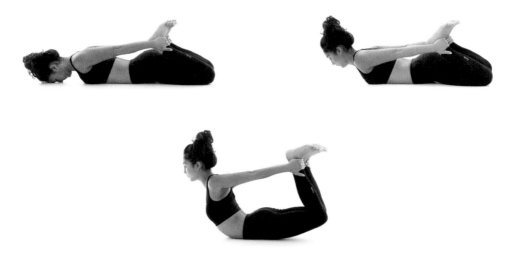

Photo series 7.3.12 b-d

WORKING IN THE POSE

» Take calm and steady belly breaths.

» Pull the shoulders back and down; elbows remain straight.

» Try to extend your knees in the pose. It deepens the back bend.

» Pull the knees towards each other to maintain hip-width alignment while simultaneously pulling the outside edges of the feet towards the outside of the knees, and rotate the feet out (which will ultimately move the into neutral alignment).

VARIATIONS

» If it is not possible to reach the ankles with the hands, rest your fingertips on your buttocks and pull the elbows towards each other and lift the sternum. Lift the knees and flex the feet (soles of feet face the ceiling/dorsal flexion). Then lift the upper body as in *cobra* while also lifting the thighs to suggest a bow (PS 7.3.12 e).

» In some traditions it is customary to rock back and forth in this pose, which is facilitated primarily by deep belly breaths.

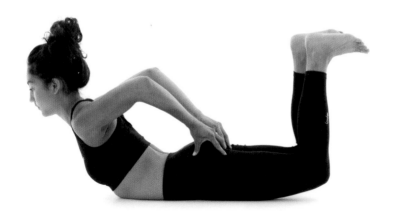

Photo series 7.3.12 e

ACTIVE AND STABILIZING MUSCLES

Shoulder girdle/arms

» Rhomboids – pull the shoulder blades together.

» Lower trapezius muscles – pull the shoulder blades down.

» Posterior deltoids – pull the arms back.

» Triceps – extend the arms.

Trunk

» Erector spinae muscles – extend the back into the backbend.

» Quadratus lumborum – extend the back/backbend.

» Gluteus maximus – extends the hips (and externally rotates the thigh, which is however not desirable in this pose).

Legs/feet

» Large adductor muscle – moves the thighs toward each other.

» Ischiocrural muscles (back of thighs) – bend the knee.

» Quadriceps femoris – extends the knee (while working in the pose).

» Tensor fasciae latae and gluteus medius - internally rotate the thigh.

» Tibialis anterior (front of the shin) and the long toe extensors (extensor hallucis and digitorum longus) – flex the foot towards the shin/dorsal flexion.

» Peroneus longus and brevis (calf bone) – externally rotate the foot.

STRETCHED MUSCLES

» Anterior deltoids

» Pectoralis major

» Biceps

» Brachialis

» Rectus abdominis

» Iliopsoas

» Pectineus

» Adductor longus and brevis

» Sartorius

» Rectus femoris

PREPARATORY EXERCISES

Stretching the hip flexors, front of thigh, front of shoulders. Loosen up the spine, hips, and shoulder joints.

COUNTERPOSE

Relaxed prone position, Child's pose (Balasana), Wind-relieving pose (Apanasana)

7.3.13 JANU SHIRSASANA – HEAD-TO-KNEE FORWARD BEND

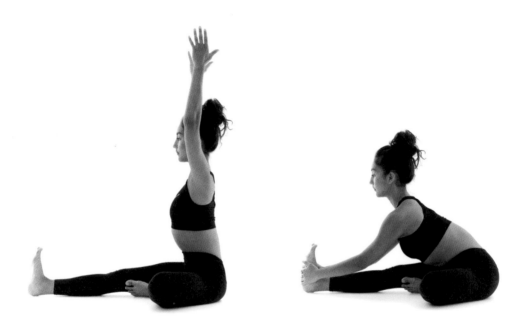

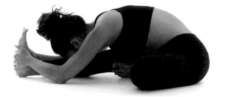

Photo series 7.3.13 a-c

SYMBOLISM/IMPACT

Janu = knee/ Shirsa = head / Asana = pose

Janu Shirsasana, Head-to-knee Forward Bend, is a seated forward bend. It is an asymmetrical stretch of the back and back of the extended leg. This pose can be practiced in forward extension as well as a forward bend. *Janu Shirsasana* is generally practiced in combination with a series of forward or side bends. It is also used as preparation for the seated twist. The bent leg gives the pose a hip-opening effect.

Like all forward bends, *Janu Shirsasana* has a purifying effect on the mind and a cooling effect on our emotional experience. The parasympathetic nervous system is activated in this pose, which is why *Janu Shirsasana* is considered one of the stress-reducing poses. The deep forward bend in the final position stimulates the digestive organs. It activates Apana Vayu, the aspect of Prana that represents the elimination of spent energy as well as letting go.

From an energy standpoint, *Janu Shirsasana* is a grounding pose. It activates the root center (*Muladhara*), and when combined with deep, even breaths, has a harmonizing effect on the sacral center in the low abdomen (*Svadhisthana*).

POSE STRUCTURE

» In *Dandasana* (Staff pose), bend one leg and pull the knee to the outside. Pull the heel towards the perineum and place the sole of the foot against the inside of the thigh. The angle between the bent lower leg and the extended leg should ideally be 90°.

» Keep the extended leg straight; kneecap and tips of toes point upward.

» As you inhale, lift the spine via axial extension and raise the arms as an extension of the trunk, shoulder-width apart.

» As you exhale, bend forward from the hip and move into a forward bend. Grip the foot of the extended leg with your hands (alternatively the ankle or calf).

» Extend the upper body along the extended leg.

WORKING IN THE POSE

» Take long, even breaths.

» Press the hip and the knee of the bent leg into the floor.

» Press the hip and back of the extended leg into the floor. In cases of shortened muscles at the back of the leg, the extended leg can be bent, or you can place a folded blanket under it.

» Allow the shoulder on the side with the bent leg to drop towards the floor so both shoulders are parallel.

» Keep the low back as flat as possible.

» In the pose, slightly open the elbows to open the chest.

» You can work dynamically to deepen the pose: Lift the sternum and extend the back as you inhale, then lower the sternum towards the shin as you exhale.

VARIATIONS

» Maha Mudra – The Great Seal: Here you set Bandhas in the pose (forward extension with a slight backbend) in combination with the breath. Maha Mudra is considered one of the very advanced Hatha Yoga practices.

» Parivritta Janu Shirsasana – Revolved Head-to-knee pose (PS 7.3.13 d-f).

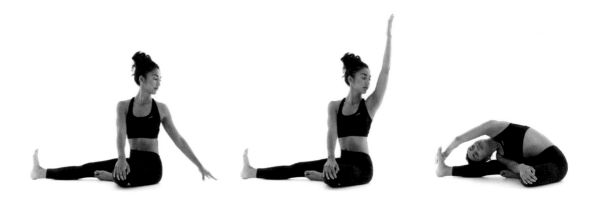

Photo series 7.3.13 d-f

ACTIVE AND STABILIZING MUSCLES

Pelvis/legs

» Piriformis – external rotation – bent knee

» Upper and lower gemellis muscle – external rotation – bent knee

» Obturator internus – external rotation – bent knee

» Quadratus femoris – external rotation – bent knee

» Sartorius muscle – flexes the hip – bent knee

» Biceps femoris – flexes the knee – bent knee

» Hip flexor: Iliopsoas muscle – flexes the hip – both legs

» Rectus femoris − flexes the hip − both legs

» Quadriceps femoris − for knee extension − extended leg

» Tibialis anterior flexes the foot (dorsal flexion) − extended leg

Shoulders/arms

» Trapezius muscle, lower section − pulls the shoulder blade down.

» Infraspinatus muscle − pulls the shoulders to the outside.

» Teres minor − pulls the shoulders to the outside.

» Anterior deltoids − raise the arms.

» Biceps − slightly bends the arms.

» Brachialis muscles − slightly bend the arms.

STRETCHED MUSCLES

» Erector spinae

» Quadratus lumborum

» Gluteus maximus − extended leg.

» Ischiocrural muscles (back of the thigh − extended leg.

» Gastrocnemius (calf) − extended leg.

» Soleus (calf) − extended leg.

» Quadriceps femoris − bent leg.

PREPARATORY EXERCISES

Stretch the back of the legs (*Supta Padangustasana*), stretch the inside of the thighs / adductors (e.g. *Baddha Konasana*), loosen up the hip joints, loosen up the spine, place the spine in an upright position, loosen up the shoulder joints.

COUNTERPOSE

Relaxed supine position (Shavasana), Shoulder Bridge (Setu Bandha).

7.3.14   MAKARASANA – CROCODILE POSE

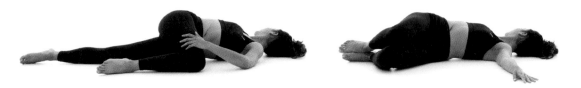

Photo series 7.3.14 a-b

SYMBOLIK/BEDEUTUNG

Makara = crocodile, sea monster / Asana = pose

Makarasana is the umbrella term for a group of poses. All of them have a spinal twist in common.

The poses are called *Crocodile poses* because as the crocodile hunts, it is able to spin nimbly and smoothly around its own axis. *Makarasana* is also known as a rejuvenating pose because people appear very youthful when they are able to flexibly twist their spine, particularly at an advanced age. Many seniors have lost this ability over the course of their life, which can have dire consequences, for instance while cycling or driving (looking over the shoulder).

By rotating the individual vertebrae, *Makarasana* keeps the entire length of the spine flexible. The deep muscles around the spine as well as the superficial muscles of the abdomen and back are simultaneously strengthened and stretched. The twists can relieve muscle tension in the back, while also having a very positive effect on the elasticity of intervertebral discs. Since the pose is practiced in a supine position, the skeletal muscles can largely relax. The breath is particularly important during Makarasana. The twists alternately compress both sides of the ribcage, which stimulates respiration (deeper inhalation and exhalation).

Purposeful breath control can generate different effects:

》   Deep belly breathing during rotation causes the diaphragm to drop during inhalation, massaging the internal organs (which has a stimulating effect on the metabolism). At the same time, the abdominal wall and the pelvic floor relax, which can relieve muscle tension in the entire low back.

》   When moving into the twist while exhaling the diaphragm lifts, which can have a loosening effect between the ribs and spine and thereby deepens the twist.

Since *Makarasana* includes a number of variations and modifications, Crocodile poses are well suited as preparatory, introductory, and counterposes, especially in beginning classes or in cases of limited flexibility.

Unlike all seated twists in which the upper body rotates over a fixed pelvis, in *Makarasana* the lower body moves against the upper body, while the shoulder girdle remains fixed in most variations. Depending on the leg position of the respective variation, the twist can be very deep or simply suggested to adapt it to the participant's abilities.

From an energy standpoint, the pose stimulates mainly *Samana Vayu*, the aspect of Prana that is responsible for converting food into energy. *Makarasana* is a grounding and cooling pose (when it is not practiced dynamically). Since it is practiced in a supine position it supports the aspects of letting go, perception, and internalization.

POSE STRUCTURE

Two very simple, preparatory introductory modifications that are practiced dynamically:

Variations 1 – with feet and knees open wide

» On your back, the body forms a straight line, a horizontal axis between the back of the head and the tailbone (PS 7.3.14 c).

» The arms are extended to the sides at shoulder level palms down.

» Feet are planted significantly more than hip-width apart; calves are in a vertical position.

» Now allow the legs to rock from side to side like windshield wipers (PS 7.3.14 d-e).

» This exercise loosens up the hip joints, stretches the inside of the thighs, and initiates a gentle spinal twist.

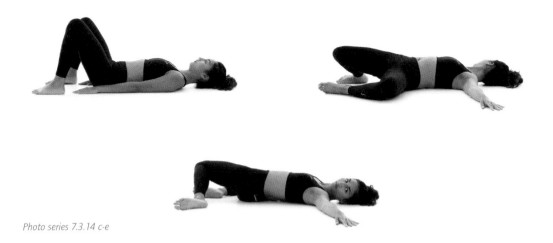

Photo series 7.3.14 c-e

183

Variation 2 – with legs closed and lower legs in a vertical position

» Pose structure as in variation 1.

» Feet are planted; the calves are in a vertical position, and the inside of the legs touch. Now allow the closed legs to rock side to side.

» This exercise generates a significantly deeper rotation of the spine (PS 7.3.14 f-g).

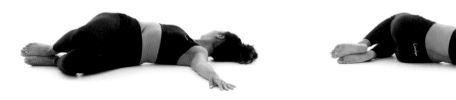

Photo series 7.3.14 f-g

The following variation can be prepared dynamically. Afterwards the Asana is held in the final position and refined.

Variation 3 – with bent knees in tabletop position

» On your back, the body forms a straight line, a horizontal axis between the back of the head and the tailbone.

» Legs are bent into tabletop: the thighs are in a vertical position, calves are horizontal, and knees are closed (PS 7.3.14 k).

» Shoulders and shoulder blades rest on the floor. Arms are either in goalpost position or straight out to the sides at shoulder-level, palms on the floor.

» In the dynamic version of this pose, lower the closed legs to one side while exhaling, raise them again while inhaling, alternating sides (PS 7.3.14 i-j).

» In the static version, the closed legs are lowered to the floor on one side at a level with the hips, the spine maintains its axial alignment, and the shoulders remain on the floor (if possible). The head turns in the direction of rotation.

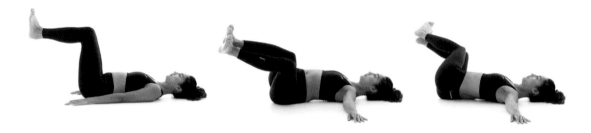

Photo series 7.3.14 h-j

Extending one or both legs further deepens the twist:

Variation 4 – the lower leg is extended in extension of the trunk, the upper knee is bent.

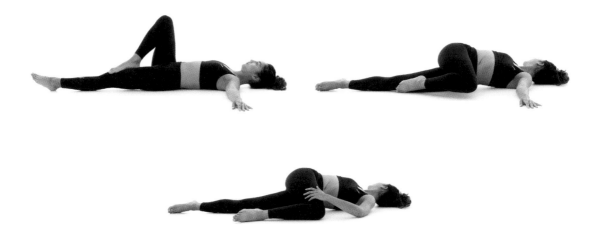

Photo series 7.3.14 k-m

Variation 5 – both legs are extended (in extension of the trunk, the upper leg at hip-level) or both legs are extended on the floor at hip level.

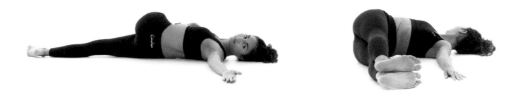

Photo series 7.3.14 n-o

WORKING IN THE POSE

» Breathe deeply and relax on the inside, meaning give in to gravity. Direct the breath deeply into the trunk's breathing spaces, and release muscle tension as you exhale.

ACTIVE AND STABILIZING MUSCLES

Trunk

» Erector spinae muscles – only slightly engaged due to supine position.

» Hip flexors – bend at the hip.

STRETCHED MUSCLES

Trunk

» Erector spinae muscles – extend the spine.

» Short and long rotators (rotatores thorax longus and brevis) – rotate the spine.

» External and internal obliques – rotate the spine.

» Gluteus maximus

» Pectoralis major

Shoulder girdle and neck

» Rhomboid major (stabilizes the shoulder blade) – head rotation.

» Sternocleidomastoid – head rotation.

» Splenius capitis – head rotation.

» Upper section of the trapezius muscle – head rotation.

PREPARATORY EXERCISES AND COUNTERPOSES

Wind-relieving poses (Apanasana and Eka Pada Apanasana), Table (Prasarita Padasana), Shoulder Bridge (Setu Bandha).

7.3.15   MARJARYASANA – CAT POSE

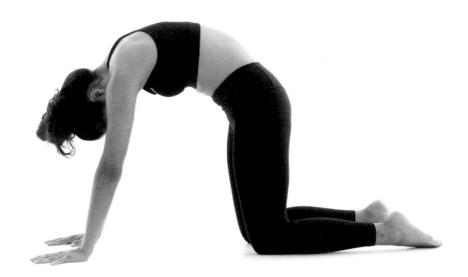

Photo series 7.3.15 a

SYMBOLISM/IMPACT

Marjary = cat / Asana = pose

Marjaryasana is a forward bend on all fours. It loosens up the spine and stretches the entire length of the back. Due to the rounded back in the pose this Asana is also known as *Chakravakasana* (chakra = wheel). Some traditions also refer to this pose as *Bidalasana* (Bidala = Cat).

A cat's movements are soft, light, and sleek, which also describes the execution of this Asana. Since this exercise in its execution is considered one of the more simple Asanas, it can be used almost universally to improve the spine's supple mobility in all its sections.

Marjaryasana offers a number of variations. All of them loosen up the spine, which includes axial extension (neutral spine), as well as *Cat*'s opposing movement *Cow* (hyperextension of the spine/backbend). When combining *Cat* with a balance pose (diagonal arm/leg extension) it is called *Extended Tiger*. These varied modifications are particularly valuable during the preparatory phase of a yoga unit to incrementally work towards more intense poses.

From an energy standpoint, combining *Cat/Cow* stimulates both Prana as well as Apana Vayu. It can also relieve excessive tension in the back muscles. This effect can be intensified by remaining and stretching in this pose.

POSE STRUCTURE

» Starting position on all fours: Hips are stacked over knees, shoulders are stacked over wrists. The spine is in neutral position (neutral curve of the spine). The gaze is downward (PS 7.3.15 b).

» Press hands and knees into the floor as you exhale and pull the lower abdomen in while rounding the entire length of the spine, particularly the lower back (lumbar spine) (PS 7.3.15 c).

» Continue to breathe evenly in the pose and deepen the back's harmonic c-curve.

» Make sure that the cervical spine is also integrated into this harmonic curve. The gaze shifts to the navel.

» Pull shoulders away from ears; arms remain extended.

» If you have tender knees, place a folded blanket under the knees.

» If you have tender wrists, you can rest on your forearms instead (parallel forearms, elbows are propped directly below shoulders).

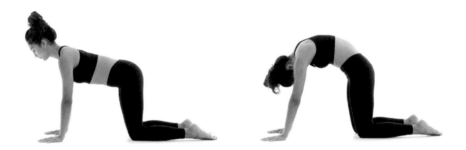

Photo series 7.3.15 b-c

WORKING IN THE POSE

» If exercise execution is dynamic, inhale into *Cow* (backbend). As you do so, make sure the spine stays long and shoulders are away from ears. Avoid "sagging" in joints and spine.

» Alternately exhale into *Cat*/inhale into *Cow*.

VARIATIONS

Extended Tiger 1

» On all fours, working on a diagonal, extend the right arm forward in extension of the trunk. As you do so, externally rotate the right arm so the thumb points to the ceiling. Pull the humeral head into the shoulder joint so both shoulders are lined up.

» At the same time, extend the left leg back at hip-level in extension of the trunk. Make sure hips stay parallel.

» As you inhale, lengthen the diagonal from the middle of the body.

» As you exhale, return to all fours, or rather *Cat*, and repeat on the opposite side.

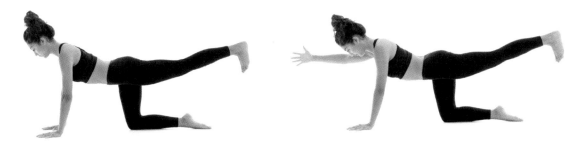

Photo series 7.3.15 d-e

Extended Tiger 2

» Instead of Cat, bring the right elbow and left knee together as you exhale and round the entire length of the back as in Cat.

» Return to Extended Tiger as you inhale.

» Repeat several times and then switch to the opposite diagonal.

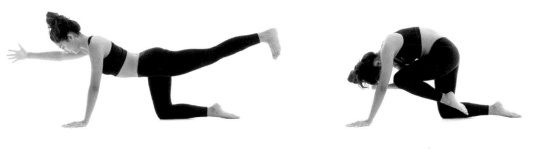

Photo series 7.3.15 f-g

ACTIVE AND STABILIZING MUSCLES

Trunk

» Rectus abdominis – flexes the spine and gives it support.

» Transverse abdominals – stabilize.

» Gluteus maximus – extends the leg.

» Searratus anterior muscle – stabilizes the shoulder blade.

Arms

» Triceps – stabilizes the elbow.

STRETCHED MUSCLES

Trunk

» Erector spinae

» Quadratus lumborum

» Trapezius (upper and lower section)

PREPARATORY EXERCISES

Loosen up the wrists (circles), strengthen the fingers and forearms (spread fingers and make a fist), loosen up the shoulder girdle, *wind-relieving pose* (*Apanasana*), *Child's pose* (*Balasana*).

COUNTERPOSE

Wind-relieving pose (Apanasana), Child's pose (Balasana).

7.3.16 NAVASANA – BOAT POSE

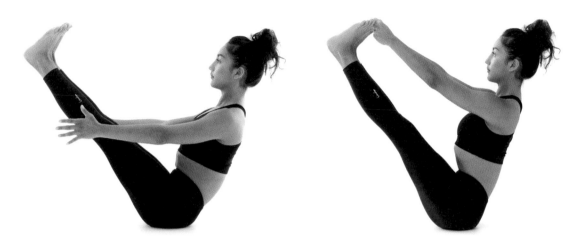

Photo series 7.3.16 a-b

SYMBOLISM/IMPACT

Nava = boat / Asana = pose

Navasana combines an axial extension of the spine with a seated forward bend and a balance pose. As forward bends go *Navasana* is an exception, because unlike the classic forward bends, the main goal of this exercise is not stretching the back of the body. Rather *Navasana* is more of a strength pose since the abdominal and core muscles must be extremely engaged in this pose. Viewed from the side, the pose looks similar to a boat. Just like the hull of a boat must be sturdy to withstand the elements during a storm on the high seas, so does this Asana, if performed over a certain amount of time, give one the ability and strength to maintain good alignment in the midsection, as well as an erect and centered posture.

Like all balance poses, *Navasana* is a grounding pose, promotes stability and a steady, clear alignment on all planes. For instance, if the focus wanes and the back starts to round, the pose loses its structure and the practitioner rolls backwards.

Navasana primarily strengthens the iliopsoas muscles and abdominals, which protects and unburdens the low back. Its great muscular intensity gives the pose a stimulating, warming effect. From an energy standpoint, the pose primarily targets the *Muladhara chakra* (grounding) in the lower pelvic area, and the *Manipura chakra* (warmth, will, power) in the solar plexus area. The pose improves abdominal perfusion, stimulates digestion and metabolism, and thus Samana and Apana Vayu.

POSE STRUCTURE

» In a seated posture, bend the knees, grip the back of the thighs with your hands, straighten the spine and evenly distribute your weight between the sit bones and tailbone (PS 7.3.16 c).

» Now shift your center of gravity backward, keeping the spine erect, abdominals and erector spinae muscles engaged, and lift the bent knees.

» Align the calves with the floor; knees form a right angle. Release the arms and extend them horizontally (*Half Boat – Ardha Navasana*) (PS 7.3.16 d).

» If mobility permits, extend the legs to move into Full Boat pose.

» If the muscles at the back of the legs and low back are extremely shortened, it will prevent a complete extension of the spine. In this case remain in *Half Boat*.

» A lack of abdominal strength causes the iliopsoas muscles to work harder, which can result in cramping. In this case also remain in *Half Boat* (or use a strap to be able to enjoy the sensation of the balancing effect).

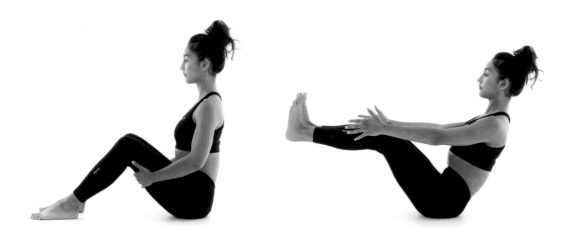

Photo series 7.3.16 c-d

WORKING IN THE POSE

» Breathe slowly and steadily during the exercise.

» First pull the shoulder blades back and down, then push them towards the chest to lift the sternum while pulling the bottom ribs in for stability.

» Make sure the back of the neck is an extension of the spine.

» As you inhale, lengthen the legs from the pelvis and straighten the entire length of the spine.

» As you exhale, imagine drawing strength from the body's periphery inward towards the body's core: engage the core muscles to straighten the back.

VARIATIONS

» *Ardha Navasana* (*Half Boat*) – as described in item 2 of the pose structure.

» *Ubhaya Padangusthasana* (*Hands-to-toes pose*) – Grip the big toes with your fingers (yogi toe lock) (or use a strap) to extend the legs (PS 7.3.16 e).

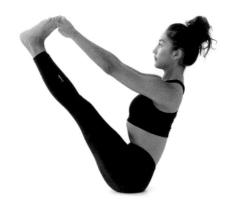

Photo series 7.3.16 e

ACTIVE AND STABILIZING MUSCLES

Pelvis/legs

» Quadriceps femoris – extends knees and bends the hip.

» Tensor fasciae latae – bends the hip, internal rotation of the thighs.

» Long and short adductors (adductor longus and brevis) – pull the legs towards each other.

Trunk

» Rectus abdominis – flex the trunk, stabilize, prevent hyperextension of the lumbar spine.

» External and internal obliques – stabilize, prevent hyperextension of the lumbar spine.

» Transverse abdominals – stabilize, abdominal pressure, prevent bulging out of the intestines.

» Iliopsoas muscle – flexes the hips, keeps the spine in neutral position.

» Erector spinae muscles – aligns the spine and bends it slightly backward.

» Quadratus lumborum muscles – support the lumbar spine.

Shoulders/arms

» Serratus anterior muscle – fixes the shoulder blades.

» Rhomboids – fix the shoulder blades.

» Infraspinatus muscle – externally rotates the upper arms.

» Teres minor muscle – externally rotates the upper arms.

» Anterior deltoids – lift the arms.

» Triceps – extend the elbow.

STRETCHED MUSCLES

Ischiocrural muscles

PREPARATORY EXERCISES

Dynamic and static abdominal strength exercises (e.g. in supine position), stretching the back of the legs, loosening up and extending the spine.

COUNTERPOSE

Balasana, Makarasana, Dwi Pada Pitham, Setu Bandha.

7.3.17 PASCHIMOTTANASANA – SEATED FORWARD BEND

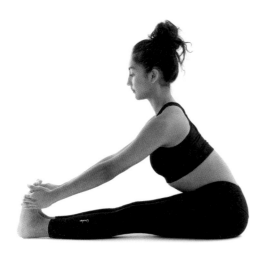 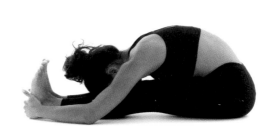

Photo series 7.3.17 a-b

SYMBOLISM/IMPACT

Pashima = part of the back, west side/ Tan (Uttana) = expansion, extension / Asana = pose

Paschimottanasana is a forward bend as well as a symmetric stretch of the back of the body. This Asana is sometimes also called *Pose of the Pliers*. A main characteristic of the pose is the deep stretching of the back of the thighs. This intense and deep forward bend counts among the devotional poses, also called *submissive poses*. The gaze is downward or rather inward, and awareness is subtilized in the pose as long as one is able to let go and give in to the intensity of the stretch and the associated internal processes.

If the pose is practiced strictly with willpower, the deeper aspects of the pose will hardly reveal themselves. As paradoxical as it may seem, here opposites unite: Experiencing the inner vastness and expansion are closely linked to the external tightness and limitation of the pose.

From an energy standpoint, Apana Vayu, the aspect of Prana that stands for letting go, is stimulated during all forward bends. On the one hand the compression resulting from the deep forward bend stimulates the internal organs, and on the other hand one can let go of everything on the mental-emotional level. The pose represents cooling and calming. *Paschimottanasana* is also a very grounding pose. The energy exchange with the earth takes place via the root chakra (*Muladhara*) in the lower pelvic area. Legs and feet, which are in direct contact with the ground in everyday life, are energized in this Asana.

POSE STRUCTURE

» Starting position *Dandasana* (*Staff pose*). If muscles at the back of the legs or along the back's kinetic chain are shortened, place a folded blanket under the pelvis/sit bones (PS 7.3.17 c).

» Properly ground the pelvis via the sit bones; legs are extended, feet are flexed, the outside edges of the feet pull towards the outside of the hips.

» As you inhale, extend the arms overhead in extension of the trunk, lift the back and stretch the flanks (PS 7.3.17 d).

» As you exhale, tilt the pelvis forward from the hips so you can extend the spine as far forward as possible when you come into the forward bend. Only then move into the forward bend, reach for your feet or calves, and let the upper body drop as close to the legs as your body allows. As you do so, continue lengthening the spine.

» Breathe slowly and evenly (PS 7.3.17 e-f).

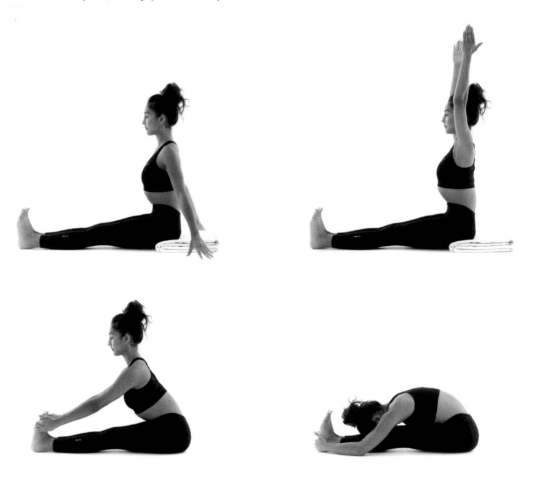

Photo series 7.3.17 e-f

WORKING IN THE POSE

» Make sure your shoulders stay down. Many people unconsciously pull the shoulder girdle up to be able to reach their feet, which can cause tightness in the shoulders and back of the neck.

» To deepen the stretch at the back of the legs, tighten the quadriceps, meaning pull up your kneecaps (reciprocal inhibition).

» Pull the thighs and knees towards each other. The forward bend causes the legs and feet to fall open slightly.

» In the pose take slow, deep breaths and expand your awareness to the entire body. Where can you let go a little more?

» Take your awareness deep inside and experience all aspects of letting go meditatively.

VARIATIONS

» As you inhale, lift the back and move into the forward extension while holding on to your feet or legs. As you exhale, move into the forward bend. Do several dynamic repetitions (PS 7.3.17 g-h).

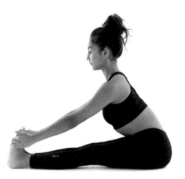 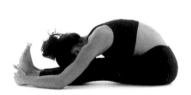

Photo series 7.3.17 g-h

» Place a yoga strap around your feet if the muscles along the back of the body are shortened, which makes a forward bend very difficult (PS 7.3.17 i).

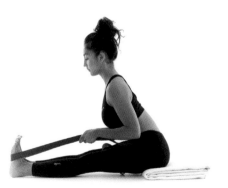

Photo series 7.3.17 i

ACTIVE AND STABILIZING MUSCLES

Shoulders/arms

» Trapezius muscles, upper section – pulls the shoulder blade down.

» Infraspinatus muscle – pulls the shoulders to the outside.

» Teres minor muscle – pulls the shoulders to the outside.

» Anterior deltoids – lift the arms.

» Biceps – slightly bend the arms.

» Brachialis muscles – slightly bend the arms.

Trunk/legs

» Rectus abdominis – bends the trunk forward.

» Iliopsoas muscle – flexes the hip.

» Rectus femoris – flexes the hip.

» Tensor fasciae latae – flexes the hip.

» Quadriceps femoris – helps extend the knee.

» Adductors – pull the legs towards each other.

» Tibialis anterior – flexes the foot (dorsal flexion).

STRETCHED MUSCLES

» Erector spinae

» Quadratus lumborum

» Gluteus maximus

» Ischiocrural muscles

» Gastrocnemius

» Soleus muscles – extended leg.

PREPARATORY EXERCISES

Table (Prasarita Padasana), leg stretches in supine position (Supta Padangustasana A), Downward-facing Dog (Adho Mukha Svanasana), Staff pose (Dandasana).

COUNTERPOSE

Relaxed supine position (Shavasana), Shoulder Bridge (Setu Bandha).

7.3.18 PRASARITA PADOTTANASANA – STANDING STRADDLE FORWARD BEND

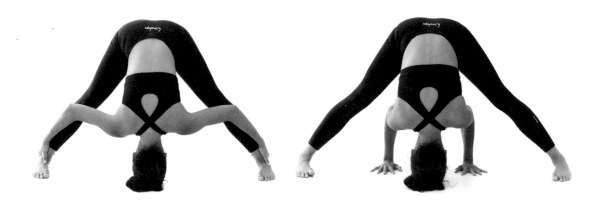

Photo series 7.3.18 a-b

SYMBOLIK/BEDEUTUNG

Prasarita = stretched, spread / Pada = foot/leg/ Ut = intensive /Tan = widen, expand

Prasarita Padottanasana combines a forward bend with an inversion from a straddle position. The solid connection of the feet with the ground and simultaneous downward head position makes this Asana a very grounding, calming pose. The leg muscles are simultaneously stretched (back and inside of legs) and strengthened (front of legs), while the pelvic floor, back, and spine stretch, or rather relax.

The structure of the pose promotes deep exhalation because gravity pulls the diaphragm and the internal organs towards the head. Conversely, as you inhale the diaphragm pushes against the internal organs towards the pelvis, which has a gently massaging effect on the internal organs and has a regulating effect on digestion. Deep, long exhales always have a deacidifying, purifying effect, which stimulates Apana Vayu. The forward bend also has a calming, cooling effect on the mind, blood pressure, and the nervous system because the head is below the heart and the pressure receptors in the large blood vessels are being stimulated.

Due to the immediately noticeable effects combined with the Asana's relatively simple structure this pose is well suited for beginning classes.

POSE STRUCTURE

» Stand in a wide straddle. Depending on the length of your legs, feet are placed about 3.5 – 4.5 feet apart. The outside edges of the feet are parallel to the outside edges of your mat. In this position, the legs feel slightly rotated inward (PS 7.3.18 c).

» The balls of the big and little toes, as well as the outside and inside of the heels press into the floor and raise the arch of the foot. The ankle is aligned with the center of the arch.

» Hands rest just below the hips, knees and hips are flexed. Move the spine into axial extension and let the shoulders drop.

» Rotate the thighs slightly inward as you initiate the forward bend from the hips.

» Making your spine really long, first move the trunk into a horizontal position and then move into a full bend from the low back and allow the crown of the head to sink towards the floor. Keep the back as long as possible during this exercise (PS 7.3.18 d-e).

» Place your hands on the floor shoulder-width apart (fingertips are lined up with toes, and if possible press the palms into the mat and pull them slightly to the outside) (PS 7.3.18 f).

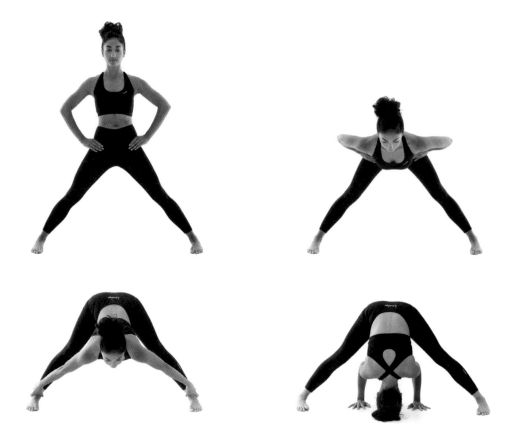

Photo series 7.3.18 e-f

WORKING IN THE POSE

» Take long, slow breaths.

» Relax the back of the neck, and pull the shoulders and shoulder blades away from the ears and towards the pelvis.

» Slightly bend the knees to initially relax the ischiocrural muscles, and then straighten them again to deepen the stretch.

» Pull the kneecaps up to deepen the stretch in the back of the legs and stabilize the posture.

» Add pressure in legs and feet from the pelvis and shift your weight to the balls of the feet without lifting the heels (deepens the stretch in the back of the legs and aligns the pelvis over the ankles).

» Tighten your abdominal muscles as you exhale to deepen the stretch in the antagonists at the back of the body.

» Energy control during the holding phase: As you inhale, gather energy through the feet and hands and direct it to the heart. As you exhale, spread the energy across the entire body.

VARIATIONS

» If the muscles at the back of the legs are severely shortened, begin by keeping the knees bent and let them support the arms (PS 7.3.18 g).

» Alternate several times between the forward extension (table top) and forward bend, working with your breath.

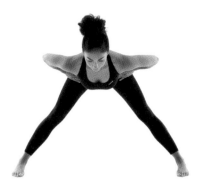 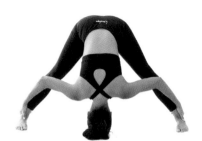

Photo series 7.3.18 g-h

ARM VARIATIONS

» Place your hands against the ankles and deepen the stretch by pulling the elbows to the outside (PS 7.3.18 h).

» Very flexible individuals may choose to extend the arms back between the legs and "palm" the floor to deepen the stretch further.

» Interlace the fingers behind your back, draw the shoulder blades together and move into a forward bend. This bind provides an additional stretch in the ribcage and the front of the shoulders (PS 7.3.18 i).

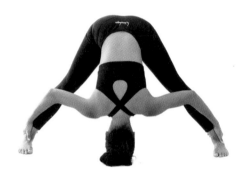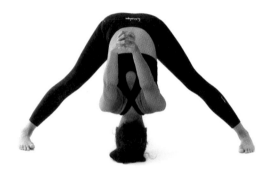

Photo series 7.3.18 h-i

ACTIVE AND STABILIZING MUSCLES

Pelvis/legs

» Quadriceps femoris – extends the knees.

» Tibialis anterior and posterior – rotate the feet slightly inward and raise the arches.

Trunk

» The lower third of the trapezius muscle – pulls the shoulder blades down.

» Teres minor – externally rotates the upper arms.

» Infraspinatus muscle – externally rotates the upper arms.

Shoulders/arms

» Biceps – bend the elbows (when arms are in an erect position on the floor).

STRETCHED MUSCLES

Pelvis/legs

» Gastrocnemius (calf)

» Soleus (calf)

» Ischiocrural muscles (back of thigh)

» Adductor magnus, longus, brevis (inner thigh)

» Gluteus maximus

Trunk

» Erector spinae

» Quadratus lumborum

PREPARATORY EXERCISES

Stretching the back of the legs, inside of the legs, gluteal muscles, low back, and flanks.

COUNTERPOSE

Tadasana, Balasana, Setu Bandha.

7.3.19   SETU BANDHA SARVANGASANA – BRIDGE POSE

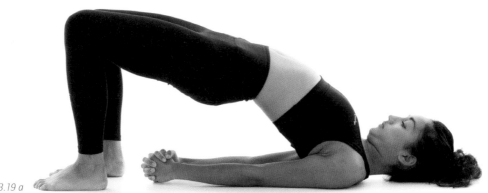

Photo series 7.3.19 a

SYMBOLISM/IMPACT

Setu = bridge / Bandha = structure / Sarvanga = all limbs / Asana = pose

Setu Bandha Sarvangasana (*Setu Bandhasana*) translates to: *bridge-structure-all-limbs pose*. It is a backbend and supine, slight inversion pose, whereby the body arches like a bridge. The term *Bandha* is also translated as *bound* or *link* or *bundling*. The bind refers to the hands linked under the low back, which pulls arms and shoulder blades towards each other, facilitating a deeper backbend in the pose.

In some traditions, it is customary to practice a hand-foot Bandha, whereby the hands encircle the ankles (more difficult for people with long torsos and short arms).

During *Setu Bandha Sarvangasana*, three additional Bandhas are passively activated inside the body via the deep backbend, which can be further deepened with active contractions in the pose: *Mula Bandha* (contraction of pelvic floor muscles), *Uddiyana Bandha* (the "upward lock" in the abdomen after exhalation), and Jalandhara Bandha (the chin lock in the throat area that occurs automatically due to the structure of the Shoulder Bridge).

They are further deepened by holding the breath for a moment after exhaling while lowering the pelvis, which lifts the pelvic floor and abdomen almost automatically.

In terms of energy, the Asana stimulates the chest (*Anahata chakra*) and throat areas (*Vishuddha chakra*). The backbend deepens the breath in the chest, which activates Prana Vayu (the aspect of Prana that is responsible for energy absorption).

Setu Bandhasana is often used in preparation for the Half *Shoulder stand* (*Viparita Karani*) and *Supported Shoulder stand* (*Salamba Sarvangasana*). It is also an alternative to inversions when those cannot be practiced due to health reasons.

POSE STRUCTURE

» Lie on your back with arms extended alongside the body. Feet and knees are hip-width apart, calves are in vertical position, and knees are lined up with the ankles (PS 7.3.19 b).

» Slightly tuck your tailbone, evenly press your feet into the floor, and lift the pelvis as you inhale (PS 7.3.19 c).

» Squeeze the shoulder blades together, lift the sternum, and extend the arms under your back and clasp your hands.

» Keep the back of the neck long and breathe evenly.

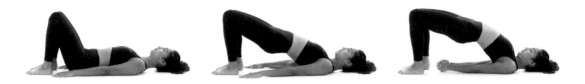

Photo series 7.3.19 b-d

WORKING IN THE POSE

» As you deepen the backbend, slightly tilt your pelvis (lengthening the lumbar spine) to extend the lumbar spine a little.

» Build up isometric tension in the legs by firmly pressing your feet into the floor while simultaneously initiating extension in the legs/knees, which deepens the backbend.

» Press the balls of the feet into the mat and pull the firmly planted feet slightly to the outside (this prevents the knees from splaying out in this pose).

» Pull the shoulders down and out and externally rotate the upper arms. Actively press the arms, which are extended under the back into the floor. Internally rotate the forearms.

VARIATIONS

» To further deepen the grounding and stabilizing aspect, extend one leg up into a vertical position (PS 7.3.19 e).

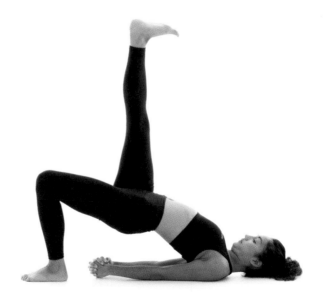

Photo series 7.3.19 e

»   *Dwi Pada Pitham: Dwi Pada Pitham*, which translates to *Two-legged Table*, is a very similar pose. The difference between it and *Setu Bandha* is in the execution. While *Setu Bandhasana* is held for a longer period of time, *Dwi Pada Pitham* is an Asana that is practiced dynamically with the breathing rhythm, and can be further intensified by lifting the arms during the inhale phase. The backbend is not nearly as deep as *Setu Bandhasana*. *Dwi Pada Pitham* is a form of Shoulder Bridge that is particularly well suited for beginning yoga students, as it can release tension in the back and respiratory system (PS 7.3.19 f-g).

Photo series 7.3.19 f-a

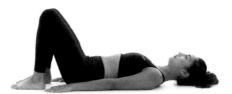 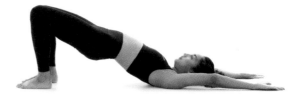

»   *Dwi Pada Pitham* with vertical forearms. Here the elbows and upper arms are pulled close to the trunk and the elbows form a right angle. During the exercise press the upper arms into the floor while simultaneously squeezing the shoulder blades together, which deepens the backbend in the thoracic spine (PS 7.3.19 h-i).

Photo series 7.3.19h-i)

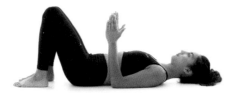 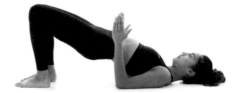

ACTIVE AND STABILIZING MUSCLES

Pelvis/legs

»   The large, medium, and small gluteal muscles – flex the hip/lift the pelvis.

»   Back of the thighs (ischiocrural muscles) – hip extension and knee flexion.

»   Adductors (longus, magnus, brevis) – stabilize; prevent knees "splaying out".

»   Muscle at the front of the shin (tibialis anterior) – flexes the foot (dorsal flexion).

Trunk

» Erector spinae muscle – extends the spine into the backbend.

» Quadratus lumborum – helps extend into the backbend.

» Large and small rhomboids – pull the shoulder blades together.

Shoulders/arms

» Triceps – extend the arm.

» Posterior deltoids – pull the arms back.

» Infraspinatus muscles – externally rotate the shoulders.

» Teres minor muscles – externally rotate the shoulders.

STRETCHED MUSCLES

» Chest muscle (pectoralis major, medius, minimus)

» Biceps brachii

» Rectus abdominis

» External and internal obliques

» Iliopsoas

» Serratus anterior

» Rectus femoris

PREPARATORY EXERCISES

Hip flexor stretches, loosen up the shoulders, loosen up the back, *Cat* (*Marjaryasana*), Dynamic Shoulder Bridge (*Dwi Pada Pitham*).

COUNTERPOSE

Wind-relieving pose (Apanasana), Child's pose (Balasana), all forward bends.

7.3.20 SHALABHASANA – LOCUST POSE

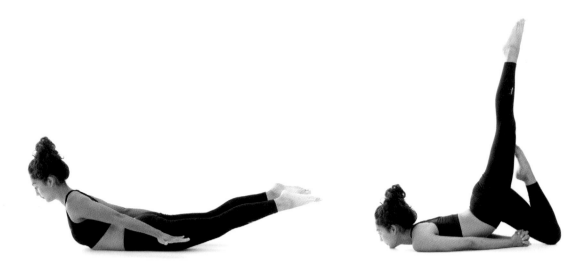

Photo series 7.3.20 a-b

SYMBOLISM/IMPACT

Shalaba = locust / Asana = pose

Shalabhasana, *Locust Pose*, is a prone backbend. There are varying degrees of difficulty: from *Half Locust* (*Ardha Shalabhasana*) all the way to *Full Locust* (*Viparita Shalabhasana*) and countless modifications. In the classic *Shalabhasana* pose, the chin rests on the floor while the legs, pelvis, and much of the trunk are lifted into a backbend. How deep the backbend is depends on the back's strength and mobility. The chin-on-the-floor variation is not appropriate for novices or for people with neck, nape, or shoulder problems. Here it would be best to practice one of the modifications to incrementally build up the flexibility and stability the pose demands.

Shalabhasana strengthens the back muscles and stretches the front of the body. The prone position causes the bodyweight to compress the stomach as well as the abdominal organs. The diaphragm must therefore breathe against resistance, which strengthens the diaphragm, deepens the breath, and opens up the breathing spaces in the chest. This Asana massages the internal organs and stimulates the metabolism, the digestive system, and gut motility. In terms of energy, the pose affects the *Manipura chakra*, in the solar plexus area, which represents transformation, willpower, self-confidence, and perseverance. Practicing Full Locust stimulates primarily the *Vishuddha chakra* (throat chakra) because of the hyperextension of the neck and corresponding opening of the throat.

POSE STRUCTURE

» Supine position: Rest your forehead on the floor, the back of the neck is long, the back is long, the arms rest on the floor alongside the body with palms facing the ceiling, the legs extend from the hips (hip-width apart), tops of feet rest on the floor, toes are pointed.

» Begin by alternating lifting the legs, making sure the hips remain parallel (PS 7.3.20 c).

» Then lift and lower both legs several times (PS 7.3.20 d).

» Now allow the legs to remain on the floor and do several repetitions of Cobra (*Bhujanghasana*) (PS 7.3.20 e). Then hold the upper body up and raise both legs (knees are bent approx. 10°). Arms remain on the floor.

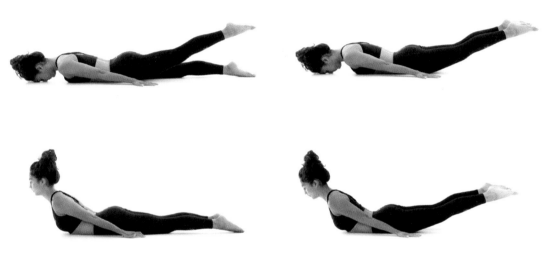

Photo series 7.3.20 c-f

WORKING IN THE POSE

» In the pose, breathe slowly and evenly.

» Make sure the head is an extension of the spine and avoid hyperextending the back of the neck.

» Pull shoulders away from ears, pull the shoulder blades down and squeeze them together, and lift the sternum. Press the backs of the hands into the floor to lift the chest higher. Later, lift the arms.

» To stabilize the pose and protect the lumbar spine, activate the rectus abdominis and oblique abdominal muscles (pull in and up).

» Contract the *Mula Bandha*: Activate the pelvic floor muscles to stabilize the spine.

>> Squeezing the knees and inside of the legs together in the pose increases the contraction particularly at the back of the thighs and in the gluteal muscles.

VARIATIONS

>> This Asana can also be practiced with the arms extended forward: Arms are extended forward shoulder-width apart at ear-level (PS 7.3.20 g).

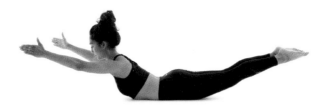

Photo series 7.3.20 g

>> Another classic variation is to clasp the hands below the trunk. They then act as a lever intended to help the leg- and pelvic lift. In this version, the chin rests on the floor (PS 7.3.20 h-i).

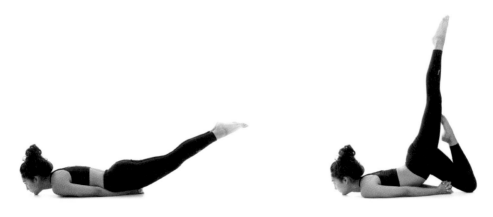

Photo series 7.3.20 h-i

ACTIVE AND STABILIZING MUSCLES

Shoulders/arms

>> The infraspinatus muscles externally rotate the shoulders.

>> The teres minor muscles externally rotate the shoulders.

» The trapezius muscles, lower section, pull the shoulder blade down.

» The triceps extends the arms.

» The anterior deltoid muscles press the back of the hands into the floor.

» The posterior deltoid muscles lift the arms.

Trunk

» The erector spinae muscle extends the back, lifts the ribcage.

» The quadratus lumborum muscles extend the back.

» The pubococcygeus muscles stabilize the pelvis and tilt the tailbone forward (helps lift the thoracic spine higher).

Pelvis/legs

» The quadriceps muscle extends the knee.

» The tensor fasciae latae muscle stabilizes.

» The gluteus maximus extends the hips.

STRETCHED MUSCLES

» Latissimus dorsi

» Pectoralis major

» Biceps brachii

» Rectus abdominis

» Iliopsoas

PREPARATORY EXERCISES

Loosen up the spine, stretch the hip flexors (ilipsoas), stretch the front of the shoulders, strengthen the back muscles. As an introduction, practice *Sphinx*, *Cobra*, and different leg variations.

COUNTERPOSE

Marjayasana (Cat), Child's pose (Balasana).

7.3.21   SHAVASANA – CORPSE POSE

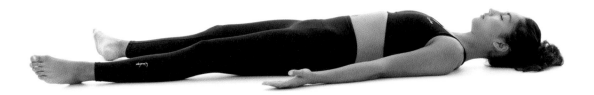

Photo series 7.3.21 a

SYMBOLISM/IMPACT

Sava = dead man, corpse / Asana = pose

Shavasana, *Corpse pose*, is one of the rest and relaxation poses. The body lies motionless on the floor, and the mind comes to rest in a state of clarity and detachment. The externally quiet posture is meant to support the mind in finding perfect tranquility. Some call Shavasana the most demanding Asana of all. This is in reference to the mental and emotional movement inside us coming to a rest.

Shavasana, also called *relaxed supine position*, can help the practitioner get in the right frame of mind by shifting the focus to body and breath awareness. *Shavasana* is often used as a rest and reflection pose during a practice (depending on the emphasis of the practice), particularly when practicing seated or reclined poses.

Shavasana is generally practiced 12-15 minutes before the end of a yoga unit, most often in combination with a guided whole-body relaxation or visualization exercise followed by Pranayama counterposes and meditation.

POSE STRUCTURE

Shavasana is an Asana with specific alignment criteria:

» The body lies symmetrically on the floor, knees and feet are slightly more than hip-width apart, toes point to the outside.

» The spine forms a vertical line from tailbone to the back of the head.

» Arms rest at a 45° angle from the body, palms face the ceiling, fingers are relaxed and slightly furled.

WORKING IN THE POSE

» Transfer all of your weight to the floor, allow yourself to melt into the floor, so the contact points and surfaces grow larger and feel wider.

» Establish a sense of pleasant heaviness and warmth.

» Allow your facial features to grow soft and permeable.

» Breathe deeply and slowly; feel the breathing rhythm in the body, in the belly and the ribcage.

VARIATIONS

» In case of back pain or muscle tension in the lower back, place a rolled-up blanket or a yoga cushion under your knees. If neither is available, simply bend the knees, plant your feet hip-width apart and allow the knees to touch.

» To relax the neck and nape, place a blanket or pillow under the head.

ACTIVE AND STABILIZING MUSCLES

» The muscles are relaxed; only gravity is active.

PREPARATORY EXERCISES

» Exercises that loosen up the spine, shoulders, and hips can help the body relax in *Shavasana*.

COUNTERPOSE

» *Apanasana, Balasana*

7.3.22 SUKHASANA – EASY POSE

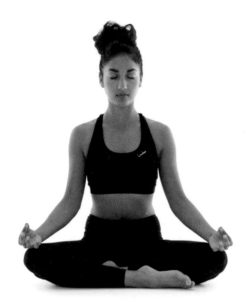

Photo series 7.3.22 a

SYMBOLISM/IMPACT

Sukha = easy, gentle, pleasant, comfortable / Asana = pose

Sukhasana means *Easy*, *Upright Seat* and is also called cross-legged seat. There are a number of upright-seated poses with varying degrees of difficulty depending on leg position. The upright seat is the basis for advanced Pranayama exercises and meditation.

The *Upright-seated pose* is the only Asana mentioned in Patanjali's *Yoga Sutra*. In chapter 2, verse 46, it says: "sthira sukham asanam", which means: The seated pose should be stable and comfortable. Strictly speaking all other Asanas are only preparations for the relaxed, Upright-seated pose, as the "quieting of the mind" (*Yoga Sutra*, chapter 1, verse 2) describes the yogic state. *Shavasana*, the relaxed supine position, is less well suited to the practice of meditation because here the mind becomes sleepy, and it is more of a preparation for meditation.

Unlike in India, in our Western culture it is unusual to just sit on the floor, which means that many people have to relearn to sit on the floor. It also means that muscles, ligaments, and joints have to be properly prepared (stretched and warmed up). Aids like rolled up blankets or pillows should be used for the upright-seated pose. When the knees are higher than the hips in the seated pose, the pelvis inevitably tilts backward, which can cause quite a bit of muscle tension.

From an energy standpoint, the pose stimulates the root chakra (*Muladhara chakra*) via its connection to the earth. In this case the crown chakra (*Sahasrara*) is the opposite pole due to its connection to the cosmic plane, which is why this pose is ideal for meditation.

POSE STRUCTURE

» Choose a blanket or pillow according to your individual seat height, and ground the pelvis on the cushion over the sit bones and the tailbone.

» The lower legs are crossed. Make sure the knees are on a gentle downward slope relative to the hips.

» Straighten the spine along its natural curves.

» Gently push the shoulders back and down; hands rest on thighs or in the lap.

WORKING IN THE POSE

» Breathe slowly and evenly.

VARIATIONS

» Virasana (Hero pose) (PS 7.3.22 b).

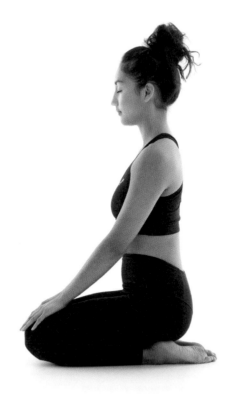

Photo series 7.3.22 b

» In case of knee problems or a lack of flexibility in the hips, Hero pose (Japanese seated pose) can be practiced on a meditation bench (PS 7.3.22 c).

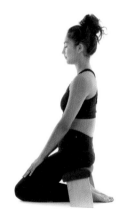

Photo series 7.3.22 c

» *Siddhasana* (*Half Lotus*) (PS 7.3.22 d).

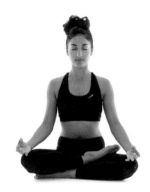

Photo series 7.3.22 d

» • *Padmasana* (*Full Lotus*) (PS 7.3.22 e).

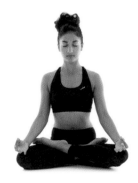

Photo series 7.3.22 e

ACTIVE AND STABILIZING MUSCLES

Trunk

» Erector spinae muscle – extends the spine.

» The multifidus muscles – extend the spine.

» The serratus anterior muscle and the rhomboids must work equally hard to stabilize the shoulder blades at the ribcage.

Arms

» The biceps slightly bend the elbows.

Pelvis/legs

» Piriformis muscle – external rotation.

» Upper and lower gemelli muscle – external rotation.

» Obturator internus – external rotation.

» Quadratus femoris – external rotation.

» Iliopsoas muscle – flexes the hip.

» Rectus femoris – flexes the hip.

» Sartorius muscle – flexes the hip. But when these three are severely shortened, they will pull the knees upward and inhibit an upright posture in the pose.

» Biceps femoris – flex the knee.

STRETCHED MUSCLES

Pelvis/legs

» All three adductors (longus, magnus, brevis).

» Gracilis muscle.

» Pectineus muscle.

» Gluteus medius and minimus.

» Tensor fasciae latae muscle.

PREPARATORY EXERCISES

Stretching the inner thighs, loosening up the hips, erecting the spine.

COUNTERPOSE

Shavasana

7.3.23 SUPTA PADANGUSTHASANA – RECLINING HAND-TO-BIG-TOE POSE

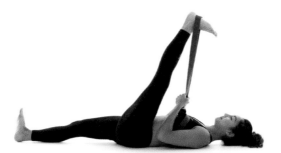

Photo series 7.3.23 a

SYMBOLISM/IMPACT

Supta = reclining / Pada = foot / Angustha = big toe / Asana = pose

Supta Padangusthasana means *Reclining Hand-to-big-toe pose*. This exercise is also called *Scissor Legs*. Traditionally it is combined with a forward bend. The more moderate version is the leg stretch without the trunk extension. If there is a lack of flexibility in the back of the body, the stretch is easier when using an aid such as a strap. When done in a reclining position, the exercise promotes focus on and awareness of the parts of the body that are being stretched.

Supta Padangusthasana 1, 2, and *3* (see variations) is one of the hip opening poses as it increases hip mobility in every way, and thus does not only deeply stretch the leg muscles but can also relieve muscle tension in the lower back and hips. This in turn helps the body achieve better alignment during all standing poses.

From an energy standpoint, *Supta Padangusthasana* stimulates primarily the root chakra (*Muladhara*) because pelvis, legs, and feet are able to form the basis for a strong rootedness.

POSE STRUCTURE

» On your back, plant both feet on the ground. Extend the leg that will be stretched straight up and grip it with both hands, or use an aid (e.g. yoga strap). Make sure the hips, pelvis, and the entire back lie symmetrically on the floor. Shoulders, neck, and head should be relaxed (PS 7.3.23 b).

» Slightly deepen the stretch with gentle dynamic pulses (PS 7.3.23 c).

» Then hold and intensify the exercise by extending the bent leg on the floor as you exhale, creating a scissor shape (PS 7.3.23 d).

» Keep the leg that is extended on the floor engaged, meaning flex the foot and place as much area as possible on the floor.

» To practice the pose in the traditional way in order to increase the stretch, lift the upper body.

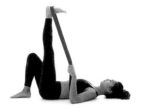 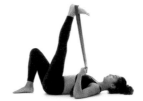 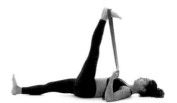

Photo series 7.3.23 b-d

WORKING IN THE POSE

» In the pose you can stretch statically or dynamically.

» When activating the antagonists, in this case the front of the thigh (quadriceps) and the abdominal muscles, the stretch in the back of the body deepens (reciprocal inhibition).

» Rotate the leg that is resting on the floor slightly to the inside and press the heel into the mat for support as it has a tendency to lift off the floor and externally rotate.

» Keep the elbows slightly bent and rotated out; pull the shoulder blades down.

» Breathe slowly and evenly, and be careful not to overstretch the leg.

VARIATIONS

» *Supta Padangusthasana 2* (stretch with simultaneous abduction of the "working leg" (PS 7.3.23 e).

» *Supta Padangusthasana 3* (stretch with simultaneous adduction of the "working leg" combined with a spinal twist) (PS 7.3.23 f).

» *Supta Padangusthasana 1* is the basis for both variations.

Photo series 7.3.23 e-f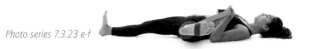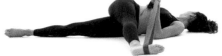

ACTIVE AND STABILIZING MUSCLES

Shoulders/arms

» Trapezius muscle, lower section – pull the shoulder blade down.

» Infraspinatus muscle – pulls the shoulders outward.

» Teres minor – pulls the shoulders outward.

» Anterior deltoids – lift the arms.

» Biceps – slightly bend the arms.

» Brachialis – slightly bend the arms.

Trunk/legs

» Rectus abdominis – bends the trunk forward.

» Iliopsoas – flexes the hip.

» Rectus femoris – flexes the hip.

» Tensor fasciae latae – flexes the hip.

» Quadriceps femoris – extends the knee.

» Adductors – pull the resting leg to the inside.

» Tibialis anterior – flexes the foot of the resting leg (dorsal flexion).

STRETCHED MUSCLES

» Gluteus maximus

» Ischiocrural muscles at the back of the leg.

» Iliopsoas

» Adductor magnus

» Gastrocnemius

» Soleus

PREPARATORY EXERCISES

Wind-relieving pose (Shavasana), Wind-relieving pose (Apanasana), Child's pose.

COUNTERPOSES

Relaxed supine position (Shavasana), wind-relieving pose (Apanasana), child's pose (Balasana)

7.3.24   TADASANA – MOUNTAIN POSE

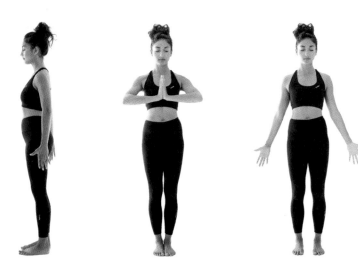

Photo series 7.3.24 a-c

SYMBOLISM/IMPACT

Tada = mountain
Pronounced: Tad-aaasana

Tadasana is *Mountain pose*, the upright standing pose and also the basis for all standing poses. *Tadasana* is also called *Samasthiti*, which means *mindfulness in all places (of my Self)*. Although *Tadasana* looks simple at first glance, it requires a certain amount of awareness, concentration, and mindfulness to internally control, build up, and hold the many muscle contractions. When first practicing yoga, it generally takes some time to develop the necessary awareness for what a firmly grounded and upright stance means.

And how much inner clarity is created when one consciously assumes a pose and is present. In our daily lives we generally stand with our weight shifted to the left or right hip, the spine and ribcage are casually pushed in some direction, and the shoulders are rarely parallel. Just practicing *Tadasana* makes us aware of the inner presence we can develop by standing correctly.

Due to the structure of the vertical axis, *Tadasana* stimulates all energy centers, but particularly the first chakra in the lower pelvis area (*Muladhara*: grounding, stability, trust) and the seventh chakra, the crown of the head (*Sahasrara*: the doorway to cosmic consciousness).

There are various forms and executions of *Tadasana*:

» Feet hip-width apart (PS 7.3.24 c).

» Closed form of *Tadasana* (feet and legs touch) (PS 7.3.24 b).

» Active form of *Tadasana* (the muscular system is consciously engaged) (PS 7.3.24 a).

» Relaxed form of *Tadasana* (upright, but permeable stance, reflection phase).

POSE STRUCTURE/WORKING IN THE POSE

» All standing poses require a solid base, which is built from the feet up. The points of contact of the feet are: outside and inside of the ball of the foot, outside and inside of the heel, the arch is mentally targeted and "pulled up".

» The outside edges of the feet are parallel to the outside edges of the mat; the second toe ("pointer toe") points forward.

» Weight is equally distributed between both legs and feet.

» During the active form, the kneecaps are pulled up to extend the knees. Hyperextension of the knees should be avoided.

» Depending on which misalignments need to be corrected, the thigh muscles are pulled up; the gluteal muscles, and muscle on the inside and outside of the leg are engaged.

» The back maintains its natural curve. Correcting the posture via pelvic alignment is done according to the respective physical structure: For instance, in cases of extreme lumbar curves ("sway back") it is corrected with the pelvic position. In the active form of Tadasana the lower abdomen and pelvic floor are pulled slightly in and up to support the upright posture.

» The joints are stacked vertically on top of each other, as well as the pelvic floor, diaphragm, and the roof of the mouth. The vertex, the crown of the head, reaches upward. The lower jaw is relaxed, and the eyes are soft and look straight ahead. Shoulders are pulled slightly back, down, and to the outside. The body is quiet, grounded, and evenly aligned.

Opinions differ in different yoga traditions when it comes to actively engaging the gluteal muscles. On the one hand doing so is credited with creating stability, while others see a narrowing/tightening in the low back. Most likely the answer to this question lies somewhere in the middle; it depends on what one wishes to achieve and actuate.

VARIATIONS

Urdhva Hastasana (*Extended Mountain pose*) – arms are extended overhead (PS 7.3.24 d).

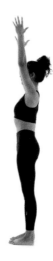

Photo series 7.3.24 d

ACTIVE AND STABILIZING MUSCLES

All of the muscles in the body participate in the pose and are activated according to their stabilizing function:

Legs/pelvis

» Quadriceps femoris – extends the leg.

» Adductors – pull the legs towards each other / stabilize.

» Tensor fasciae latae – stabilize.

» Gluteus maximus, medius, and minimus – extend the hip, externally rotate the thigh.

Trunk

» Quadratus lumborum – stabilizes the back.

» Erector spinae – extends the spine.

» Rhomboid major and minor – stabilizes the shoulder blades, pulls them together.

» Serratus anterior – stabilizes.

» Lower third of the trapezius muscle – pulls the shoulder blades down.

» Rectus abdominis – stabilizes.

Shoulders/arms

» Posterior deltoid – pulls the arm back slightly.

» Teres minor – stabilizes.

» Triceps – extends the arm.

PREPARATORY EXERCISES

Loosen up feet and toes, hip joints, spine, shoulders, cervical spine. Stretch the flanks.

COUNTERPOSES

Uttanasana, Apanasana, Balasana

7.3.25   URDHVA HASTASANA – UPWARD HANDS POSE

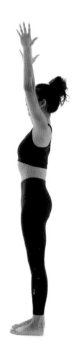

Photo series 7.3.25 a

SYMBOLISM/IMPACT

Urdhva = high, raises / Hasta = hand

Urdhva Hastasana is the *extended mountain pose*, a variation on *Tadasana*. The arms are extended overhead in extension of the trunk. In the classic Mountain pose, the palms touch, which is meant to facilitate inner and outer composure as well as the balancing of the polar forces. The structure of the pose is vertical; the arm posture symbolizes the ethereal, the higher power.

POSE STRUCTURE/WORKING IN THE POSE

See description of *Tadasana*.

VARIATIONS

Another form of execution is with the arms extended overhead and the joints in vertical alignment (PS 7.3.25 a). Shoulders, elbows, and wrists are lined up, and hands are open shoulder-width apart. The shoulder-width position is initially gentler for people with severe tension in the shoulders and back of the neck. This arm position also trains awareness of joint alignment.

ACTIVE AND STABIIIZING MUSCLES

Legs/pelvis

»   Quadriceps femoris – extends the leg.

»   Adductors – pull the legs towards each other/stabilize.

»   Tensor fasciae latae – stabilizes.

»   Gluteus maximus, medius, and minimus – extend the hip, externally rotate the thigh.

Trunk

»   Quadratus lumborum – stabilizes the back.

»   Erector spinae – extends the spine.

»   Serratus anterior – fixes the shoulder blades.

»   Lower third of the triceps muscles – pull the shoulder blades down.

»   Rectus abdominis – stabilizes the trunk.

Shoulders/arms

»   Deltoids – lift and externally rotate the arm.

»   Infraspinatus muscle – external rotation.

»   Triceps – extends the elbow.

STRETCHED MUSCLES

»   Latissimus dorsi

»   Rhomboids

PREPARATORY EXERCISES

Loosen up the shoulder girdle; loosen up the feet and toes, hip joints, spine, shoulders, cervical spine; stretch the flanks.

COUNTERPOSES

Uttanasana, Apanasana, Balasana

7.3.26 URDHVA PRASARITA PADASANA – TABLE POSE

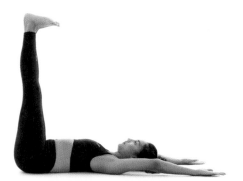

Photo series 7.3.26 a

SYMBOLISM/IMPACT

Urdhva = upright, upward / Prasarita = extended, stretched / Pada = foot/leg

Urdhva Prasarita Padasana (UPP), also called *Table pose*, is a supine pose in which the legs are extended vertically. Depending on its execution, this Asana can be performed as a stretch for the back of the body, as a static strength exercise for the core muscles, as part of a flow, or as a preparatory/introductory exercise. All variations share the deep stretching of the ischiocrural muscles (back of the thigh) as well as a major strengthening and stabilizing effect on the core muscles. Moreover, it also serves as preparation for and introduction to all standing and seated forward bends with extended legs.

POSE STRUCTURE

» On your back, extend the spine along its axis on the mat.

» Bend the knees, then extend the legs up one at a time (PS 7.3.26 c-e).

» Extend the arms overhead shoulder-width-apart in extension of the trunk (PS 7.3.26 f).

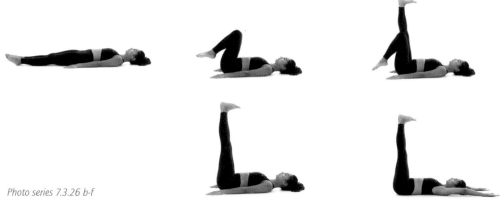

Photo series 7.3.26 b-f

WORKING IN THE POSE

» Tuck the chin so the back of the beck is long and neutral.

» Keep the arms long and allow the lower ribs to sink into the mat and pull the lower abdomen in to avoid arching the back (hyperlordosis of the spine).

» Breathe slowly and evenly into the ribcage.

» Lengthen the inside of the legs upward while simultaneously pulling the outside edges of the feet towards the outside of the hips (pronation).

» Push the heels up and pull the toes towards the shins (calf stretch).

» Engage the muscles at the front of the thighs (pull the kneecaps towards the hips) to deepen the stretch in the back of the legs.

VARIATIONS (DYNAMIC)

Variation 1

» From Apanasana ((11)) to Table (UPP): Exhale: – Apanasana / Inhale: Table (UPP) (PS 7.3.26 h).

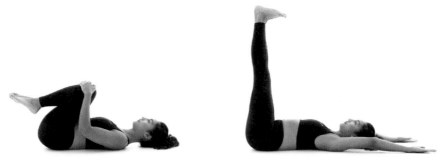

Photo series 7.3.26 g-h

Variation 2

» Strengthening the core muscles: Inhale: – UPP (PS 7.3.26 i) / Exhale – extend arms at 180° next to the hips and lift the upper body (crunch) (PS 7.3.26 j).

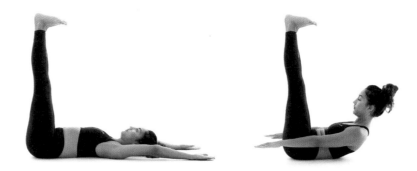

Photo series 7.3.26 i-j

Variation 3

» Alternate raising and lowering the legs (PS 7.3.26 k-l).

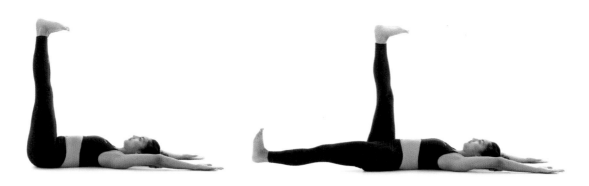

Photo series 7.3.26 k-l

Variation 4

» Raise and lower both legs (only do this if your core muscles are very strong and you can keep your back stable during the exercise).

ACTIVE AND STABILIZING MUSCLES

Trunk

» Iliopsoas muscle – flexes the hip joint.

» Rectus abdominis – flexes the trunk.

» Transverse abdominals – stabilize.

» Internal and external obliques – stabilize.

» Erector spinae – extends the spine, stabilizes.

Legs

» Quadriceps femoris – flexes the hip, extends the knee.

» Tibialis anterior – flexes the foot.

Shoulders/arms

» Deltoids – all parts.

» Triceps – extends the elbow.

STRETCHED MUSCLES

Trunk

» Latissimus dorsi

» Pectoralis major

Legs

» Ischiocrural muscles

» Gastrocnemius

Shoulders/arms

» Biceps

PREPARATORY EXERCISES

Apanasana, supine leg stretches (*Supta Padangustasana 1*)

COUNTERPOSES

Apanasana, Setu Bandha, Makarasana

7.3.27 UTTANASANA – STANDING FORWARD BEND

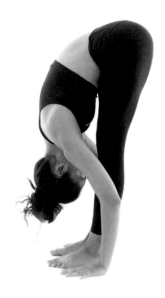

Photo series 7.3.27 a

SYMBOLISM/IMPACT

Ut = intensive / Tan = stretching oneself / Uttana = stretched / Asana = pose

Uttanasana is a standing forward bend combined with an inversion. It is also called *Intensive Forward Stretch*. As the name of the pose suggests, it is a deep stretch that stretches the kinematic chain of the entire back of the body. With respect to its physical structure, *Uttanasana* can be compared to *Paschimottanasana* if it were turned 90° to the left, but also includes the inversion aspect since the heart is above the head. *Uttanasana* can be performed by itself, but it is also an important part of all Sun Salutations and Vinyasa flow variations. Like all forward bends, it is one of the devotional or humility poses. Its effect on the emotional experience and the nervous system is calming and cooling.

Form an energy standpoint, *Uttanasana* is connected to the root chakra (*Muladhara*) and like all standing poses has a grounding effect.

POSE STRUCTURE

» *Tadasana*: Feet are planted hip-width apart with the outside edges of the feet parallel to the outside edges of the mat. Toes are extended and the arch of the foot is up (PS 7.3.27 b).

» As you inhale, move the spine into axial extension and assume extended mountain pose (*Urdhva Hastasana*) (PS 7.3.27 c).

» As you exhale, place your hands just below your hips and move into forward extension from the hip. Maintain the forward extension of the spine as long as possible while the upper body moves closer to the floor (PS 7.3.27 d).

» When you have arrived in the final pose, allow the crown of the head to sink towards the floor and rest your hands/palms next to your feet (PS 7.3.27 e).

» Breathe slowly and evenly.

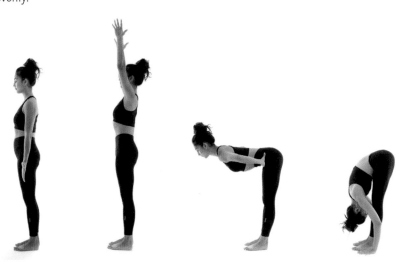

Photo series 7.3.27 b-e

WORKING IN THE POSE

» If the muscles in the back of the legs are severely shortened (or in case of back injuries) it is advisable to initially practice the pose with knees bent (PS 7.3.27 f-g).

» Shift your body weight to the front of the feet without lifting the heels so hips and ankles are lined up vertically.

» Contract the muscles at the front of the thighs (quadriceps) for support (Visualization: Imagine pulling your kneecaps up).

» Keep neck and nape relaxed in this pose. The forehead moves towards the shins. Make small yes/no motions with the head to make sure the neck is relaxed.

» Breathe slowly and evenly.

» When exiting the pose, first lift the back into axial extension (*Ardha Uttanasana*) and then come up.

» If the muscles at the back of the legs are shortened, bend the knees as you come up to lengthen the back and prevent rolling up.

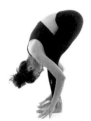 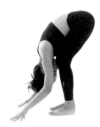

Photo series 7.3.27 f-g

VARIATIONS

» *Ardha Uttanasana* (Ardha = half), Forward Extension (PS 7.3.27 h).

» The linking of *Uttanasana* and *Ardha Uttanasana* is dynamic, meaning it is done in time with the breathing rhythm. Exhale: *Uttanasana* – Inhale: *Ardha Uttanasana*, hands remain on the floor (PS 73.27 h-i).

» If the backs of the legs aren't flexible enough yet, keep the knees bent in the beginning (PS 7.3.27 j).

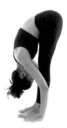 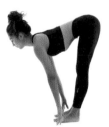 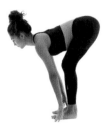

Photo series 7.3.27h-j)

ACTIVE AND STABILIZING MUSCLES

Shoulders/arms

» Trapezius muscles, lower section – pull the shoulder blade down.

» Infraspinatus muscle – pulls the shoulders to the outside.

» Teres minor – pulls the shoulders to the outside.

» Anterior deltoids – lift the arms.

» Biceps – flex the arms.

» Brachialis muscles – flex the arms.

Trunk/legs

» Rectus abdominis – bends the trunk forward.

» Iliopsoas muscle – bends the hip, the trunk forward.

» Rectus femoris – flexes the hip.

» Pectineus muscles – flex the hip.

» Tensor fasciae latae muscle – flexes the hip.

» Quadriceps femoris – extends the knees.

STRETCHED MUSCLES

» Erector spinae

» Quadratus lumborum

» Gluteus maximus

» Ischiocrural muscles

» Gastrocnemius

» Soleus – extended leg.

PREPARATORY EXERCISES

Supine leg stretches (Supta Padangusthasana)

COUNTERPOSES

Wind-relieving pose (Apanasana), Child's pose (Balasana)

7.3.28 UTTHITA PARSHVAKONASANA – EXTENDED SIDE ANGLE POSE

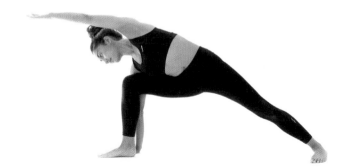

Photo series 7.3.28 a

SYMBOLISM/IMPACT

Utthita = extended, stretched / Parshva = side / Kona = angle / Asana = pose

Utthita Parshvakonasana is an asymmetrical standing pose with lateral flexion (side bend) on the side of the bent knee. This Asana is a continuation of *Virabhadrasana 2*. It combines the sturdy base of the legs and pelvis with the flexibility and length of the trunk and arms. It deeply stretches and opens the flanks and chest area, particularly on the upper side, which opens up the breathing spaces. On the side that faces the floor the deep side bend stimulates the internal organs and the diaphragm.

POSE STRUCTURE

» From *Tadasana*, step into a wide straddle. Hips and feet are parallel.

» Laterally raise the arms to shoulder level and let the shoulder girdle drop.

» Move the spine into axial extension.

» The leg that will be the back leg for the remainder of the exercise is rotated in on the ball of the foot, 15° at the hip; the foot is grounded. The front leg is rotated out on the heel, 90° at the hip, and the outside edge of the foot is now parallel to the edge of the mat. The front heel and back arch should be on an imaginary line (PS 7.3.28 b-c).

» Make sure both feet are well grounded (stance/arches push up).

» Now bend the front leg until the knee is lined up with the ankle; the back of the knee forms a right angle (PS 7.3.28 d).

» The spine forms a straight line. Make sure the center of the eyebrows, the sternum, the navel, and the pubic bone form a vertical line.

» The shoulders form a vertical line over the hips.

» The front knee does not swing in or out; the calf is vertical.

» As you exhale, bend your trunk towards the front leg. Make sure both sides of the trunk lengthen. Bring the lower arm to the floor on the outside of the front calf next to the foot.

» Extend the top arm over the top ear in extension of the trunk. Either hold the head in a neutral position (in case of shoulder or neck problems) or gently turn the head towards the top hand (PS 7.3.28 e).

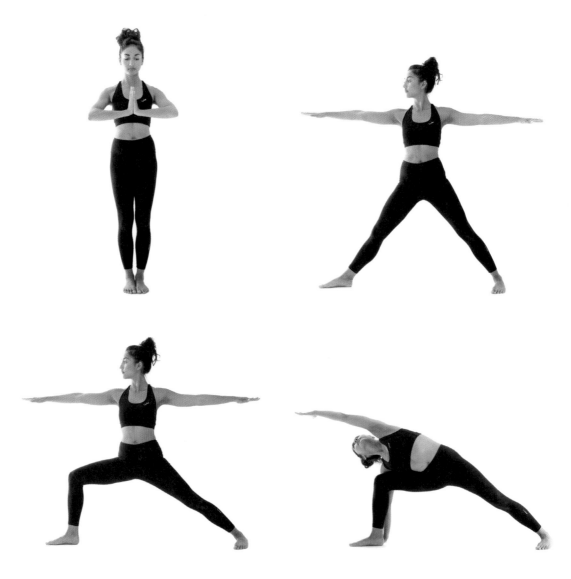

Photo series 7.3.28 b-e

WORKING IN THE POSE

» Press the sole and outside edge of the back foot into the floor, and keep the back leg steady and long.

» Pull the buttock of the front leg and the tailbone forward (towards the pubis) to keep the pelvis from tilting back.

» Pull the navel and lower ribs in to stabilize the trunk.

» To keep the upper body from sagging, push the bottom side of the trunk forward and up and pull the bottom side of the trunk back and down.

» Lengthen the top arm as you exhale and widen the armpit.

» Release the bottom arm to check the amount of weight placed on it.

» As you exhale, direct energy/strength from the low back into the legs and trunk.

» As you inhale, absorb energy via the legs and trunk and direct it to the heart.

People who are very flexible must be careful in this exercise not to "hang in their joints". It causes the pelvis to sink too low, below the knees. If this is the case, increase stability by pulling the legs isometrically towards each other on the mat.

VARIATIONS

» *Utthita Parshvakonasana* can be performed at different intensities. If the legs are not yet strong and stable enough for intense, deep side bends, the "forearm-to-thigh" variation is a suitable modification. Here it is important to make sure that the weight of the upper body does not rest on the arm and the shoulder doesn't slide over to the ear (PS 7.3.28 f).

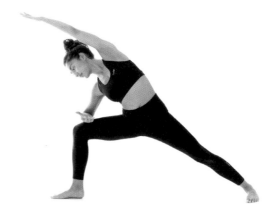

Photo series 7.3.28 f

» Parivritta Parshvakonasana combined with deep side bend with a twist (PS 7.3.28 g-h).

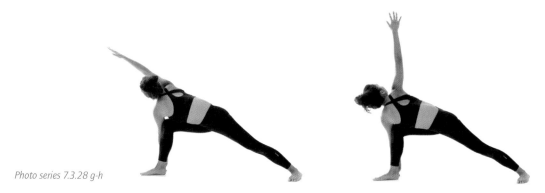

Photo series 7.3.28 g-h

ACTIVE AND STABILIZING MUSCLES

Legs/pelvis

Front leg

» Iliopsoas muscle – bends the front hip.

» Pectineus muscle – bends the front hip.

» Quadriceps femoris – bends the hip.

» Sartorius muscle – bends hip and knee.

» Ischiocrural muscles – bend the knee.

» Tensor fasciae latae muscle – stabilizes, external rotation.

» Gluteus medius – stabilizes, external rotation.

» Tibialis anterior – flexes the foot.

Back leg

» Tibialis anterior – flexes the foot.

» Quadriceps femoris – extends the knee.

» Gluteus maximus – extends the hip.

» Tensor fasciae latae – stabilizes.

Trunk

» Erector spinae muscle – erects the spine.

» Rectus abdominis – stabilizes the trunk.

» Transverse obliques – stabilize.

» Quadratus lumborum – stabilizes the back.

Shoulders/arms

» Deltoids – abduct and lift the arms.

» Triceps – extend the elbow.

» Serratus anterior – stabilizes and abducts the bottom shoulder blade.

» Rhomboids major and minor – pull the top shoulder blade to the center.

» Infraspinatus muscle – externally rotates the upper arms.

» Teres minor – externally rotates the upper arms.

» Lower third of trapezius muscles – pulls the shoulder blades down.

STRETCHED MUSCLES

» Back of thighs/hamstring (ischiocrural muscles – both legs.

» Gastrocnemius – back leg.

» Soleus – back leg.

» All adductors (adductor group) – both legs.

» Gluteus maximus – front leg.

» Iliopsoas muscle – back leg.

» Serratus anterior – top side of trunk.

» Erector spinae – top side.

PREPARATORY EXERCISES

Loosen up joints: shoulders, hips, ankles, stretch adductors, ischiocrural muscles, calves, flanks, stabilization exercises for the trunk.

COUNTERPOSES

Tadasana, Uttanasa with slightly bent knees, Adho Mukha Svanasana, Balasana

7.3.29 UTTHITA TRIKONASANA – TRIANGLE POSE

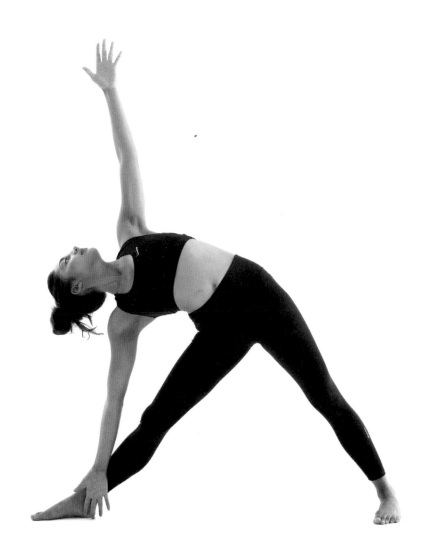

Photo series 7.3.29 a

SYMBOLISM/IMPACT

Utthita = extended / Tri = three / Kona = angle / Asana = pose

Utthita Trikonasana means *Extended Triangle pose*. It is a standing pose in a straddle with lateral flexion. It is asymmetrical. The deep stretches that extend across the body's muscle chains make this a demanding pose. We therefore differentiate *Trikonasana* (side bend of the trunk is less deep) and *Utthita Trikonasana* (side bend of the trunk is nearly parallel to the floor).

The number *three* symbolizes the three inseparable Hindu trinities: creation, preservation, destruction – *Satchitananda* (being-consciousness-bliss) – *Sattva*, *Rajas*, *Tamas*. These qualities are expressed in the pose via the many *Kona* (angles) or *triangles* the body forms in this pose.

Its stable stance makes *Trikonasana* a very grounding pose. It stimulates primarily the first chakra (*Muladhara*: grounding, stability, trust) in the lower pelvic region. But the pose also stimulates the fourth chakra in the heart space (*Anahata*: higher heart, wide heart space).

This Asana requires much preparation with respect to pre-stretching and strengthening of the leg and trunk muscles. It is not necessarily recommended for beginning students and should be worked up to with a suitable practice over a longer period of time. Feeling pain in the pose should always be seen as the body's warning of overstretching or improper joint alignment.

POSE STRUCTURE

» From *Tadasana*, step into a wide straddle. Hips and feet are parallel (PS 7.3.29 b).

» Laterally raise arms to shoulder level. Allow the shoulder girdle to drop.

» Move the spine into axial extension.

» Internally rotate the leg that will remain the back leg 30° at the hip on the ball of the foot and ground the foot. Externally rotate the front leg 90° at the hip on the heel. The outside edge of the foot is now parallel to the edge of the mat. The front heel and the back arch should be on an imaginary straight line (PS 7.3.29 c).

» Make sure both feet are well grounded (four-point stance/arches push up).

» Legs are extended, but avoid hyperextension of the knees.

» Imagine the body being parallel to a wall. First pull the upper body far over the front leg and lengthen the lower flank.

» As you do so, pull the front thigh into the hip joint and push the back hip back and up. The pelvis will tilt sideways. This process can be aided by temporarily bending the front knee.

» Simultaneously initiate the side-bend of the trunk until the front arm touches the shin (floor or yoga block) (PS 7.3.29 f).

» The front arm is now in a vertical position; hand, elbow, and shoulder form a straight line. The back arm is an extension of that vertical line, reaching upward (PS 7.3.29 g).

» Either hold the head in a neutral position in extension of the spine (in case of neck problems), the nose/gaze points to the top hand.

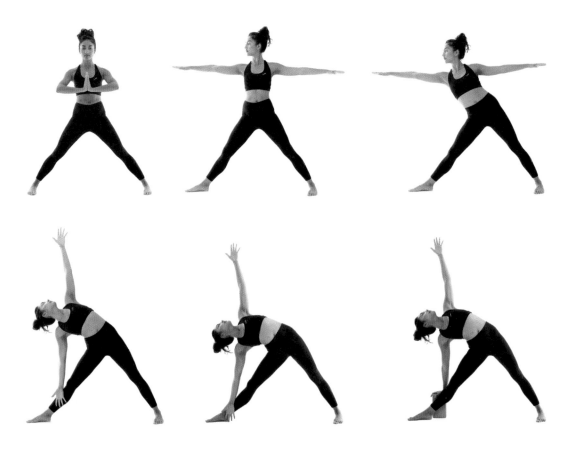

Photo series 7.3.29 b-g

One of the most common mistakes in this pose is allowing the body to tilt too far forward in the side bend (usually in an attempt to reach the floor with the hand). The pelvis is then pushed back and the upper arm bent back, which makes the pose completely crooked.

» To avoid doing so, line up the shoulders with the front leg. The hand of the lower arm can then rest on the shin (PS 7.3.29 e), but without adding the weight of the upper body. Therefore only place the fingertips lightly against the shin. The holding force should come primarily from the legs and the stable trunk.

WORKING IN THE POSE

» Keep an eye on the feet's points of contact with the ground.

» Slightly rotate the thigh of the front leg out (kneecap points towards the middle of the foot). Remember the calf's correcting compensating motion.

» Pull up the kneecaps, but don't hyperextend your knees.

» Tilt the tailbone forward and lengthen the low back.

» Pull the lower ribs and abdomen in for stability.

» Rotate the bottom side of the ribcage forward/up until the flanks are stacked.

» Pull the shoulder girdle away from the ears.

» As you inhale, lift the sternum and open the entire chest and back.

» As you exhale, direct strength/energy from the pelvic area into the legs and along the spine up to the upper extremities.

» As you inhale, pull the feet isometrically towards each other and direct energy/strength along the legs and up to the pelvis and heart space.

» Remain internally permeable in spite of the deep pose, and feel and lengthen the breath.

VARIATIONS

» Not stretching the flanks quite as deeply is a good way to incrementally build up strength and the stretch in this pose.

The following three variations are advanced and require lots of strength and flexibility:

» *In Utthita Trikonasana*, extend the top arm parallel to the floor (deepens the flank stretch in the upper side).

» *In Utthita Trikonasana*, extend both arms into an extension of the trunk (increases stability).

» *Parivritta Trikonasana* – Revolved Triangle (PS 7.3.29 h with block), (PS 7.3.29 i without block).

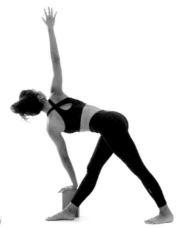 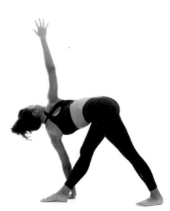

Photo series 7.3.29 h-i

ACTIVE AND STABILIZING MUSCLES

Legs/pelvis

Front leg

» Iliopsoas – bends the front hip.

» Pectineus muscle – bends the front hip.

» Quadriceps femoris – bends the hip, extends the knee.

» Sartorius muscle – bends the hip.

» Tensor fasciae latae – stabilizes.

Back leg

» Tibialis anterior – flexes the foot.

» Quadriceps femoris – extends the knee.

» Tensor fasciae latae – stabilizes.

» Gluteus maximus – extends the hip.

Trunk

» Erector spinae – erects the spine.

» Internal/external obliques – tilt the trunk, stabilize.

» Rectus abdominis – stabilizes.

» Transverse obliques – stabilize.

» Quadratus lumborum – stabilizes the back.

Shoulders/arms

» Middle deltoid – abducts the arms.

» Triceps – extends the elbow.

» Serratus anterior – stabilizes and abducts the bottom shoulder blade.

» Rhomboids major and minor – pull the upper shoulder blade to the center.

» Infraspinatus muscle – externally rotates the upper arms.

» Teres minor – externally rotates the upper arms.

» Lower third of trapezius muscle – pulls the shoulder blades down.

STRETCHED MUSCLES

» Back of thighs/hamstring (ischiocrural muscles) – both legs.

» Gastrocnemius – back leg.

» Soleus – back leg.

» All adductors (adductor group) – both legs.

» Gluteus maximus – front leg.

» Iliopsoas muscle – back leg.

» Internal/external obliques – upper side of trunk.

» Serratus anterior – upper side of trunk.

» Rhomboids – lower side of trunk.

PREPARATORY EXERCISES

Loosen up all joints, stretch adductors and backs of legs, stretch flanks, erect the spine.

COUNTERPOSES

Tadasana, Uttanasana with knees slightly bent, Balasana.

7.3.30   UTKATASANA – CHAIR POSE

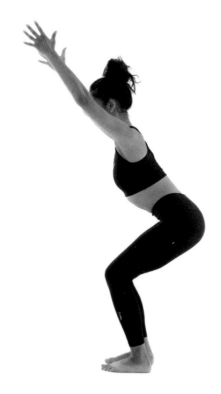

Photo series 7.3.30 a

SYMBOLISM/IMPACT

Utkata = high, mighty, wild / Asana = pose

Utkatasana, *Chair pose*, is a standing pose on both feet with bent knees and an extended spine. The pose is also known as the *Fierce pose*. This pose is sometime also called a *squat*, particularly when the pose is modified and lacks the intenseness of the arms extended overhead.

There are different modifications for *Utkatasana*, that can easily be adapted to every practice level in terms of intensity. The pose symbolizes grounding and rootedness via the lower extremities, while the arms in extension of the erect and stable spine point like arrows up to heaven, thus forging the connection to the cosmic plane.

Depending on the execution of the exercise, *Utkatasana* can have a warming effect and also promote circulation. The deep knee bend facilitates a stable stance. When the arms are extended overhead it opens up the breathing spaces, allowing the breath to flow more freely. From an energy standpoint, *Utkatasana* is linked to the *Muladhara chakra* (grounding, trust), the *Manipura chakra* (warmth, strength, energy), and the *Sahasrara chakra* (link to the cosmic source).

POSE STRUCTURE

There are different executions of *Utkatasana* with respect to foot and leg position. Standing with feet hip-width apart corresponds with anatomical joint alignment. But this Asana is also practiced with closed legs, which lends lots of stability and steadiness to the lower extremities. Choosing one of the two options depends on whether *Utkatasana* is practiced as a transitional Asana within a flow or is practiced by itself.

» *Tadasana*: Place your feet hip-width apart. Pay attention to the four-point stance of the feet and lift the arches.

» Slightly shift your weight back towards the heels, but don't lift the toes.

» While the spine remains in axial extension, bend your knees, tilt the pelvis forward, and do a deep knee bend (PS 7 3. 30 c).

» Extend the arms forward and overhead in extension of the spine, shoulder-width apart, and externally rotate the upper arms: palms face each other, thumbs point behind (PS 7.3.30 c)

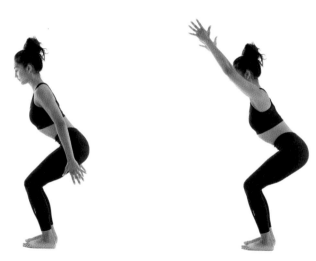

Photo series 7.3.30 b-c

WORKING IN THE POSE

» To avoid overloading the knee joints, shift the knee's center of gravity farther back.

» Direct strength from the pelvis to the feet via the legs, while also directing energy along the spine up into the arms.

» As you exhale, drop the pelvis deeper into chair pose, as you inhale move the back into a more upright position.

» Actively pull the shoulder girdle down while lifting the sternum.

» Pull the lower abdomen and lower ribs in.

VARIATIONS

Ardha Utkatasana – Half Chair pose

» In *Half Chair pose* the arms/hands are raised only to shoulder level. This is recommended for people with tightness in the shoulder girdle and back of the neck. This allows the shoulder girdle to stay down. The knee bend and upright back position can be as intense as in the previous exercise.

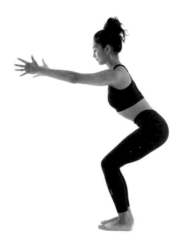

Photo series 7.3.30 d

Parivritta Utkatasana – Twisted Chair pose

» Stabilize the legs and rest the left upper arm on the right thigh.

» Place the palms together, build up isometric tension, and move into a twist (PS 7.3.30 e-f).

» Push the lower left rib towards the right thigh.

» Keep your hips parallel; if necessary, correct the left hip by pulling it back slightly.

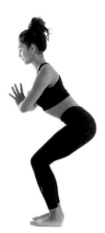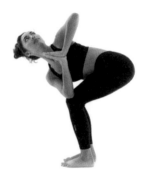

Photo series 7.3.30 e-f

ACTIVE AND STABILIZING MUSCLES

Legs/pelvis

» Quadriceps femoris – eccentric*.

» Hamstring (ischiocrural muscles) – eccentric* in combination with the quadriceps femoris.

» All adductors (adductor group) –pull the legs towards each other, stabilize and support hip flexion.

» Pectineus muscle – flexes the hip.

» Gluteus medius and minimus – are synergists in all movements except adduction.

» Tibialis anterior – flexes the ankle.

» Soleus – eccentric*.

The muscle is stretched during contraction.

Trunk

» Iliopsoas muscle – flexes the hip.

» Quadratus lumborum – stabilizes the back.

» Erector spinae – erects the spine.

» Rectus abdominis – stabilizes.

» Serratus anterior – fixes the shoulder blades.

» Trapezius, lower third – pulls the shoulder blades down.

» Trapezius, middle section – fixes the shoulders.

Shoulders/arms

» Anterior deltoids – lift the arms.

» Infraspinatus muscle – external rotation.

» Triceps – extends the elbow.

STRETCHED MUSCLES

» Latissimus dorsi

» Rhomboids

» Gluteus maximus

PREPARATORY EXERCISES

Loosen up shoulders and hips as well as the spine; stretch the front of the shoulders and the back of the legs; strengthen abdominal and back muscles for stability.

COUNTERPOSE

Uttanasana, Tadasana, Setu Bandha or hip flexor stretches.

7.3.31   USTRASANA – CAMEL POSE

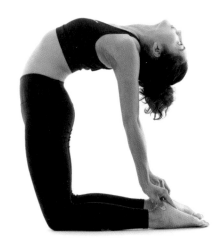

Photo series 7.3.31 a

SYMBOLISM/IMPACT

Ushtra = camel / Asana = pose

Camel pose is a deep, kneeling back bend. Like Bow pose, it combines arms and legs, and based on its structure it is a bow (*Dhanurasana*) that is rotated 90°. But the execution of *Camel* is more challenging because leg and trunk muscles and the entire support apparatus must work much harder, particularly to enter and exit the pose.

Like all backbends, it stretches the front of the body. Chest and throat are stretched deeply, which deepens the breath and increases lung volume. *Ustrasana* strengthens the back muscles and the spine and has a stimulating effect on the internal organs, and thus also on the metabolism. In terms of energy, it stimulates the throat chakra (*Vishuddha*: communication, connection between heart and brain), and the heart chakra (*Anahata*: love, empathy). On an emotional level, *Ustrasana* has a major effect on our trust and self-confidence because in order to enter the pose we must allow ourselves to "blindly" sink backward while leaving our heart and abdomen unprotected.

POSE STRUCTURE

» On your knees (place a folded blanket under tender knees), tops of the feet rest on the floor. Hips are stacked vertically over the knees (PS 7.3.31 b).

» Place your hands on your hips and pull the elbows towards each other.

» Stabilize the hips and thighs or push them forward.

» As you inhale, lift the sternum, pull the shoulders further back, and initiate the backbend (PS 7.3.31 c)

» Now lower the hands to the feet and place the palms on the soles or the heels.

» The head is an extension of the spine.

  • When exiting the pose, come straight up, that is make sure to avoid any rotation that could injure the spine in this deep backbend.

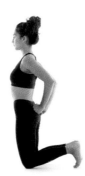 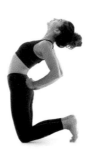 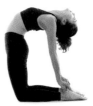

Photo series 7.3.31 b-d

WORKING IN THE POSE

» Take long, even breaths into the chest.

» Push the hips and pelvis forward during the entire exercise sequence to maintain the vertical knee-hip axis.

» Avoid clenching your buttocks: To support your return to an upright position, press the shins and tops of the feet into the mat like you are trying to straighten your knees.

» Rotate the thighs in slightly, so the sacroiliac joints remain stable.

» To deepen the back bend, actively pull the shoulder blades together and externally rotate the upper arms.

» To stabilize the pose, contract the pelvic floor (*Mula Bandha*) and the rectus abdominis muscle.

VARIATIONS

» To shorten the distance between hands and heels, modify the pose by tucking the toes (PS 7.3.31 e).

» If the body is not ready for such a deep backbend (if the hips try to drop back), the practitioner should initially perform the easier version and keep hands on hips.

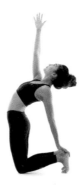

Photo series 7.3.31e

ACTIVE AND STABILIZING MUSCLES

Legs/pelvis

» The tensor fasciae latae muscle stabilizes the hips.

» The ischiocrural muscles bend the knees and tilt the pelvis.

Trunk

» Erector spinae – extends the back into the backbend.

» Quadratus lumborum – extends the back/backbend.

» Gluteus maximus – flexes the hips.

» Trapezius, lower section – pull the shoulder blades down.

» Rectus abdominis – works post-isometric.

Shoulders/arms

» Posterior deltoids – extend the shoulder.

» Infraspinatus muscles – externally rotate the shoulders.

» Teres minor – externally rotate the shoulders.

» Triceps – extends the arms.

STRETCHED MUSCLES

» Quadriceps

» Iliopsoas

» Rectus abdominis

» Pectoralis major and minor

» Anterior deltoids

» Biceps

» Brachialis muscle

PREPARATORY EXERCISES

Stretch the hip flexors (iliopsoas) and front of the thighs (quadriceps), stretch the front of the shoulders, loosen up the spine, the shoulder and hip joints, *Cobra (Bhujangasana)*

COUNTERPOSE

Child's pose (Balasana)

7.3.32   VRIKSHASANA – TREE POSE

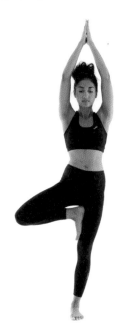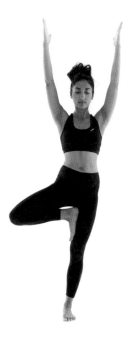

Photo series 7.3.32 a-b

♦ HATHA YOGA

SYMBOLISM/IMPACT

Vriksa = tree / Asana = pose

Vrikshasana combines a standing with a balance pose. Hardly any other Asana has as much symbolism as tree pose. The pose symbolizes the aspect of grounding (rootedness) as well as a connection to the higher power. The roots lend stability to the tree and supply it with nutrients all the way up into the crown, where it also absorbs energy from the power of the sun. The polarities, top and bottom, earth and cosmos, tangible and ethereal, are represented here in perfect balance.

When a tree is healthy, supple, and flexible, it can weather even severe storms. It may sway in the wind, but it remains upright and sturdy. Thus, the tree is a symbol of balance, and it reminds us that we are all equally nurtured by the earth and the cosmos.

The focus on physical stability on the one hand, and the simultaneous awareness of the vertical inner axis on the other hand, trains and promotes our mental stability. At the same time we practice permeability in Tree pose, because when we are too rigid and tense we quickly lose our balance. We need alert awareness to allow subtle movement and swaying without letting it throw us off balance.

The structure of the vertical axis facilitates stimulation of all energy centers in the pose, particularly the lower chakra (*Muladhara chakra*: grounding, stability, trust) and the upper chakra (*Sahasrara chakra*: the doorway to cosmic consciousness).

POSE STRUCTURE

» In *Tadasana*, engage the muscles of the feet and lift the arches; weight is equally distributed.

» Become aware of the inner/ vertical axis along the spine; lift the spine to give the pose length.

» Shift your weight to the supporting leg and slightly lift the playing leg, bend the knee, externally rotate the leg and pull it upward along the inside of the supporting leg (use the hand for support).

» Place the foot of the playing leg against the inside of the supporting leg's thigh. The heel points towards the perineum, the toes point down (avoid "banana foot", the supination of the supporting foot).

» Pull the shin slightly towards the navel to add length to the low back and prevent the hip from pushing out on the side of the supporting leg.

» Lift the spine, let the shoulders drop, and place the palms together in front of the chest in *Anjali Mudra*.

» Once balance has been established, the arms can be extended up shoulder-width apart in extension of the trunk; thumbs point behind. This arm variation is recommended for people with tightness in the shoulder girdle and back of the neck.

» The classic *Tree* variation: With arms extended overhead, place palms together and look up.

» Reflect before switching sides and notice the difference.

WORKING IN THE POSE

» To stabilize the pose, press the playing leg firmly into the inside of the supporting leg's thigh, and vice versa (build up counter-pressure, isometric tension).

» Direct pressure/energy from the pelvis through the supporting leg and into the foot and floor while simultaneously lengthening the spine in the opposite direction. Visualization: The body lengthens in both directions.

» Lift the sternum, let the shoulder girdle drop, engage the core muscles, and pull the abdomen and lower ribs in slightly.

VISUALIZATION AIDS AND ENERGY CONTROL

» Imagine a beam of light along the spine's vertical axis that stretches into the sky as well as deep into the ground. Extend your body along this beam of light.

» Imagine growing strong roots from the supporting foot deep into the earth.

» Imagine your body as a tree: Foot, leg, and trunk form the tree trunk; shoulders and arms are the crown. Arms and hands (the branches) reach towards the light.

» If the posture is very shaky: Remember that trees also sway, sometimes more and sometimes less, and that a tree swaying in the wind is perfectly fine.

VARIATIONS

» People who struggle with balance can remain in *Tadasana* and place their hands in *Anjali Mudra*, imagining a tree with a sturdy trunk. Here, too, the image of a beam of light along the spine can be helpful.

» If the hip opening is too small for the external rotation, the ball of the playing foot can remain on the floor and the heel can rest above the ankle.

» The playing leg can also be placed against the calf. However, to protect the knee, no direct pressure should be applied to the knee joint.

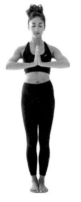 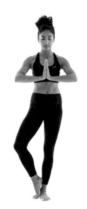 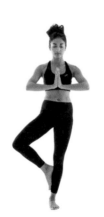 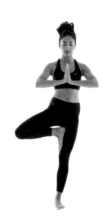

Photo series 7.3.32 c-f

ACTIVE AND STABILIZING MUSCLES

Legs/pelvis

Supporting leg

» Muscles in the foot and toes.

» Calf muscles – stabilize.

» Tibialis anterior (front of shin) – stabilize supporting leg and foot.

» Quadriceps femoris – extends the knee.

» Gluteus maximus and medius – extend, stabilize.

» Tensor fasciae latae – stabilizes.

» Adductors – isometric/stabilize.

Playing leg

» Iliopsoas muscle – bends the leg in the hip.

» Sartorius muscle – externally rotates the leg, bends the knee.

» Gluteus maximus, medius, and minimus – abduction, external rotation.

» Tensor fasciae latae – abduction.

Trunk

» Erector spinae – erects the spine.

» Quadratus lumborum – stabilizes the back.

- » Serratus anterior – fix the shoulder blades.
- » Rectus abdominis - stabilizes the trunk.
- » Lower third of trapezius – pulls the shoulder blades down.

Shoulders/arms

With arms extended overhead:

- » Deltoids – lift the arms and external rotation.
- » Infraspinatus muscle – external rotation.
- » Triceps – extends the elbow.

STRETCHED MUSCLES

- » All adductors (playing leg).
- » Latissimus dorsi
- » Rhomboids

PREPARATORY EXERCISES

Stretch the adductors, loosen up the ankles and toes, loosen up the hips in various ways, loosen up the spine and work on spinal stability, activate the pelvic floor, strengthen the core muscles, loosen up the shoulder girdle.

COUNTERPOSES

Forward bend with knees bent (modified Uttanasana), Adho Mukha Savasana, Balasana, Apanasana.

7.3.33   VIRABHADRASANA II – WARRIOR II POSE

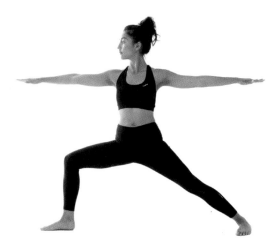

Photo series 7.3.33 a

SYMBOLISM/IMPACT

Vira = courageous/heroic / Bhadra = beautiful, good / Asana = pose

Virabhadra is the name of a mythical warrior. The *Warrior pose* is an asymmetrical standing pose with one leg extended and the other knee bent. There are three warrior poses total, and they are referred to as *Warrior I, II, and III.*

The *Warrior* symbolizes someone who is ready to do battle. This generally refers to internal conflicts that are bravely confronted and closely observed to take action at the right moment. This requires the skill of being alert and present, a clear internal and external alignment, and the ability to wait, to practice patience and serenity, to be at peace with oneself. We can learn all of these qualities in the warrior poses when we take our gaze outside as well as inside.

Warrior II is the easiest of the three poses. When looking at it in terms of logical progression, *Warrior II* expresses composure and inner alignment. In *Warrior I* the arms, which can be seen as arrows or swords, are extended upward and moved into position as the body turns towards its target. The action or attack follows in *Warrior III* (*standing balance*). The (arms) arrows, swords reach towards the target. The body could even be viewed as a flying arrow.

Like all standing poses, *Warrior II* is very much a grounding Asana, and is linked to the first chakra (*Muladhara*: grounding, stability, trust). The qualities of the third chakra (*Manipura*: strength, power, energy, courage), the fourth chakra (*Anahata*: love, empathy, wide-open heart), the sixth chakra (*Ajna*: intuition), and the seventh chakra (*Sahasrara*: link to the plane of higher consciousness) are aspects that can be helpful on the warrior's path and are allowed to blossom.

The challenge in *Warrior II* is opening the hips while simultaneously bending in the hip and maintaining an erect spine. When first practicing this pose, many participants tend to reach for the forward leg with the trunk, which takes the trunk out of its axial extension.

POSE STRUCTURE

» From *Tadasana*, step into a wide straddle. Hips and feet are parallel (PS 7.3.33 b-c).

» Laterally raise the arms to shoulder-level and let the shoulder girdle drop.

» Move the spine into axial extension.

» Internally rotate the leg that will be the back leg throughout this exercise on the ball of the foot 15° from the hip, and ground the foot. Externally rotate the front leg on the heel 90° from the hip. The outside edge of the foot is now parallel to the outside edge of the mat. The front heel and back arch should be lined up on an imaginary line (PS 7.3.33 d).

» Make sure both feet are well grounded (four-point stance/lift the arches).

» Now bend the front knee until the knee is lined up with the ankle and the back of the knee forms a right angle (PS 7.3.33 e).

» The spine is in a straight vertical line. Make sure the space between the eyebrows, the sternum, navel, and pubic bone form a vertical line.

» The shoulder joints are vertically lined up with the hips.

» The front knee does not swing out or in; the calf is in a vertical position (PS 7.3.33 f).

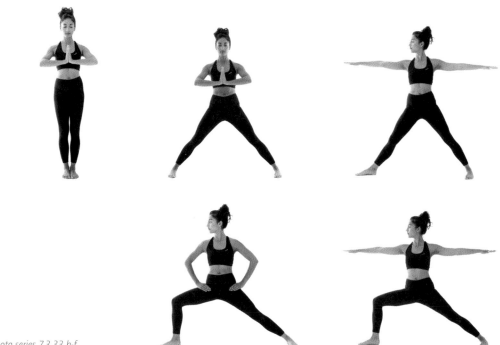

Photo series 7.3.33 b-f.

WORKING IN THE POSE

» Slightly rotate the thighs out (lift the inner thighs; pull the muscles in the right buttock towards the tailbone). Remember the correcting compensating movement in the calves, knee alignment, and the grounding points of the feet.

» Allow the pelvis to drop lower and pull up the kneecap of the back leg.

» As you exhale, direct energy/strength from the pelvis down into both legs while simultaneously pulling the spine up in an opposing movement.

» As you inhale, draw energy/strength from the feet up into the pelvis, direct it to the heart, open the chest and lengthen the arms.

» Let the shoulder girdle drop back and down.

» Rotate the upper arms out and the forearms in; palms face the floor.

» Direct the gaze along the front arm into the distance.

VARIATIONS

» The pose can be modified by resting the back knee on the floor. This helps to open the hips.

» *Virabhadrasana I* – the body turns 90° towards the front leg; hips are parallel and arms are extensions of the spine; slight backbend (PS 7.3.33 g).

» *Virabhadrasana II* – standing balance pose; hips are parallel and arms are extensions of the spine (PS 7.3.33 h).

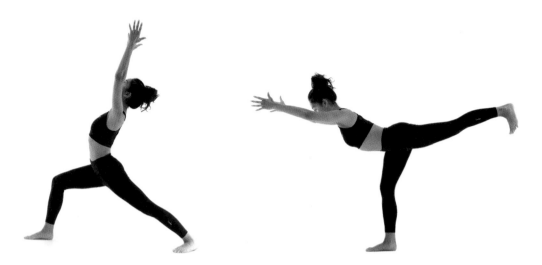

Photo series 7.3.33 g-h

ACTIVE AND STABILIZING MUSCLES

Legs/pelvis

Front leg

» Iliopsoas – bends the front hip.

» Pectineus muscle – bends the front hip.

» Quadriceps femoris – bends the hip.

» Sartorius muscle – bends hip and knee.

» Ischiocrural muscles – bend the knee.

» Tensor fasciae latae – stabilizes, external rotation.

» Gluteus medius – stabilizes, external rotation.

» Tibialis anterior – flexes the foot.

Back leg

» Tibialis anterior – flexes the foot.

» Quadriceps femoris – extends the knee.

» Gluteus maximus – extends the hip.

» Tensor fasciae latae – stabilizes.

Trunk

» Erector spinae – erects the spine.

» Rectus abdominis – stabilizes the trunk.

» Transverse obliques – stabilize.

» Quadratus lumborum – stabilizes the back.

Shoulders/arms

» Lateral and posterior deltoids – lift the arms.

» Infraspinatus muscle – externally rotates the upper arms.

» Teres minor – externally rotates the upper arms.

» Lower third of trapezius – pulls the shoulder blades down.

» Serratus anterior – stabilizes and abducts the lower shoulder blade.

» Rhomboids – pull shoulder blades together.

» Triceps – extends the elbow.

STRETCHED MUSCLES

» Ischiocrural muscles – front leg.

» Iliopsoas – back leg.

» Gastrocnemius – back leg.

» Soleus – back leg.

» Tensor fasciae latae – back leg.

» Pectoralis major

» Biceps

» Adductors

PREPARATORY EXERCISES

Loosen up all joints and the spine, pre-stretch the back and inside of the legs, stretch the hip flexors, extend the spine, stretch the flanks.

COUNTERPOSES

Tadasana, Uttanasana with knees slightly bent, Balasana.

7.3.34 VIPARITA KARANI – LEGS-UP-THE-WALL POSE (HALF SHOULDER STAND)

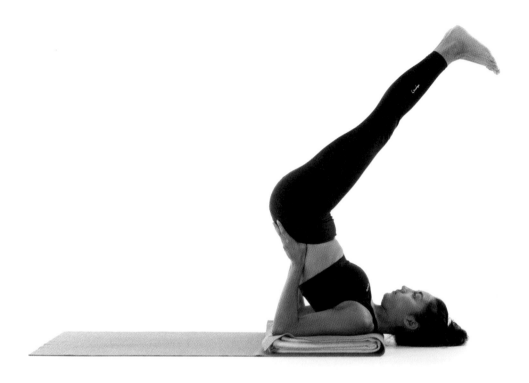

Photo series 7.3.34 a

SYMBOLISM/IMPACT

Viparita = reverse, turned inward / Karani = shape

Viparita Karani, Half Shoulder stand, is an inversion. It is a meditative pose that allows the mind to come to a rest and has a harmonizing effect on the energy experience. When combining *Viparita Karani* with breath- and energy control as well as *Bandhas* (using muscle contractions to direct energy), it is called *Viparita Karani Mudra*. *Mudra* means *seal*.

Viparita Karani is a perfect transition after a yoga unit because the Asana can guide us to a state of rest: to gently allow the mental experience to fade away and direct the gaze inward. For *Viparita Karani* to take full effect one should allow plenty of time for this Asana and properly prepare it with the appropriate practice. Most writings emphasize the aspect of inner reversal that can result from the practice of *Viparita Karani*.

The pose structure of "feet up, head down" can give us the incentive to view life's concerns from the opposite perspective. The pose might also be an inspiration to reverse a path one has chosen in the course of one's life because it has proven to be a dead end or is no longer passable.

On a physical level, the pose promotes the backflow of venous blood and lymphatic fluid from the legs, which is particularly beneficial in cases of varicose veins or swelling of the legs. Moreover, gravity causes the internal organs to sink into the dome of the diaphragm. Deep, steady belly breaths push the organs back towards the pelvis, which has a massaging and stimulating effect on digestion and metabolism.

From an energy anatomy perspective, the pose stimulates *Samana Prana Vayu*.

Viparita Karani is a stand-alone Asana, but is very well suited as an alternative or preliminary step for more challenging Asanas like, for instance, the Shoulder stand (*Salamba Sarvangasana*).

POSE STRUCTURE

» From Shoulder Bridge, plant the slightly bent elbows close to the ribs, squeeze the shoulder blades together and lift the sternum.

» Now place your hands against the lower back like shallow cups making sure the lumbar spine maintains its lordotic curve. The lower ribs and hipbones should be lined up. It will lift the sternum closer to the chin and opens the heart space.

» Now place the legs, one at a time, into a vertical position. Legs are extended, but knees are not locked. The energy should be able to flow.

» If this style of execution is too stressful for the hands/arms, one of the below variations should be practiced as an alternative.

Another option for entering the pose is using a little bit of momentum, as with a half backward-roll, and then place the hands against the low back. You can first roll back and forth a few times on the mat with a rounded back. Many people initially find the momentum version easier, but the amount of momentum should be moderate and not too vigorous (to avoid stressing the neck and nape).

WORKING IN THE POSE

» Breathe slowly and evenly and remain permeable.

» Allow the mind to come to a rest.

» To exit the pose, lower the feet to the floor one at a time and then gently unwind the back.

VARIATIONS

Variation 1: A very easy modification in cases of shoulder and neck problems: rest the vertically extended legs against a wall.

Variation 2: Place a folded blanket under your shoulders to take pressure off the neck (PS 7.3.34 b).

Variation 3: Place a thick pillow, several folded blankets, or some yoga blocks under your bottom. As you do so, make sure the lumbar spine maintains its lordotic curve. The lower ribs and hipbones should be lined up. It will lift the sternum closer to the chin and opens the heart space. Make sure the pose feels relaxed. Rest the arms on the floor alongside the body or are prop them on the floor with the elbows bent and shoulder blades squeezing together (PS 7.3.34 c).

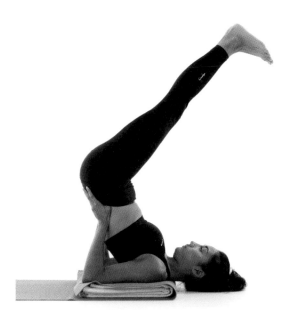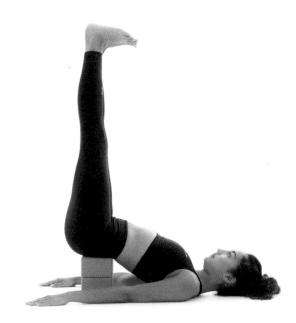

Photo series 7.3.34 b-c

ACTIVE AND STABILIZING MUSCLES

Legs/pelvis

» Iliopsoas muscle – bends the hips.

» Pectneus muscle – bends the hips.

» Quadriceps femoris – bends the hips, extends the knees.

Trunk

» Erector spinae – erects the spine and backbend.

» Quadratus lumborum – supports the backbend.

Shoulders/arms

» Rhomboids major and minor – pull the shoulder blades together.

» Middle and lower trapezius muscles – pull the shoulder blades down.

» Infraspinatus muscle – externally rotates the upper arms.

» Teres minor – externally rotates the upper arms.

» Posterior deltoids – pull the upper arms back.

» Triceps – pulls the upper arm back.

» Biceps – bends the elbows.

STRETCHED MUSCLES

» Ischiocrural muscles

» Gastrocnemius

» Soleus

» Gluteus maximus

» Rectus abdominis

» Pectoralis major and minor

PREPARATORY EXERCISES

Loosen up the hips, shoulders, spine, wrists; stretch the back of the legs and the gluteal muscles; work on strengthening/stabilizing the back muscles, arms and hands.

COUNTERPOSES

Apanasana, Balasana

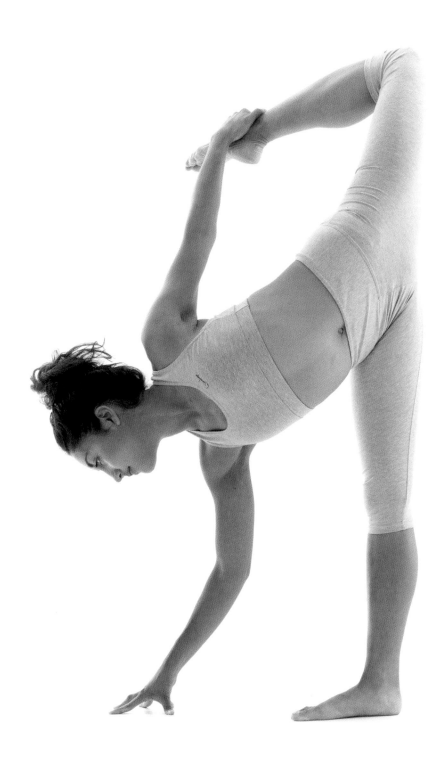

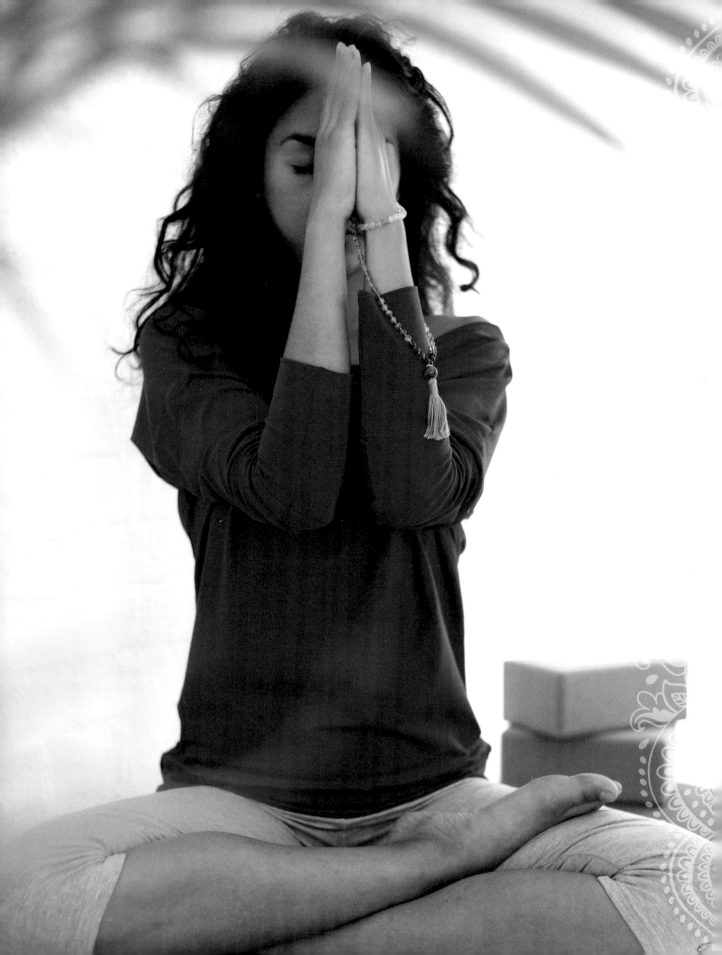

8 SIGNIFICANCE OF KARANA AND SURYA NAMASKAR

8 SIGNIFICANCE OF KARANA AND SURYA NAMASKAR

8.1 KARANA/VINYASA FLOW

The Western term for *Karana* is *flow*, or *Vinayasa flow*. *Vinyasa* is translated as *with movement, position, linking*. *Vinyasa flow yoga* (also known as *power yoga*) is the term for a type of yoga that combines all of the Asanas in the practice into flows (Karanas). The primary goal is to build heat that will have a purifying effect on the system (body and mind), as well as making the body strong and supple, whereby body and mind should come to rest during the flow.

There are *Karanas* or *flows* for all levels of practice with different focus areas. They warm up the body and prepare it for the Asana practice. All of them are practiced with conscious breathing.

Sample Karana "Breathing Cat":

Starting position – Utthita Balasana – PS 8.1 a

Inhale – lift the head, extend the back – PS 8.1 b

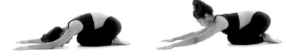

Exhale – Marjaryasana – PS 8.1 c

Inhale – long back – PS 8.1 d

Exhale – Adho Mukha Svanasana – PS 8.1.e

Inhale – All-fours position – PS 8.1 f

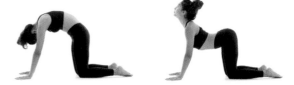

Exhale – Utthita Balasana – PS 8.1 g

Photo series 8.1 a-g

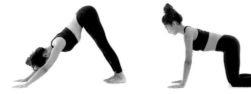

8.2   SURYA NAMASKAR – SUN SALUTATION

"By focusing on the sun, the yogi achieves knowledge about the universe."
(*Yoga Sutra*, 3.27[60])

Surya = sun / Namaskar = greeting, reverence

Das wohl bekannteste Karana ist der Sonnengruß, Surya Namaskar.

"From time immemorial, the sun with its light- and warmth-giving power has acted as a source of fertility, vitality, and joy. Each day, it appears in the sky with absolute regularity and is considered a symbol of eternal life. Surya means sun and is also the name of the Vedic Sun God who has represented the power of the sun as a higher light and divine revelation. In many Vedic rituals and sacrificial cultures the Sun God was asked for benevolent support.

The Sun Salutation is also called the sun prayer. It is assumed that the sun prayer harkens back to a Parsi religious group and their prophet and founder Zarathhustra. They, too, revered the sun and fire as archetypical symbols of the divine. When the Parsi ethnic group settled in India during the mass migration, the Hindus over time adopted their special worship ritual into their own religious customs and possibly adapted it to their own purposes."[61]

In India, the *Sun Salutation* is traditionally performed with the rising of the sun to greet the dawning day with deference, gratitude, and meditative concentration. One focuses internally on the higher power and connects with the transformative and nurturing power of the light, the sun.

Over the years, different traditions have developed different *Sun Salutations* with different levels of intensity. But all of them include the dynamic alternation between forward- and back bends, which place alternating pressure on the area of the solar plexus. The classic *Sun Salutation* includes seven Asanas, five of which are practiced twice. It consists of 12 movements in total.

During the standing phase, one initially collects oneself in the heart and directs one's consciousness to the inner light. Then one stretches towards the sun, opens up to its power, embraces it and bows to it. This is followed by prostration during which one bows in humility to the sun, the earth, and the entire cycle of creation. After the bow, one returns to an upright posture and again collects oneself in the heart, until the start of the next cycle. One set consists of two repetitions during which first the left side and then the right side (or vice-versa) is practiced. The number of sets can vary, between 3 - 6 -12 - 24 - 108 repetitions.

On the physical plane, during the *Sun Salutation* the body is warmed, strengthened, and kept supple. Muscles, tendons, and ligaments in the front and back of the body alternately contract and stretch. Respiration, circulation, the nervous system, and the endocrine glands are stimulated. The body enters a state of well-being, because *Tamas* and *Rajas* (see *Gunas*) are equally decreased.

---

60 Skuban, R. (2011), pg. 194.
61 Surya Namaskar, The meditative experience of the Sun Salutation Kirti Peter Michel

On the ethereal plane, the vital center in the middle of the body (*Manipura chakra*) is activated, and *Agni*, the digestive fire, the fire of transformation is activated.

Preparatory exercises and the execution of Surya Namaskar can be found in chapters 11 and 12.

8.2.1 SUN SALUTATIONS AND MANTRAS

The spiritual effect of *Surya Namaskar* is intensified and made more vivid when the respective mantras are sounded. Every mantra represents one of the many different aspects of light.

1.		Tadasana/Anjali Mudra • Inner composure • Inhale and exhale. Palms together at the heart	**OM MITRAYA NAMAHA** Greetings to every friend.
2.		Tadasana with backbend • Inhale • Open towards the light	**OM RAVAYE NAMAHA** Greetings to the radiant one.
3.		Uttanasana • Exhale • Bow to the sun	**OM SURYAYA NAMAHA** Greetings to he who bestows vitality.

4.		**Lunge** • Inhale • Get grounded and lift the higher heart towards the sun.	**OM BHANAVE NAMAHA** Greetings to he who enlightens.
5.		**Adho Mukha Svanasana** • Exhale • Get grounded	**OM KHAGAYA NAMAHA** Greetings to he who permeates all spaces.
6.		**Prostration/humility pose that expresses gratitude:** • Fluid movement into the eight-point stance • Inhale • Exhale	**OM PUSHNE NAMAHA** Greetings to he who nurtures us and gives us strength.
7.		**Bhujangasana** • Inhale • Get grounded and lift the higher heart towards the sun	**OM HIRANYAGARBHAYA NAMAHA** Greetings to the golden seed.
8.		**Adho Mukha Svanasana** • Exhale • Get grounded	**OM MARICAYE NAMAHA** Greetings to the radiant one.
9.		**Lunge** • Inhale • Get grounded and lift the higher heart towards the sun	**OM ADITYAYA NAMAHA** Greetings to the son of Aditi, the cosmic mother.

10.	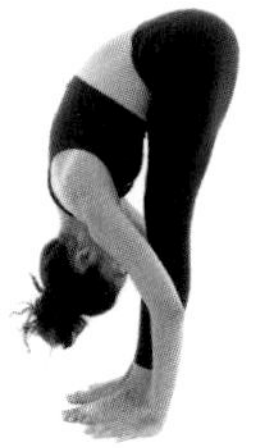	Uttanasana • Exhale • Bow to the sun	**OM SAVITRE NAMAHA** Greetings to the conscious creative power.
11.	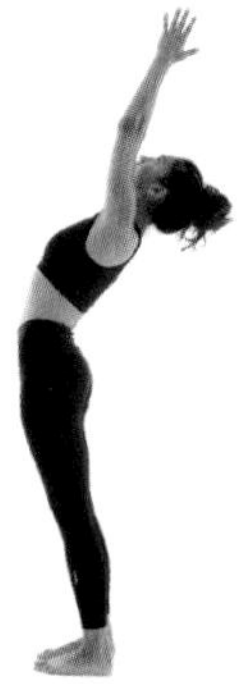	Tadasana with backbend • Inhale • Open up to the light	**OM ARKAYA NAMHA** Greetings to the venerable one.
12.	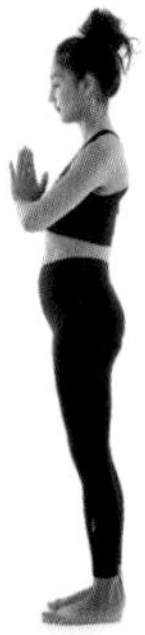	Tadasana • Exhale • Gather yourself	**OM BAHASKARAYA NAMAHA** Greetings to the one who fills everything with his radiance.

8.2.2   SURYA NAMASKAR MODIFICATIONS

The complete cycle as shown above should only be practiced after becoming familiar with the individual Asanas and their transitions. Paying attention to joint alignment to avoid yoga injuries is of particular importance.

Here are two examples:

a) Small Sun Salutation (without prostration)

Surya Namaskar is often referred to as a *yoga warm-up*, but it is recommended to do some preparatory exercises beforehand, such as loosening up shoulders and hips, as well as the spine, to pre-stretch the muscles at the back of the legs and hips, and to prepare the body for the backbends with the appropriate preliminary exercises.

The components of *Surya Namaskar* can be separated into small bites and taught step-by-step. This is particularly helpful in cases of restricted range of motion such as extreme shortening, muscle imbalances, or joint problems.

The following variation, which is an introduction to the classic *Sun Salutation*, emphasizes an erect spine, its axial extension, and hip flexor stretches. The lunge is practiced and the participants can initially focus on safe knee- and foot alignment.

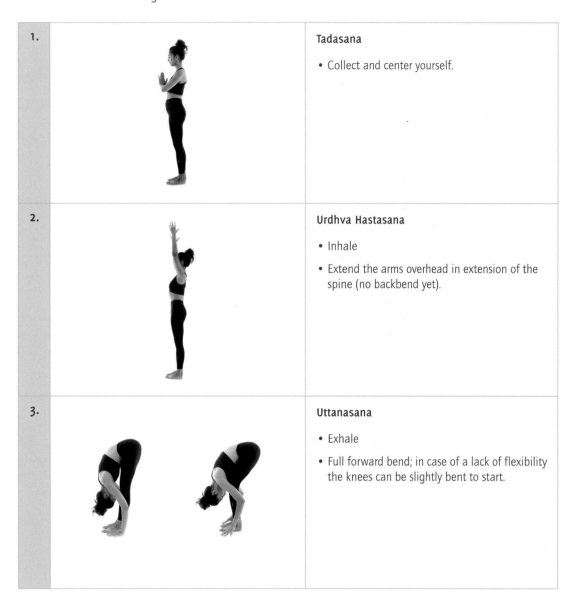

1.		**Tadasana** • Collect and center yourself.
2.		**Urdhva Hastasana** • Inhale • Extend the arms overhead in extension of the spine (no backbend yet).
3.		**Uttanasana** • Exhale • Full forward bend; in case of a lack of flexibility the knees can be slightly bent to start.

4.		**Ardha Uttanasana** • Inhale. • Extend the spine; in case of a lack of flexibility the knees can be slightly bent to start. (In this variation the participants learn the difference between a flexed and an extended spine.)
5.		**Anjaneyasana variation** • Inhale • Still without backbend with emphasis on hip flexor stretch and an erect spine.
6.		**Uttanasana** • Exhale • Full forward bend; in case of a lack of flexibility the knees can be slightly bent to start.
7.		**Urdhva Hastasana** • Inhale • Extend the arms in extension of the spine (no backbend yet).

8.	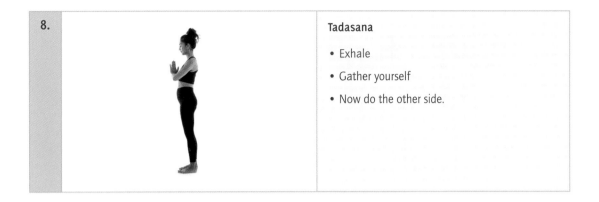	**Tadasana** • Exhale • Gather yourself • Now do the other side.

b) The second example

Here is an incremental approach to the prostration, the *floor Vinyasa*. Steps 1-4 are identical to the *Small Sun Salutation*. The breathing rhythm of the motion sequence on the floor (the prostration) is such that it can be repeated several times before returning to a standing position.

1.		Tadasana
2.		Urdhva Hastasana
3.		Uttanasana

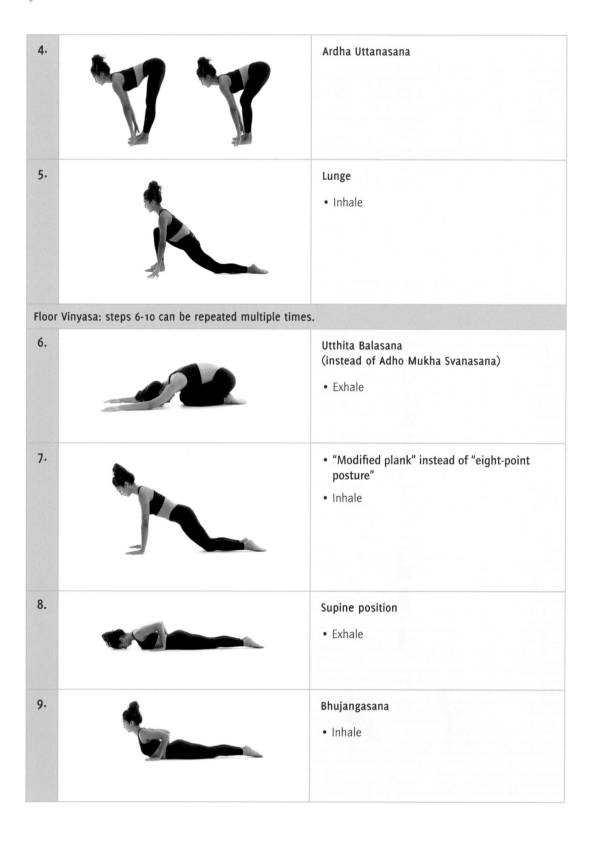

| 4. | | Ardha Uttanasana |
| 5. | | Lunge
• Inhale |

Floor Vinyasa: steps 6-10 can be repeated multiple times.

6.		Utthita Balasana (instead of Adho Mukha Svanasana) • Exhale
7.		• "Modified plank" instead of "eight-point posture" • Inhale
8.		Supine position • Exhale
9.		Bhujangasana • Inhale

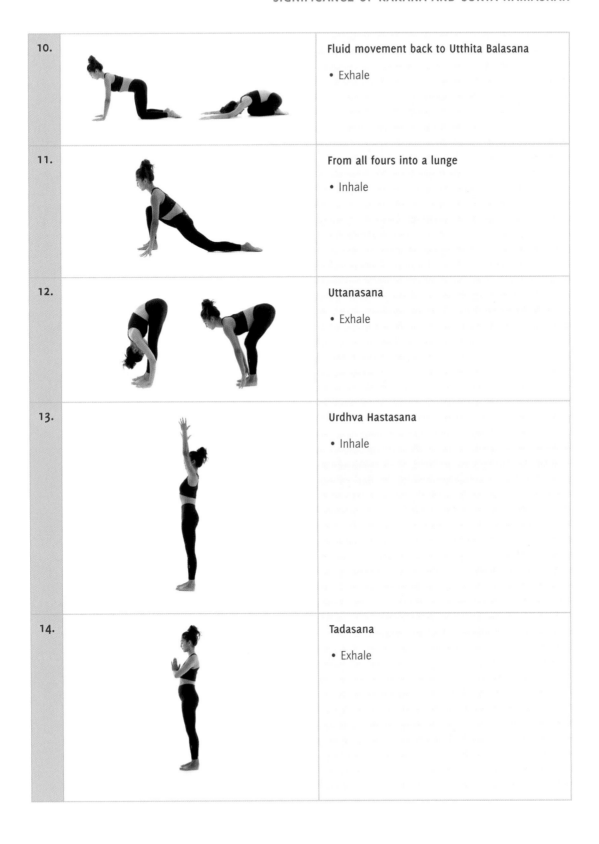

10.		Fluid movement back to Utthita Balasana • Exhale
11.		From all fours into a lunge • Inhale
12.		Uttanasana • Exhale
13.		Urdhva Hastasana • Inhale
14.		Tadasana • Exhale

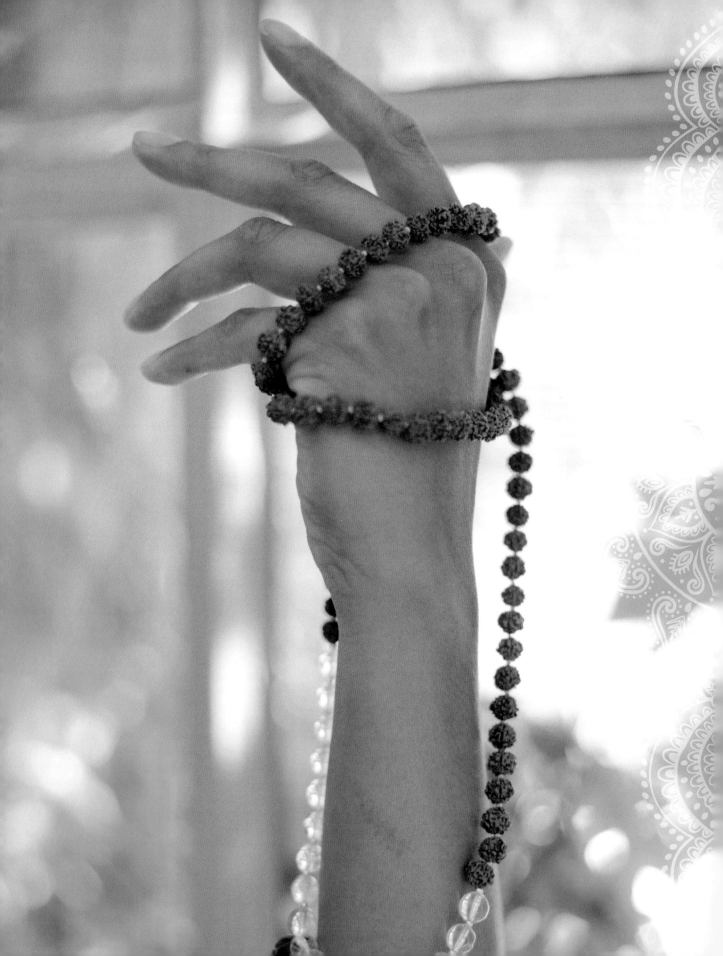

9 YOGIC BREATHING

9   YOGIC BREATHING

"With each inhale I am born, with each exhale I die. On the threshold to the unknown, every moment is a new universe."
Kirti Peter Michel (The Final Curtain)

9.1   IMPORTANCE OF BREATHING

The old German word *Odem* means *breath*, and in the Bible is translated as *what God has breathed into us*. The Hebrew meaning of the word *Ruach* is *breath*, *wind*, *waft*, or *spirit*. The old Indian Sanskrit word *Atman* stands for the *eternal essence of the spirit in the individual*, and the Sanskrit word *Prana* is translated with *breath* and *universal vital energy*.

These terms from different cultures express the coherences of the different dimensions and connections between body, mind, and breath. They also show that the breath is far more important than the purely physical process of breathing by taking in oxygen and releasing spent energy (carbon dioxide).

Conscious breathing is an essential part of the yoga practice. A deep and conscious breath connects us with vital energy, clarity, and strength. A long, slow, and even breath has a calming effect on the mental experience and the mind. An irregular, shallow, and fast breath is often a sign of nervous anxiety or emotional turmoil. The yogis observed the relationship and reciprocity between the breath and the emotional, energy-related, mental, and physical processes early on. In the famous work *Autobiography of a Yogi*, Paramahansa Yogananda explains:

"Prolonged attention is always subject to slowed breathing. By contrast fast or irregular breathing is an unmistakable sign of damaging emotions such as fear, lust, or rage. The restless ape breathes 32 times per minute, but the average human only 18 times. The respiration rate of elephants, turtles, snakes, and other animals known for their longevity is even lower than that of humans. The giant tortoise, for instance, which can reach an age of 300 years, breathes only four times per minute."[62]

---

62 Paramahansa Yogananda (1993). *Autobiography of a Yogi* (chapter 26, pg. 257, paragraph 2). Bern und Munich: Scherz Publishing.

These and similar observations may have prompted early yogis to experiment with the breath. This resulted in a system of complex and highly effective breathing exercises, which in yoga are called Pranayama.

Prana = ethereal, universal vital energy / Ayama = expansion, stretching, distribution

Pranayama is translated as *the distribution of vital energy. Breath control* and *breath regulation* are also common names.

Pranayama in the classical sense is comprised of breathing techniques that are practiced in combination with physical poses (Asanas) or Bandhas (energy locks) and greatly affect the subtle body.

9.2 THE BREATH IN EVERYDAY LIFE

Most people breathe unconsciously in their daily lives, which is primarily because the breath has accompanied us from birth as a matter of course. The body breathes without our having to do anything, which on the one hand is a big advantage because otherwise we would be unable to sleep at night for extended periods of time.

Compared to people, dolphins for instance, breathe consciously and are therefore only able to sleep with one half of their brain while the other half controls their breathing. But it is precisely the unconscious breathing that often causes the breath to grow shallow and unnoticed. This is particularly true during exclusively seated activities. The consequences are a lack of energy, fatigue, loss of concentration, usually combined with various digestive problems.

When someone is under mental and emotional strain, under time- or performance pressure, the breath is generally not just short but also fast and irregular. In the worst-case scenario, this sends danger signals to the nervous system (fight-or- flight reflex) and results in the release of stress hormones. If these cannot be reduced through exercise or other suitable means it results in a self-perpetuating stress spiral.

"Take a deep breath", or "Hold your breath", or "I need a breather", all are statements we hear in every life whenever we need to find inner calm, need to reflect, focus, gain clarity, or strength.

People who have paid little attention to or ignored their breath all their lives would most likely be overwhelmed by a complete seated breathing meditation if neither concentration nor awareness and their power of observation have previously been sufficiently trained. Beginning with a practice that combines breathing and Asanas would offer some valuable opportunities here that would pave the participant's way to more breath awareness and more advanced Pranayama:

1. Becoming aware of the breath.

2. Observing the breath.

3. Being aware of the breathing spaces.

4. Directing the breath to different breathing spaces.

5. Introduction to complete yogic breathing.

6. Finding one's own pace.

7. Lengthening the breath.

8. Ujjayi breath

As with all things in life, the dose is important. Attention to the breath requires a certain amount of calm and time. When setting the mood for a yoga class it helps to initially direct the attention to the body and then to breath awareness (from tangible to ethereal). How long this process takes depends on how much experience the students already have.

Experienced yoga practitioners can concentrate considerably longer while novices tend to become distracted, or when an exercise is practiced in a supine position they may sink into Tamas (fatigue or lethargy). Particularly with novices, the attention should periodically be gently directed back to breath awareness so the breathing experience can gradually manifest itself in the consciousness.

9.2.1   BREATH AWARENESS

Breath awareness is the first step towards deeper breathing consciousness. It is about liberating the breath from the cellar of unconsciousness and developing a sense for the opportunities that come with conscious breathing. Breath awareness also means self-awareness.

With breath awareness the aspects of daily life (How am I doing? Is something pinching somewhere? Is my stomach, back, or neck tense? Am I hungry or thirsty? Do I need a break?) can also be felt much more keenly. Breath awareness means mindfulness.

9.2.2   WATCHING YOUR BREATH

An essential part of the yoga practice is learning to observe, which is also the basis for all meditation. During the practice we initially learn to observe the body, our thoughts, and emotions, and one of the very first steps in the yoga practice is to observe the breath, the breathing process. Here many people learn right away that just observing the breath is enough to allow the breath to flow longer and calmer.

For most yoga novices, simply observing the breath for a while is a new experience. Being aware of how the breath wants to flow by itself. When we are at rest, but also when the body is moving. Being fully aware of the breath without trying to regulate it right away when the movements become more intense. Internally moving with the breath and witnessing where the breath travels, its rhythm, how long or how deep it flows. Breath awareness and observation create an inner understanding of the entire breathing process, and is also the basis for all forms of breath control all the way to the more subtle forms of yoga, energy control.

Experiencing breath observation can initially be practiced in a relaxed supine position to subsequently be integrated into the practice and the rest- and reflection phases. Observing the breath during the Asana practice, before and after, takes the practitioners deeper into self-awareness and themselves. And the participant will most certainly experience again and again that he forgets to breathe when his attention is focused on the movement and body alignment. Continuously "remembering the breath" is part of the yoga practice and it is the yoga instructor's job to integrate these aspects into yoga instruction.

The breathing process is broken down as follows:

» Inhalation –> inspiration (Puraka),

» Exhalation –> expiration (Rechaka).

» Breathing pause –> (Kumbhaka). After every natural inhale and exhale there is a brief pause. The natural pause is slightly longer after exhalation than after inhalation.

By calmly shifting attention to the breathing process we can become aware of these brief pauses. Being aware of the breathing pauses makes the breaths calmer and deeper.

Advanced Pranayama techniques teach us to greatly lengthen these natural pauses. Within a harmonic practice these pauses should only be extended gradually. Some forms of meditation are based on the natural pauses between breaths. Since our thoughts also come to a rest during these pauses, they are also referred to as "gaps between our thoughts" or "leaps into infinity".

9.2.3 AWARENESS OF BREATHING SPACES

Awareness of breathing spaces is closely linked to breath observation. Breathing spaces are those areas of the body in which we can perceive breathing movement. When the breath is shallow, we feel it primarily in the upper chest area or rather the area around the collarbone. When the breath flows deeper and longer, we can feel it in the following areas:

» Chest (in the front towards the sternum; to the sides into the costal arches; in the upper back to the shoulder blades, and up to the collarbone area);

» Abdomen (depending on perceptive ability, all the way down to the pelvic floor);

» Flanks (lateral expansion between ribs and iliac crest);

» Back (expansion in the middle and lower back).

The noticeable breathing movements in the trunk are a result of the raising and lowering of the ribcage (sternum and ribs) and the moving of the diaphragm, which drops as we inhale, putting gentle pressure on the internal organs, and rises again as we exhale.

9.2.4 DIRECTING THE BREATH TO DIFFERENT BREATHING SPACES

To be better able to feel the breathing movements, in the beginning it is helpful to rest the palms for a while first on the stomach, then the side of the ribcage in the area of the costal arches, and on the collarbone area. By breathing into the palms we can develop an awareness of the respective areas and breathing spaces.

This can be amplified by mentally directing the breath to the lower pelvic region, the low back, the flanks, the area of the higher heart, and under/between the shoulder blades.

The somewhat subtle breathing movements in the different breathing spaces (especially the back and pelvic floor) can be amplified and felt more intensely through a targeted Asana practice. This allows the participants to feel more keenly into the different areas of the body, resulting in improved cognition and differentiation of different sensory impressions.

Conscious breathing is energy control. Wherever we shift our attention, energy begins to flow there at the same time. Energy always follows mindfulness. This can easily be verified by focusing for a few moments on your relaxed palms while mentally directing energy there. After a short while, most people feel a slight prickly sensation or warmth in their palms.

a) Breathing physiology

The main function of respiration is to supply our cells with oxygen, as well as the elimination of carbon dioxide. But from a yoga perspective, we don't just take in oxygen with our breath, but also Prana, universal vital energy.

When we inhale (inspiration –> Puraka), oxygen-rich air makes its way from the outside via the nose, the trachea, the bronchial tubes, all the way to the alveoli (air sacs in the lungs where a gaseous exchange takes place). The lungs expand in the ribcage. The intercostal muscles lift the costal arches, the ribcage widens and the diaphragm drops.

When we exhale (expiration –> Rachaka), used up, carbon-dioxide-rich air is expelled. Lungs and ribcage contract, the intercostal muscles relax and the diaphragm rises again. Some of the previously inhaled air always remains in the lungs. By actively engaging the respiratory muscles, exhalation can be further accelerated.

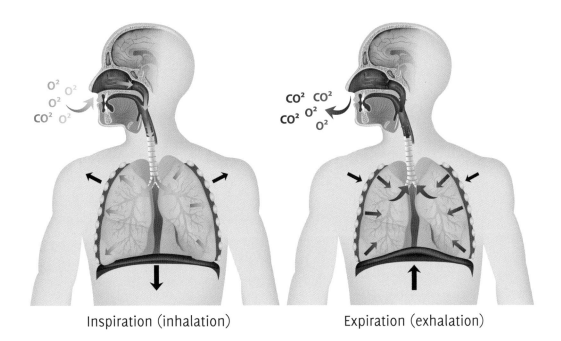

Inspiration (inhalation)   Expiration (exhalation)

Fig. 12 a/b: Breathing process and workings of the lungs

From a physiological standpoint we differentiate

» External breathing (lung breathing: oxygen is absorbed with inhalation and carbon dioxide is expelled with exhalation.

» Internal breathing (cellular breathing: gaseous exchange between cells and blood).

b) Mouth and nose breathing

Nose breathing is considered physiological breathing. When we breathe through the nose, the nose hairs at the nose entrance intercept foreign bodies. The inhaled air is moistened in the lining of the nose and having warmed up, moves on through the nasal cavity, the pharynx and the larynx, to the trachea, where it branches off into the two bronchial tubes.

When breathing through the mouth, the air moves from the mouth to the oral cavity, the pharynx and the larynx, and finally the trachea. In the process it is neither warmed up, nor moistened or cleaned, and has the additional disadvantage of drying out the oral cavity and pharynx. If the nose is not stuffy, like with a cold, it is definitely much healthier and advisable to always breathe through the nose.

c) Respiratory center

Respiration is controlled by the respiratory center, the *medulla oblongata*. It is the continuation of the brain stem and is part of the central nervous system. Rhythmic breathing and the depth and rate of breathing are coordinated here because chemoreceptors are constantly checking the blood for oxygen- and carbon dioxide content as well as pH-value. The blood pH-value indicates how acidic or alkaline the blood is. Respiratory drive (breathing stimulus) increases when the oxygen content goes down, carbon dioxide content goes up, and the pH-value falls. The respiratory drive weakens with increasing oxygen content, decreasing carbon dioxide content, and rising pH-value.

9.3 COMPLETE BREATHING IN YOGA

"True people draw their breath from way below, while average people breathe only with the throat."[63] (Zhuang Z.)

The breath is generally divided into *belly-*, *chest-*, and *collarbone breaths*.

Belly- or *diaphragmatic breathing*: As you inhale, the belly visibly bulges; breathing is controlled primarily by the diaphragm. Belly breathing makes up about 60% of the breath volume. This type of breathing is particularly noticeable in infants and young children. Belly breathing gently massages the internal organs because the diaphragm drops. This is the healthiest way to breathe in daily life.

Chest breathing: The ribcage visibly rises and falls, and respiration is controlled primarily by the intercostal muscles. Chest breathing makes up about 30% of breath volume. Women often breathe exclusive in the chest if they want their waist to remain small and/or due to clothing that is too tight in the stomach area.

Collarbone breathing: This is a very shallow way of breathing that takes place strictly in the upper ribcage area. Respiration reaches primarily the upper lungs, the apex of the lungs. Collarbone breathing makes up about 10% of breath volume. This form of breathing is generally used in stressful situations. Long-term shallow breathing has a negative effect on the energy supply via oxygen and the metabolism. People get tired quickly, feel weak, and most likely have digestive problems.

"Complete yogic breathing" includes all three areas.

» The breath is first directed into the belly. Breathing movement in the belly is visible due to the contracting/dropping of the diaphragm. The breath is loosely directed downward; any attempt at "pushing the breath down" should be avoided. This is where the previously mentioned breathing spaces come into play. For instance, if the breathing movement travels easily into the belly in a supine position, the expansion can also subtly be felt in the flanks, in the lower pelvic region, and in the low back.

» Still inhaling, the breath flows into the chest. Here, too, the expansion can be felt in the front, the sides, and the upper back.

» All the way at the top, the breath flows into the apex of the lungs, ventilating the collarbone area.

» Exhalation takes place in the opposite order from top to bottom.

---

63 Zhuang, Z, *The True Classic of Southern Florescence*. Düsseldorf/Köln. Eugen Diederichs Publishing.

The "complete yogic breathing" breathing process can be compared to a gentle wave moving through the body. It is also called wave of breath.

The simple, combination breath movement exercise "arm raises" can let us feel this wave more distinctly in all areas of the body. Moreover, the movement expands the chest and collarbone area.

Inhalation: The inhalation wave connects us with the aspects of admittance, acceptance, activity, vastness, expansion, and abundance.

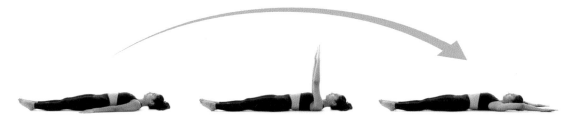

Photo left: No breath (brief, natural pause)

Photo center: The inhalation wave flows from the lower abdomen into the chest and collarbone area. The arms accompany the breath and act as a kind of "breath indicator".

Photo right: Full breath (brief, natural pause).

Exhalation: The exhalation wave connects us with the aspects of letting go, relinquishing, passivity, contracting, and emptiness.

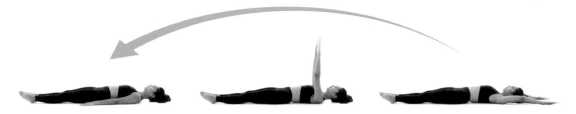

Photo right: Full breath (brief, natural pause).

Photo center: The exhalation wave flows from the top downward. Active exhalation can be supported by abdominal contractions. Here the abdominal muscles act as respiratory support muscles. In this case, the exhalation wave is felt from bottom to top, i.e. rising.

Photo left: No breath (brief, natural pause).

The natural pauses occur automatically, but they can be gently lengthened as the practice becomes more advanced.

The inhalation and exhalation wave represents life's polarities. During a breath cycle, we experience becoming and passing, coming and going, abundance and emptiness.

9.4   FINDING YOUR OWN PACE – BREATH FLOW PRACTICE

For a large portion of the population, everyday life is "jam-packed". Family, work, and leisure activities largely determine the temporal framework. One of the most common complaints is the problem of not having enough time. Sometimes it seems as though we are all rushed through our daily lives by deadlines and appointments that must be adhered to.

This alone is bad enough, but it seems that many people also rush through their free time. For many that collective haste and breathlessness has become a habit. Practicing in the breathing rhythm gently interrupts it. Not only do our movements become slower when we prioritize the breath, but they also gain in strength, intensity, and vitality.

The above exercise "arm raises" not only supports the experience of the breathing spaces, it also helps the practitioner develop a feel for his own pace that isn't dictated by someone else. Moving with the breathing rhythm sounds easy, but for many it is in fact a little challenging at first. On the one hand, one must concentrate on the body movements and on the other hand, focus on the breathing movements, and the two must be coordinated.

By focusing on the breath first and then allowing the body, the movement, to follow, we gradually build a breath-guided practice. Among other things, this type of practice is one of the many reasons why lots of yoga practitioners report getting back in touch with themselves through the yoga practice.

Even if an instructor leads breath-guided flows during a yoga class (e.g. *Sun Salutation*) and sets a certain pace that matches the breath, with respect to the own breath-guided practice it makes sense to frequently give participants the opportunity to freely practice within their own breathing rhythm. By doing so they will over time develop a sure feel for their own pace.

9.5   LENGTHENING THE BREATH

Within the yoga practice, there are breathing techniques that are based on short and very forceful puffs of breath. *Kapalabhati*, a purifying exercise, includes fast and forceful exhales. *Bhastrika Pranayama* (a warming breathing technique, primarily used in combination with a subsequent meditation) includes forceful inhalation and exhalation.

But generally the goal is to take subtle, calm, and long breaths. When someone has "a long breath", it suggests a certain amount of stamina and inner strength. In the Asana practice a long breath is valuable, especially when the Asanas are physically demanding or the movements from one Asana to the next have long levers. A long breath also creates calm, and that is the main reason to learn and practice it.

The breath can be lengthened during both the inhalation and the exhalation phase. It makes sense to first practice a longer exhalation since a long exhale has a cleansing and deacidifying effect. Inhaled air can be better taken in when the lungs have been emptied first. Besides, most people find it easier to exhale longer.

Since lengthening the breath is based on a contraction in the esophagus, when practicing with inhalation, at first it could cause unpleasant sensations like not being able to "get enough air". After a while, once breath awareness and the respiratory muscles have developed and lengthening the breath has become familiar, it becomes easier to also apply this technique to lengthening inhalations.

Sometimes lengthening the breath is also practiced in sports and to some extent in respiratory therapy by using pursed-lip breathing. Compared to pursed-lip breathing, lengthening the breath by contracting the glottis in the laryngeal area has the advantage that air accumulates behind the nearly closed vocalis muscle, which activates the respiratory muscles.[64]

Preliminary exercises such as sounding out vowels while exhaling, humming or exhaling with the mouth slightly open, can be helpful in acquiring a feel for the glottis contraction in the larynx.

Breath lengthening preliminary exercises can be practiced in combination with the exercise "arm raises":

1. As you inhale through the nose, extend the arms overhead:

2. As you exhale, sound out vowels, blow out, or hum:

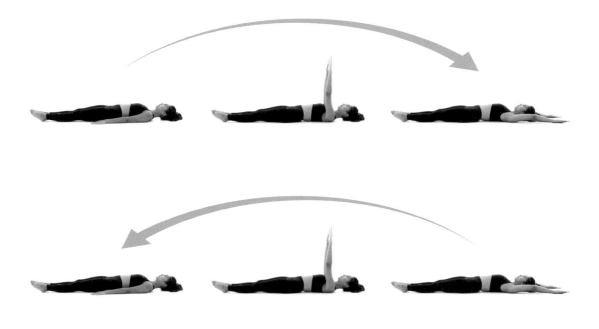

---

64 Trökes, A. (2004). *Pranayama, BDY Studienbegleitung in der Yogalehrerausbildung.* (pg. 27). Göttingen. BDY branch office.

9.6 THE UJJAYI BREATH

Ujjayi means *the victorious one*. This breath-lengthening technique is known as the *victorious turning of the inner breath*. The gentle fricative created by contracting the glottis in the laryngeal area is reminiscent of the sound of the ocean surf, which is why this breathing technique is sometimes also called *sound-of-the-ocean breathing*.

The Ujjayi breathing technique requires strictly nose breathing during both breathing pauses. The lengthened breaths supply the body with lots of energy (Prana) during inhalation, and stimulate a cleansing process in the body and the lungs during exhalation. Ujjayi breathing creates a slight vibration in the bronchial tubes, which removes dirt particles from the lungs. Moreover, the long exhalations leave less air remaining in the lungs. The larynx closure combined with the vigorous inhalation and exhalation strengthens and tones the diaphragm. The intercostal muscles are strengthened and stretched, depending on the breathing phase.

In the second chapter of the *Hatha Yoga Pradipika*, *Ujjayi* is described as one of the main Pranayamas. A number of variations are derived from the technique (*Anuloma Ujjayi*) described there.

But the basis of Ujjayi is the narrowing of the glottis. It is practiced in many yoga schools, such as *Ashtanga Yoga* or the related Vinyasa flow schools, during the Asana practice. Not only because it triggers the "body fire" (digestive fire) according to HYP II, 53, but also because the breath, when performed in this manner, flows very consciously.

The practitioner then listens over the gentle "airflow sound" in the throat during the entire practice. It makes it more difficult to forget the breath, as it is present throughout the practice. However, loud ocean sounds have no effect. In some yoga classes one may get the impression that the participants are competing against each other for the loudest throat sounds. Ujjayi needs to be only as loud as a whisper to be effective. You should only barely be able to hear just yourself.

Is there a "correct" breath?

Sometimes participants come to yoga class with rigid concepts about "the right way to breathe". People with a fitness background have learned to exhale upon exertion. Others have very firm principles when it comes to breathing and the pelvic floor.

Some people believe they must breathe very loudly to get an adequate effect, and others mentally roll their eyes when the breathing topic comes up because they consider it a bore. And occasionally participants put pressure on themselves about breathing "correctly", for instance during a *Sun Salutation*.

With all these different ideas and concepts, adding determinate yoga principles or provoking a right-and-wrong discussion isn't very helpful. Often the desire for specific breathing rules is triggered by insecurity that should not be perpetuated with additional rules.

The simplest and most effective way is to guide participants into breath awareness, to strengthen their self-awareness, and to allow them or rather their bodies to decide how the breath wants to flow.

When carefully watching the breath after a while, a logical breathing and movement pattern usually develops on its own.

There are a number of Asanas and exercises that, from a purely physiological standpoint, support exhalation. These include forward bends, twists, and half or full inversions. Backbends on the other hand support inhalation. During backbends the breathing spaces in the ribcage open, the breath flows almost automatically into the chest.

That is why, for instance, we exhale when bending forward during a *Sun Salutation* and inhale during all back extensions. But it doesn't help when this knowledge is imposed on people. Instead it is better to practice shorter sequences with close breath observation (without deliberately directing the breath). This helps develop a deeper understanding of the breathing process and bolsters faith in one's own feeling for the breath.

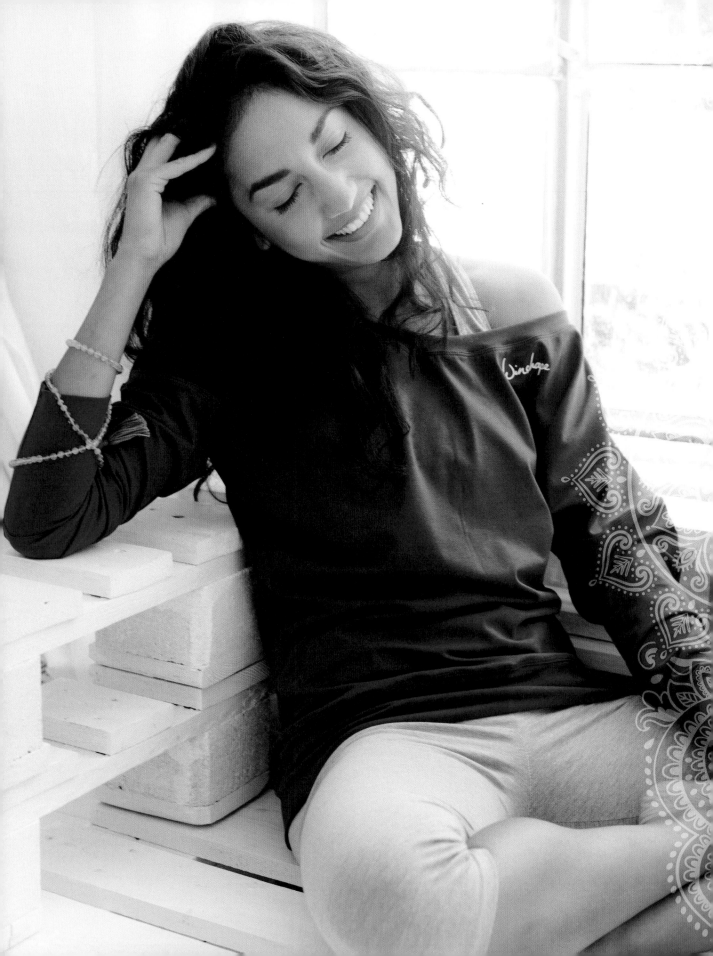

10 RELAXATION

10   RELAXATION

10.1   FROM ABSENTMINDEDNESS TO COMPOSURE

The desire to relax is one of the major themes of the day. The faster technological advances take place in nearly all areas of life, the more difficult it seems to get off the hamster-wheel of faster, higher, farther. In addition we love a certain amount of excitement. The entire entertainment industry is geared to people's appetite for action and thrills.

But the longing for inner peace, relaxed tranquility and meaning is vastly increasing in a large portion of the population, which, if nothing else, is apparent in the growing popularity of yoga and other Far Eastern disciplines.

The supply of relaxation opportunities is very diverse. There seems to be a program for every type. The palette ranges from active relaxation in nature, to sports and exercise, all the way to calm and meditative choices, which is what this chapter focuses on.

Interestingly the term *relaxation* as such does not exist in yoga terminology. It almost seems as though what we in the West consider relaxation is a kind of "by-catch" on the yoga path. Correspondingly Sanskrit names like *Yoga Nidra* (yoga healing sleep) and *Shavasana* (corpse pose/supine position for practicing deep relaxation) come closest to the term relaxation.

But what exactly is relaxation? How is relaxation defined here in the West?

The word re-LAX-ation already suggests that it must be a relatively tension-free state. What people associate with relaxation differs from person to person.

The dictionary defines relaxation as *"the feeling of being physically and mentally calm or unconstrained and tension-free."*

The German Wellness Association's definition is: *"Relaxation refers to physically and mentally noticeable and measurable state that is considered the opposite of tension".*[65]

All processes that trigger the experience of relaxation or tension and the associated noticeable and measurable symptoms are controlled by the nervous system.

---

65 http://www.wellnessverband.de/infodienste/lexikon/e/entspannung.php

10.2   THE NERVOUS SYSTEM

The central nervous system (CNS) is our vital control center and is formed by nerve structures of the brain and the medulla. The main tasks are conscious and unconscious thinking, voluntary motor activity, and stimulus processing of the sensory organs. It is closely linked to the hormonal system. The CNS controls body functions such as respiration, movement, procreation, and digestion.

The peripheral nervous system (PNS) includes all neural pathways outside the skull and the vertebral canal. *Peripher* means *away from the trunk*. Beginning at the medulla, the neural pathways permeate the body all the way to the outer extremities, similar to a large net. Here afferent neural pathways transmit information from the sensory organs to the brain and medulla, and efferent neural pathways transmit information from the CNS to the periphery.

In terms of function, the rigid delineation of CNS and PNS would not make sense, as it is a nervous system that is divided strictly by its position in the body.

10.2.1   VOLUNTARY AND VEGETATIVE NERVOUS SYSTEM

A functional classification of the nervous system is the *voluntary* (*somatic*) and the *vegetative* (*autonomic, involuntary*) nervous system.

The voluntary nervous system is subject to volition, conscious control such as specific muscle movement, while the vegetative (involuntary) nervous system functions independent of volition. This includes all vital internal activities such as heartbeat, digestion, respiration, that must continue to function, for instance, while we sleep.

The vegetative nervous system is divided into the *sympathetic nervous system* and the *parasympathetic nervous system*. Both are antagonists as they have opposite functions.

Their functions are also called *performance state* and *relaxation state*.

10.2.2   PERFORMANCE STATE – SYMPATHETIC NERVOUS SYSTEM

The *sympathetic nervous system* activates body functions that place the body in a state of heightened performance readiness. This state is also called fight-or-flight mode.

When a situation becomes so dangerous that it presents a major threat to life or safety, large strength reserves are quickly released that prompt a person to act fast and immediately.

The pituitary gland, the central hormonal control organ, causes adrenaline to be released via the adrenal gland, which results in a number of immediate reactions.

» The organism reacts with raised blood pressure.

» The heart beats faster and stronger ("heart is in the throat").

» The bronchial tubes expand.

» Breath frequency and oxygen uptake increase.

» Blood vessels in the brain, in the intestines, and in the skin contract (skin gets pale).

» Digestion slows.

» The liver releases glucose into the bloodstream for a quick energy supply.

» The pancreas works harder.

» The pupils dilate and the eyes focus on the distance.

» Increased excretion from the sweat glands cools the skin (moist hands).

» Salivary gland production decreases (dry mouth).

» Muscle tone increases.

» Metabolism is stimulated and nutrient oxidation increases, which results in depletion of strength reserves.

» The individual is in a state of tense alertness.

The performance state is a protective function that is essential to the survival of the organism in order to be able to act during danger.

10.2.3   RECOVERY STATE – PARASYMPATHETIC NERVOUS SYSTEM

The *parasympathetic nervous system* is the antagonist to the sympathetic nervous system. Once a dangerous situation has passed, the parasympathetic nervous system becomes active and the organism begins to relax. This restores inner equilibrium (homeostasis) in the body.

The parasympathetic nervous system takes care of the basal metabolism via neurotransmitters (acetylcholine). It activates body functions that serve regeneration and the building of energy reserves. The parasympathetic nervous system's activity is felt much less acutely than the activation of the performance state as these processes are much more subtle.

» Blood pressure and heart rate drop during the recovery phase.

» Blood vessels expand (warm sensation).

» Breathing rate slows down (breaths become longer and calmer).

» Salivary glands become active (water in the mouth).

» Digestive processes are stimulated (belly noises due to increased peristalsis, stomach growls).

» Excretory processes are stimulated (urge to urinate, urge to evacuate the bowels).

» Sweat gland excretion decreases.

» Pupils constrict.

» Metabolic processes and nutrient oxidation slow down.

» Muscle tone decreases; muscles relax.

In the recovery phase the body feels pleasantly warm and heavy due to the relaxed muscles and expanded blood vessels. Sleep is the most intensive form of recovery.[66]

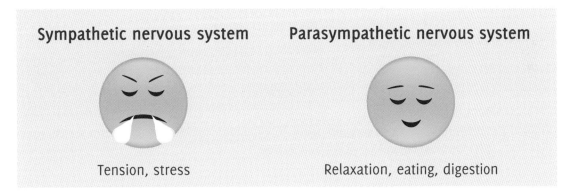

Fig. 13: Sympathetic and parasympathetic nervous systems

In a healthy and balanced system or way of life, a performance state is followed by a phase of recovery and regeneration. This switch takes time and a certain amount of tranquility. If the recovery state is blocked by too much activity or a constant state of alert, the organism is off-balance, which can manifest itself in many different stress symptoms.

10.3 STRESS

In everyday life, our attention is largely focused outward. Activities like driving, operating machinery, dealing and communicating with people, or simultaneously coordinating different activities require alert attentiveness. For instance, when you are inattentive in traffic, it can have life-threatening consequences.

---

66 Kruse, P., Pavlekovic, B. & Haak, K. (1992). *Autogenic Training*. (pg. 24). Niedernhausen. Falkner Publishing.

But when our attention is continuously focused outward, and additional factors like time and performance pressure come into play, focused, relaxed attentiveness can quickly turn to overload. Our entire Western society is geared to increased performance closely linked with an extremely high activity level. When the harmonic equilibrium between tension and relaxation is continuously disrupted, it directly affects the mental-emotional-physical wellbeing, and ultimately our health. This is called *stress*.

The word *stress* comes from the Latin word strictus and means tightened, taut, tense. In itself this is nothing negative, because many things in life must be taut or tense in order to function.

Siddharta Gautama, the founder of Buddhism, recognized approx. 500 BC: *"When you tighten one string too much it will break. If you tighten it too little you cannot play on it."*[67]

From a physiological standpoint, stress is the organism's reaction to physical or emotional stimuli that present a challenge. We experience these challenges every day. We are hungry, thirsty, tired and need some sleep, we are cold and need warmth. In this case the organism gives us the appropriate signals to regain our equilibrium (homeostasis).

There are different types and manifestations of stress. Frequent stress factors are noise, time and deadline pressure, conflict and disagreements, rivalry, perfectionism, ambition, crowds, fear of failure, fear of responsibility, lack of self-worth, an inability to delegate tasks or say "no", disorder.

Different people experience stress very differently. The founder and "father" of stress research, Hans Seyle , thus differentiated between *eustress* and *distress*.[68]

10.3.1 EUSTRESS

Eustress (eu = good) refers to all forms of stress that are felt as positive. Eustress is associated with a certain thrill. This form of stress tends to have a stimulating and motivating effect. Eustress triggers the release of happiness hormones. Being in love is an acute form of eustress. So are sports like bungee jumping, rafting, and other activities that release a pleasant-feeling hormone cocktail.

The release of stress hormones (see performance state) places the organism in a higher state of alertness and responsiveness. This allows the organism to react incredibly fast in dangerous situations. Subsequently one feels awake, alive, refreshed, and perfused. In a healthy organism the stress hormones released during eustress can be completely reduced in a short period of time.

---

67 https://www.aphorismen.de/zitat/190559
68 Seyle, H. (1976). *Stress in health and disease*. Verlag Butterworth-Heinemann.

10.3.2 DISTRESS

Distress (dis = bad) is perceived as a negative and unpleasant state of tension. Nowadays, the use of the word stress generally refers to the distress aspect. But today it is assumed that we can still develop abilities or skills under the influence of distress that will benefit the individual.

Distress is primarily experienced as strain that is inflicted externally. When we are distressed we fell physically and mentally overloaded, overburdened, constrained, pressured, powerless, worn-out. There are many stress factors and every individual experiences stress differently. Energy activation, the release of stress hormones takes place just as it does in eustress (performance state), but cannot be used in a positive way.

When this hormone cascade triggered by a stressful situation cannot be reduced via an appropriate energy release (exercise or targeted relaxation), the organism becomes overloaded. In this case the brain does all it can to return to a normal state. More stress hormones are formed and released in an effort to create a balance. This can result in feelings of inner and muscular tension, fear, and muscle tremors, elevated blood pressure, rapid heartbeat, etc.

If the stressful situation is long-term, one is in a self-perpetuating cycle. The organism's motivation is increasingly inhibited and blocked.

Stress reactions can also be triggered without external causes, meaning just by imagining a calamitous situation, e.g. extreme mental-emotional stress like test anxiety or fear of all sorts of failures. When the body is in a constant state of alert, and relaxation or regeneration are not possible, stress can result in illness.

"From an evolutionary standpoint, a state of stress should only last for a few hours as a kind of 'life insurance' and not become chronic long-term strain. But when that is the case, it can result in physical stress reactions that threaten health and cause health problems such as susceptibility to infections, chronic fatigue and chronic pain, sleep disorders, etc."[69] *(Werner Stangl).*

10.4 RELAXATION

From a physiological point of view, *relaxation* is the nervous system's switching from performance state to recovery state. Since the sympathetic and parasympathetic nervous systems are governed by the vegetative, autonomic nervous system, the tension and relaxation functions cannot be triggered voluntarily.

It is therefore not enough to cheerfully tell someone "Just relax!" when they are at the apex of the stress curve. The will or desire for relaxation does not automatically trigger an immediate state of calm. If it were that simple there would be no need for the entire wellness and relaxation industry.

---

69 http://psychologie.stangl.eu/definition/Stress.shtml@Werner Stangl

Along with recognizing the stress-triggering patterns and factors, switching from a performance state to a recovery state can be practiced as a permanent solution.

Western forms of relaxation, such as *autogenic training* (AT) or *progressive muscle relaxation* (PM) on the one hand are based on improved body awareness, and practice the recovery state via specific techniques like visualizing heaviness, warmth, and certain relaxing images (AT) and targeted tensing and relaxing (PM), so the changeover process into a state of rest is purposefully practiced.

As the term "training" already implies, relaxation training requires a certain amount of regularity and repetition. The content of the yoga practice includes far more than just relaxation training, but during the relaxation phases (deep or final relaxation, Yoga Nidra) works with the same techniques (body awareness, breath awareness, visualization, autosuggestions). Switching the organism from a performance state to a recovery state in a yoga class takes place on the one hand via active movement (e.g. *Sun Salutations/* stress reduction), via deliberate slowing of movements during the Asana practice, and though Pranayama and meditation.

According to Dr. Christian Fuchs[70], there is evidence that the founder of autogenic training, the neurologist J.H. Schultz, was inspired by individual yoga techniques during the conception of AT. Thus Schulz propagates AT as a modern and "rational" counterpart to the "mysticism-tinted" Hatha Yoga. In his article *"Oberstufe des autogenen Trainings und Raya Yoga"* (advanced autogenic training and Raya Yoga) published in 1932, the doctor compares the upper level of his autogenic training with classical yoga based on Patanjali. He concludes: "In this sense autogenic training can be described as physiologically rationalized and systematized yoga (...)."[71] In the 1960s, Schultz distanced himself from his earlier statements and announced that AT had been developed from European medical hypnosis.[72]

10.5   PERCEPTION

If one were to compare the content of a yoga unit with the recipe for a tasty and multi-course meal, perception would be one of the most important ingredients that should not be left out of any course.

Perception is defined as assimilation, observation, understanding, and *processing of sensory input.* Awareness always happens in the moment. It is the immediate experience of the present. By training awareness, the sensory organs are also being sharpened. The practitioner immerses himself in the moment, which is prerequisite for complete relaxation. When the focus is directed exclusively to awareness, mental processes instantly take a backseat. Namely, for as long as the ability to concentrate allows the focus on perception.

70 In: *Der Weg des Yoga, Handbuch für Übende und Lehrende.* pg. 532 (10.1.1). BDY, Vianova.
71 J. H. Schultz (1932). Advanced Autogenic Training and Raya Yoga. *Magazine for Comprehensive Neurology and Psychiatry, volume 139, 34.*
72 In: The Yoga Path, Manual for Practitioners and Instructors, pg. 532. BDY, Vianova.

Perceiving the environment takes place via the sensory organs:

» Eyes – visual perception (vision);

» Ears – auditory perception (hearing, listening);

» Nose – olfactory perception (smell);

» Mouth – gustatory perception (taste);

» Skin – exteroceptive perception (feel, touch).

Caring for the senses has special significance in yoga and Ayurveda. The more explicitly and subtly the senses function, the sharper is our perception of our environment. *Sensuousness* means perceiving with all our senses. When our senses are impaired, we generally don't realize it right away, as this process is very stealthy. Most of the time it is noticed due to external factors, namely when the senses require increasingly stronger stimuli to be able to function: when grandpa keeps turning up the volume on the TV and wonders why the neighbors complain.

Others require lots of salt or "hot spices" for their food because they otherwise are unable to taste it. Declining vision is usually noticed very quickly when we are no longer able to read small print. And many people develop "anosmia" and thoroughly "spoil" their fellow human beings with the creations of the perfume industry.

When the senses no longer function our experiences are also greatly restricted. We can only perceive our environment through our senses or with the physical body. The exclusive focus on one of the senses (see Dharana) allows the senses to sharpen again.

Body and breath awareness are important in the yoga practice.

Body awareness is actively focusing our perception on the body and the body's interior. Training and improving body awareness promotes:

» Perceiving the body as a whole. Someone who tends to be overly intellectual in everyday life often fails to hear or ignore the body's most basic signals.

» Detecting muscle or organ tension.

» Perceiving the position, tonicity, and movement state of the muscles and the locomotor system (proprioception).

» Perceiving equilibrium (our sense of balance coordinates our body's position in the room).

» The differentiation of properties according to the elements with respect to the body (see chapter 4 – The *Gunas*), in terms of heavy, light, permeable, warm, cold, wide, narrow, etc.

The following are suggestions for training and improving body awareness:

» Feel all of the body's contact points and surfaces.

» Notice where the body's contact points are wide and where they are just points.

» Notice which parts of the body don't touch the floor.

» Notice which parts of the body are covered with clothing.

» Notice which parts of the body are exposed to the air.

» Notice the space surrounding your body.

» Notice whether the two sides of your body feel the same, or if there are differences.

» Notice which parts of the body feel heavy (or light, wide, narrow, permeable, etc.)

» Notice these things without changing anything or interpreting your feelings.

Body awareness is about perceiving the status quo. This form of non-suggestive guidance and of feeling is well suited to the start of a yoga unit. It takes the practitioner from his head into his body, from thinking to feeling.

Breath awareness is an even finer and subtler level of perception. Before actively interfering in the breathing process one observes the breathing process. Breath awareness always follows body awareness (from tangible to ethereal). As with body awareness, the focus is initially on observing the breath and noticing its quality. Many meditation techniques build on breath awareness. Here, too, it is about looking inward.

The following suggestions serve to train and improve breath awareness:

» Shift your attention to the breath.

» Notice how the breath comes and goes without your doing anything.

» Notice how deeply the breath flows.

» Notice where your breath flows.

» Shift your attention to the breath moving in your body.

» Feel how the body expands when you inhale and contracts when you exhale.

» Notice the rhythm of your breath.

Perception with respect to the yoga practice is primarily observation. It is about learning to gradually remove oneself from identifying with the body, the breath, one's thoughts and feelings to take on an inward perspective called *eagle perspective* or *witness awareness*. The exercise is in observing and perceiving without immediately interpreting or going to the action level.

10.6   PRATYAHARA – SENSE WITHDRAWAL

Pratyahara is the fifth level of the *Ashtanga Marga* (the eightfold yoga path) according to Patanjali. *Pratyahara* is translated as sense withdrawal.

As already described in chapter 10.5, *Perception*, we perceive our environment strictly through our senses. Our senses and sensory organs are the doorways to our environment. If these doorways are always wide open we easily lose touch with our inner world. Associated sensory perceptions and enticements are very powerful.

We smell something delicious and get hungry; our mouth begins to water. One reason so many diets fail is the power our senses have over us. We may just want a tiny piece of chocolate, or just one little peanut, just for a taste, and before we know it the package is empty. We see something nice and suddenly we desire it, want to have it.[73] We receive information through our ears. When we listen more closely, much of the information we are bombarded with each day is superfluous, of little relevance to our lives, or simply immaterial.

The effects of the senses on our consciousness are explained as follows in the Katha Upanishad (approx. 1500 BC) in the famous Allegory of the Chariot:

"Think of the Self as the master of the chariot, the body as the chariot itself, the discerning mind is the charioteer, and the mind is the reins. The horses, the wise men tell us, are the senses, and the distances they travel are selfish desire (...). When someone lacks judgment and has an undisciplined mind, the senses run here and there, like wild horses."[74]

The entire advertising industry takes advantage of the fact that the senses have such enormous power over us. Advertising campaigns are largely designed to trigger strong stimuli in the potential buyer and thereby induce him to make a purchase. For instance the auto industry, which pictures expensive cars with scantily clad women.

In chapter 2.58 of the *Bhagavadgita* (yoga of the rational will) Krishna instructs the warrior Arjuna in the use of the senses:

"He who withdraws the senses from the objects of the senses as the turtle withdraws its legs into its shell, his knowledge rests on the strong foundation of wisdom."[75]

And finally the Yoga Sutra of Patanjali, chapter 2.54-55 says:

"When the senses withdraw from the objects and quasi enter the mind's own being, this state is called "withdrawal of the senses". This results in complete control of the senses."[76]

---

73 See Patanjalis Yoga Sutra, chapter 2, "Kleshas: Raga – desire, greed".
74 Easwaran, E. (2008, Katha Upanishad, 3.3-5, pg. 126-127).
75 Aurobindo, S. (2005, pg. 20).
76 Bäumer & Deshpande (1990, pg. 122).

With regard to the yoga practice, this means that we should practice deliberately closing the "doorways to the world" for a while during everyday life to reduce all external diversions and to reach ourselves, to collect ourselves.

The aspect of rest on the mat is therefore very much encouraged in a yoga class. In many yoga schools it is customary to eliminate all conversation immediately prior to a yoga class, so the mind can already gradually power down beforehand. When intense conversations about ccc-topics (complaints, consumption, children) are held from mat to mat before a yoga class, the mind tends to be preoccupied with these topics for a while longer.

Pratyahara means looking inward and consciously halting the "entertainment machine" from the outside. This also includes music, particularly when it creates powerful moods such as rock or pop music. This may seem strange to beginning yoga students because the mind is used to being busy. External silence or calm can initially seem boring, simply because it is unfamiliar.

But when perception is turned inward and we are given suggestions as to which aspects we can focus on, these "resistances" quickly dissipate and step-by-step the foundation for the higher levels of Ashtanga Marga is built. Pratyahara is practiced particularly at the beginning of a class, during the rest and reflection and deep relaxation phases of the class.

At many yoga and meditation retreats, *Pratyahara* in the form of silence (*Mauna*) is an important aspect to achieving tranquility.

10.7 SAMYAMA – THE THREE HIGHER PATHS

"He who masters Samyama gains the light of wisdom. Samyama develops incrementally" [77]
(Yoga Sutra, 3.5-6).

The Sanskrit term *Samyama* means *collection, concentration, control, self-control.*[78] In chapter 3 of the *Yoga Sutra*, Patanjali summarizes the three upper levels of the *Ashtanga Marga* under the name *Samyama. Samyama* includes:

» Dharana – concentration.

» Dhyana – meditation,

» Samadhi – consolidation, experience of oneness.

---

77 Skuban, R. (2011, pg. 166).
78 Huchzermeyer, W. (2015, pg. 168).

10.7.1 DHARANA – CONCENTRATION

"Concentration is the consciousness focusing on one point (one object one idea)"[79]
(Yoga Sutra, 3.1).

Dharana is the next level of the Ashtanga Marga. *Dharana* is *concentration* and means directing our attention exclusively to a certain object for an extended period of time.

In yoga, everyday consciousness is often called "monkey brain" because our thoughts usually change erratically, much like a troop of monkeys jumping from tree to tree. Most of the time, we only become aware of this state when we quiet down and observe our thoughts. The "restless" monkey brain is considered one of the great meditation obstacles.

Patanjali lists nine obstacles we will encounter on the yoga path. They are factors that dull our clarity and can make our mind restless: illness, rigidity (lethargy), doubt, carelessness, laziness, greed, misconception, inability to concentrate, lack of perseverance. Here one thing leads to the next. These obstacles are generally accompanied by pain, dejection (depression), physical weakness, and anxiety.

To eliminate these nine obstacles, Patanjali recommends continuously focusing on just one object. In doing so the object of the focus should be retained for an extended period of time.

Due to factors like perpetual accessibility, noise, as well as the aspiration to take care of as many things as possible at the same time, internal and external distraction, as well as information overload, many people find it increasingly difficult to focus on just one thing for an extended period of time. But concentration can be learned, whereby concentration is subject to a certain "mental effort".

In a yoga class, concentration is prepped by focusing on perception, and through Prayahara, the "withdrawal of the senses. The yoga practice includes a number of exercises that train concentration:

» Concentrating on the breath (consciously perceiving the coming and going of the breath).

» Concentrating on a part of the body (e.g. the center of the forehead, the vertex, the center of the head, the lower abdomen, or the space of the higher heart).

» Concentrating on an external image (e.g. a candle flame/Tratak, a Yantra/ritual diagram or a Mandala/spiritual symbol).

» Concentrating on an internal image (e.g. a lake that is as smooth as glass, a light beam, waterfall, Yantra).

» Sounds (e.g. sounding out vowels, humming.

» Mantra recitation (e.g. OM, Bija mantras).

» Any visualization techniques/guided imagery are also concentration exercises.

---

79 Skuban, R. (2011, pg. 162).

The organism's changeover from a performance state to a state of rest usually also causes us to get sleepy. Deep relaxation at the end of an Asana practice is generally done in a supine position. This has the advantage of body and mind being able to relax completely; however, the body's heaviness and warmth and the decreasing brain activity also make it easy to fall asleep.

When concentration exercises are practiced after deep relaxation in preparation for meditation, it is advisable to perform them (and the meditation) in an upright, seated position to be able to stay awake during the exercise.

10.7.2   DHYANA – MEDITATION

Dhyana, meditation is the seventh level of *Ashtanga Marga*

"Meditation is the uninterrupted flow of consciousness towards the object of its focus."[80]
(Yoga Sutra, 3.3)

"There (in this concentration) meditation is the joining in a single experience."[81]
(Yoga Sutra, 3.3)

Both translations of the *Yoga Sutra* (3.3) point out that *Dharana, concentration*, and *Dhyana, meditation*, are fluid processes that merge and cannot be clearly separated. During meditation the mind rests. Patanjali recommends focusing on the radiance in our inner space to calm the mind (Yoga Sutra, 1.36).

Even during meditation, thoughts periodically intrude. But during meditation we don't identify with those thoughts. We are witnesses to our thoughts; the consciousness observes itself. The ability to differentiate (Viveka) between transience and reality is trained. When someone is able to observe his thoughts, he learns that in the core of his being he is not his thoughts.

10.7.3   SAMADHI – FUSION

Samadhi, unification, fusion, is the eighth and final level of *Ashtanga Marga. The Vrittis*, the thoughts and emotions have completely quieted down. You have reached the state that Patanjali defines right at the beginning of the Yoga Sutra as "Yoga is the quieting of thoughts, the constantly changing mental patterns."[82]

"As the mental processes subside the consciousness feeds itself on transparency, called fusion. Like a crystal it reflects what lies before it: the one who sees, that which is seen, and seeing"[83] (Yoga Sutra)

---

80 Skuban, R. (2011, pg. 162).
81 Bäumer & Deshpande (1990, pg. 123).
82 See chapter 2
83 Cope, S. (2007). *The Wisdom of Yoga.* (pg. 402). München: Goldmann Arkana.

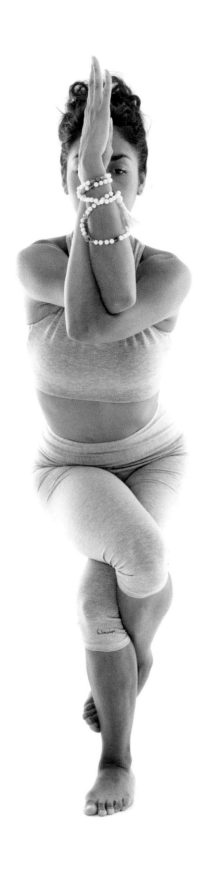

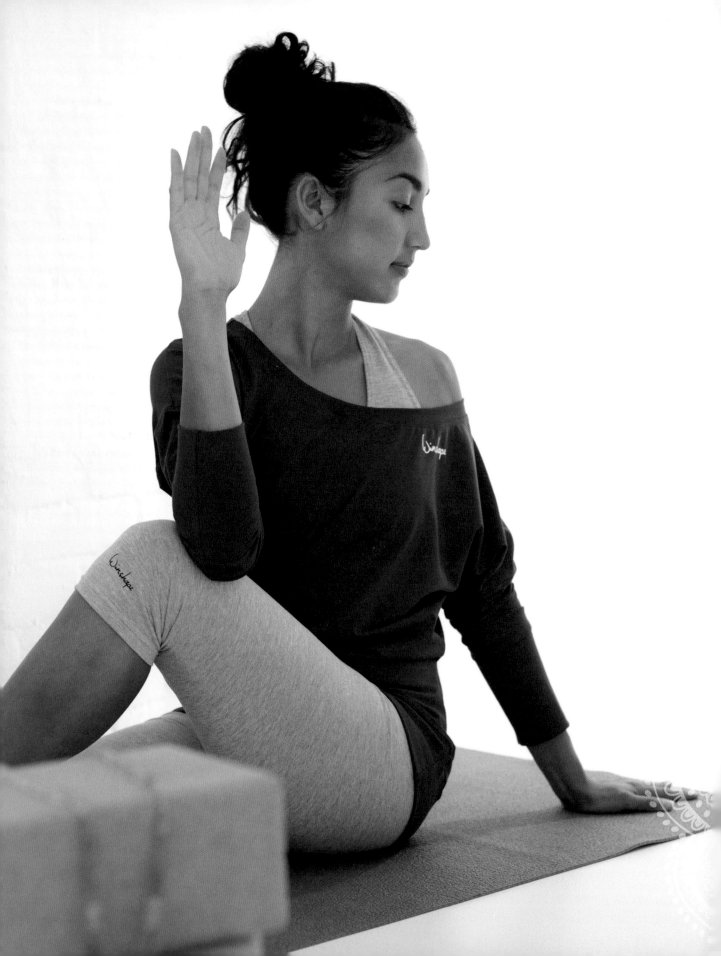

11 TEACHING YOGA

11   TEACHING YOGA

The spectrum of yoga offerings is enormous. For people interested in practicing yoga it is often a challenge to identify the style appropriate for them from the abundance of choices, particularly since the motivation for taking yoga can differ widely.

Some want to just try it first to see what this "exercise trend" is all about. Others may come because their doctor recommended yoga for tight muscles or stress. Many just come because they wish to find tranquility and their own Self. And still others have read books beforehand and immersed themselves in spirituality and view the yoga practice as part of their life's journey.

At the start of yoga training and advanced yoga training, I like to ask my participants the following question and offer different, to some extent not entirely serious, answers:

11.1   WHAT IS YOGA?

A: A type of trendy Indian gymnastics?

B: An exercise program for people who don't like to exert themselves too much?

C: An alternative healing method?

D: A spiritual journey?

Interestingly, a discussion often ensues at this point. Opinions and views vary quite a bit on each of these statements. In the end, most everyone agrees that all of the answers, each in its own way, can apply to a more or less broad public.

The yoga offerings extend from meditative awareness-oriented classes to classic Hatha Yoga formats in which either philosophical-spiritual themes or focus on the physical work set the perimeters for the Asana practice, all the way to dynamic Vinyasa variations with a rather more athletic character.

Anyone interested in teaching yoga should first have a clear idea about their own offerings, their level of knowledge, which target group they wish to reach and what they want to teach. Teaching beginners brings with it different challenges than teaching experienced participants.

Someone who practices a type of yoga in which the practice structure includes specific sequences or series, is usually linked to an organization that dictates the steps of the didactic methods and spiritual content. For the instructor this initially makes it less complicated to plan classes because he needs to primarily focus on the already specified teaching steps and their implementation.

These forms work well as long as the class participants' abilities are in line with the teaching system's requirements. But when a participant is unable to do certain parts of a practice because they may be too demanding or too complicated, there can be an associated risk of injury, particularly if the instructor was not trained to adapt the plan.

Since there is no such thing as an average participant, yoga instructors should ideally be able to easily adapt to teaching different levels. The contents of this book and the DTB yoga training program are geared to participants that want to start doing yoga or already have some previous experience. It is about providing guidance that allows the participant to gradually participate in the practice without risk of injury.

Themed classes provide options for building content that will allow the instructor to teach the physical practice step-by-step in accordance with the philosophical-spiritual aspects.

Teaching yoga requires complete immersion in the themes within one's own practice, and a deep interest in the contents. Developing one's own consciousness is the basis for quality instruction.

Teaching is a dynamic process. Every teacher is also a student. The longer you do it, the more involved you get in the content while always discovering new aspects, because yoga is so multi-layered.

Teaching isn't about perfectionism but about sharing and communicating what you yourself have experienced on the yoga path.

The following questions should help you assess which aspects apply with respect to your planned teaching activity, or must still be developed:

1. Do I have enough personal experience to teach yoga?

2. Is my knowledge of yoga philosophy sufficient to be able to place instruction and practice in the appropriate context?

3. Do I have a well-developed perceptive ability (with respect to my own body, breathing, and with respect to the energy-related, emotional, and mental aspects) to be able to communicate these experiences to participants in an appropriate manner?

4. Am I able to take the backseat to give priority to the participants and their needs?

5. Do I have valid knowledge about the structure, makeup, and effects of the most important Asanas?

6. Am I able to modify the contents and poses according to the participants' level?

7. Do I have experience in recognizing participants' skill level and plan my class content accordingly?

8. Am I able to provide space and time for participants to experience the qualities of yoga?

9. Do I enjoy teaching the content?

11.2 PLANNING A CLASS

Extensive planning of the class content and flow should ideally precede every class. This is primarily based on the participants' abilities and level of knowledge – and of course the instructor's abilities and level of knowledge.

There is controversy among yoga instructors as to class planning, that is whether the contents should be planned long-term or if it is better to orient content to the form of the day and the current interests and needs of participants. They are not mutually exclusive. Opponents of preplanned classes usually argue that the can intuitively feel what participants need on any given day.

Well-developed intuition and observation skills are a major advantage when teaching. However, purely intuitive instruction is a method that requires a lot of inner development and experience. Otherwise it can easily happen that the participants stagnate in their long-term development because the instructor's background experience and level of knowledge are not sufficiently advanced.

Systematic planning of class content over an extended period of time has the advantage that you are developing a common thread that makes it possible to synchronize different themes in a coordinated way that makes sense and is appropriate for the participants' level of development. For the instructor, this initially means more effort than an intuitive or random teaching approach.

But a well thought-out plan doesn't have to be viewed as a rigid construct that must be adhered to at all cost (see implementation).

A plan consists of preparation, implementation, and subsequent reflection.

a) Preparation
Based on the available information about the group, the instructor thinks about what the common thread of the class should be and what content would be appropriate. Which building blocks do we want to use to fill up the hour?

b) Implementation
You teach the class. But sometimes situations arise that force the instructor to deviate from the plan. Be it that the content is too easy or too difficult, or it becomes apparent that the group has different needs on that particular day. Here observation skills, intuition, and the ability to modify comes to bear, meaning this or that exercise needs to be slightly modified or substituted, or may be more time is needed than previously planned. That does not mean that the entire class concept has become obsolete. Most of the time, an appropriate adjustment to the content is sufficient.

c)   Reflection/evaluation

After the class, you evaluate how it went and then integrate that knowledge into future class planning. It might be necessary to integrate intermediate stages or change content. Reflecting on the plan also includes revising the plan.

d)   Structured and planned yoga instruction includes the following considerations:

Classroom conditions
Goal setting
Didactics and methods
Step-by-step preparation of individual theme areas based on the Vinyasa Krama principle.

11.3   STRUCTURED AND PLANNED YOGA INSTRUCTION

11.3.1   CLASSROOM CONDITIONS

Classroom conditions set the parameters for content planning. Familiarizing yourself with the conditions and analyzing them provides important information that will essentially determine planning, goal setting, and implementation. The following requirements should be taken into account during planning:

a)   Institutional conditions: Where is the class being held?

First you must determine where and in what context the class will take place:

At a fitness studio?
At an association?
At a yoga school?
At a business (business yoga or workplace health promotion)?
Is there a contracting entity or is it a course?
Is a space being rented by the hour?

The location greatly influences class planning. If you are an independent contractor and don't have a direct employer, you are largely free of external input. However, most of the time it is necessary to take into account an employer's expectations. Businesses, associations, and exercise studios sometimes stipulate that the class focuses less on the spiritual aspects.

Potential concerns regarding typical yoga content such as mantra recitation, meditation, but also just teaching philosophical content, must be learned beforehand to determine whether a basis for collaboration exists between yourself and the employer. How the course content is announced should also be determined beforehand.

b) The room

To avoid surprises that may negatively affect the course flow, it is advisable to examine the room where instruction will take place or to ask detailed questions beforehand about what conditions and facilities can be expected:

» **The size and shape of the room determine:**
   a) The number of participants
   b) Mat alignment. In a square room it is easy to arrange the mats in a circle. In a long and narrow room, a circular arrangement is usually not possible with a large number of participants.
   c) Walls: Can the walls be used for some of the exercises? Not every employer likes having hand or back prints on white walls.
   d) Where is the room located? Are there other classes in adjacent rooms at the same time? Is there audible noise from outside? How soundproof is the room?

» **Room features**
   a) How is the room ventilated? Are there windows that can be opened? Is the room air-conditioned? If yes, how is it operated? Does it make noise? Can it be turned off? Are the controls in or outside the room?
   b) How is the room heated? Is it warm enough for yoga in winter?
   c) What are the light conditions in the room? Are the light switches in or outside the room? Can the lights be dimmed? Are there multiple light sources?
   d) Is there a stereo available for use?
   e) Are there mats, blankets, blocks, straps, or other aids available for use? Or do participants need to be told beforehand what they should bring?
   f) Are there decorations? Is the use of candles allowed?

Please note: Occasionally there is that perfect yoga room that meets all of the instructor's wishes. But most rooms require some compromise. When you are really familiar with the conditions of a room, you can work towards a largely hitch-free class by planning or avoiding certain things. This prevents situations like yoga instructors who can't find the light switch before the deep relaxation phase.

c) Lesson material

» Is there material you can use? For instance anatomical charts or exercise handouts?

d) Time

» What time does class start? Morning or evening? Do participants come during their lunch break? Or in the late evening?
» How long is the course?
» How long are the individual classes?
» Are there other classes before or after?

e) Target group

» What is the composition of the group with respect to gender and age?
» Are there health restrictions that must be taken into consideration?

» Is it a newly formed group or has the group been together for some time?
» If the class has been in existence for some time:
» a) How is the class listed?
» b) What have the participants practiced so far?
» c) Are they experienced participants or beginners?
» Is it an open class or does it require registration?
» What are participants' expectations for the class content?

11.3.2 GOAL SETTING

The goals set for a class depend on participant makeup, participants' needs and wishes, as well as thematic focal points an instructor wants to teach. Both aspects -the participants' and the instructor's wishes and expectations- should be in sync. Sometimes instructors and groups aren't a good fit because their views and expectations regarding yoga instruction are too far apart.

After everything the instructor was able to learn about a group beforehand, he makes "an offer" with his themes and communicates with the participants about their content. This can be a closing communication in which participants speak out about their experience with the content or the class theme. Ideally the demand the instructor sees and has ascertained is in line with participants' wishes and expectations.

But that isn't always the case. Here the instructor's sensitivity is necessary in choosing the content and goals so the practice is in line with what he deems appropriate, while simultaneously meeting participants at their current level.

For instance, when an instructor notices that a large portion of the group ignores their breathing during the course or completes the exercises more like "gymnastics" than a conscious practice, one of his intermediate-term goals and thematic superstructure can be to improve breath and body awareness. This theme can be integrated into the yoga practice step-by-step in the form of exercises that correspond to the content and that the participants are already familiar with. You add something to what is already there and combine new points of view of your own practice and compatible exercises with already familiar content.

This is a helpful formula: 20% new content, 80% familiar content.

Learning processes require time and repetition. Even if you have a major goal, a Chinese proverb tells us: "Everything starts with the first step." It is helpful when the instructor knows the way and can specify the direction.

The following steps result for the practice:

Overriding goal or theme: "Improving breath and body awareness"

Long-term goal: What are the goals for the next 3-6 months?
E.g. experiencing a definite increase in energy and vitality through conscious breathing.
E.g. understanding the link between conscious breathing and vital energy.

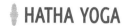

Short-term goal: What are my goals for the next 3-5 classes?
*E.g. practicing synchronization of breath and movement during simple Asanas, like **Apanasana**.*

11.3.3 DIDACTICS AND METHODS

When implementing goals the question arises about suitable content and methods that need to be taught. Here the didactic and methodological considerations come into play:

Didactics refers to the theory and practice of teaching and learning processes.
» Didactics includes the analysis of conditions and the planning of lessons (see above/classroom condition).
» Didactics poses these questions:
» a) Which theme should be taught?
» b) Which goals are being pursued by doing so?
» Didactics takes into account prior knowledge and parameters such as facilities, participants' or employer's wishes, and scheduling.
» Didactics determines the contents that are being taught.

The theme results from the analysis of all the requirements and conditions. Goals are then determined in coordination with the theme before choosing the appropriate content.

The main theme of didactics is: WHAT is taught and WHY?

Methods refers to all methods used to implement and teach the contents after the parameters have been set.

Methods that apply to yoga instruction:
» Can include the use of media like music or charts;
» Can include partner work, group or individual work to teach contents;
» Applies to corrections (tactile, verbal, as group demonstration, correction by simplifying the exercise, correction via partner work);
» Is the form of instruction (verbal or visual such as "demonstration/imitation");
» Determines the choice of aids;
» Determines the form of address (casual, formal).

The main methodological theme is: HOW is being taught and WHY?

11.3.4 VINYASA KRAMA

Vi = in a particular way / in a special way
Nyasa = placing, setting, laying, positioning
Krama = step, sequence, approach

Patanjali's Ashtanga Marga, the eightfold yoga path that is described in the *Yoga Sutra*, is based on the *Vinyasa Krama* principle.

Vinyasa Krama means incremental progression or step-by-step approach. It refers to a methodical approach that incrementally (Krama) leads to a goal:

» From simple to complex;

» From familiar to unfamiliar;

» From tangible to ethereal;

» From the outside to the inside.

The principle of *Vinyasa Krama* is always oriented to the participant, and with respect to content and theme, should meet him at his current level. On the one hand the principle is meant to prevent overextension and the associated risk of injury, on the other hand very complex content can be introduced in very small, sensible steps (usually over an extended period of time). The principle applies to a single hour as well as a period of time of 10 hours or more.

a) The common thread

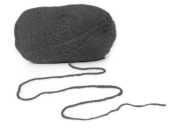

The *Vinyasa Krama* principle is always based on a goal to be achieved via a systematic and logical developmental path. One can think of this developmental path as a *common thread* whose theme stretches through the entire practice. Aspects like Asana, breathing, visualization, relaxation, and meditation can also be linked in this way.

The principle of *Vinyasa Krama* extends across the entire practice, on every plane.

With every theme that will be taught, be it an Asana, a Pranayama, or a principle, you first determine which partial aspects the theme can be broken down to and which additional aspects can be integrated into the theme from a yoga philosophy point of view, and then find a developmental path that makes sense.

With respect to an Asana, this means that you must first analyze in which category of poses an Asana belongs, what its effects, function, and methodology are. You determine which areas of the body are primarily engaged in the target Asana. They are then introduced step-by-step with the appropriate preparatory exercises (loosening up, stretching, stabilizing, strengthening) and suitable introductory exercises as described in chapter 7, until the target Asana or a modification of the Asana can be assumed.

HATHA YOGA

When preparing an entire hour class, the Asanas should be chosen so one Asana prepares for the next one, or an exercise builds on the previous one. In doing so, choose a building path that gradually increases in difficulty and intensity until the goal for that particular hour has been reached.

If you wish to teach a breathing technique like, for instance, *Ujjayi breath*, you again assess what is necessary for the safe execution of Pranayama. A possible introduction method in terms of Vinyasa Krama would be for instance:

» *Breath awareness* (being conscious of the natural breath).

» Then shifting the focus to *awareness of the breathing spaces*.

» *Leading to breath control* (complete yogic breaths, feeling the breath wave, experiencing aspects of accepting and letting go; this can be intensified via supporting, simple Asanas and movements).

» *Extended exhalation with mouth slightly open* (for instance with sounding out and humming), to feel the narrowing of the glottis.

» *Extended exhalation with mouth closed and visualization aid* (e.g. suppressing a yawn or a silent MMMMHHH).

When there is an overriding goal you wish to reach, you should break it down into partial aspects and decide with which sensible steps to approach and reach the goal over a certain time period.

If you wish to immediately teach a complex subject area such as, for instance, introducing the chakra system or an individual chakra, you again start with the familiar. After an introductory explanation from an energy and anatomy point of view, a possible building method would be, for example, the root chakra/ *Muladhara chakra* experience:

» Body- and breath awareness.

» Shifting attention to the lower pelvic region (feeling and perceiving on a physical level).

» Directing the breath to the lower pelvic area.

» Expanding the focus to the energy in the feet and legs.

» Loosening exercises for the pelvic region, legs, and feet.

» Introducing simple exercises to activate the pelvic floor.

» Preparatory exercises for the subsequent Asana- and Karana practice.

» Making it possible to experience the principle of stability and grounding via, for instance, Shoulder Bridge and suitable standing poses.

» Elucidating the principle of rootedness/grounding via simple balance poses (tree/boat).

» Capturing the sensation of pleasant heaviness and trust during guided deep relaxation.

» Intensifying the experience of grounding and rootedness in a closing visualization (e.g. imagining a *tree* whose roots reach deep into the earth and nourish the tree).

These examples are intended to show that it is possible to build a safe practice in the sense of *Vinyasa Krama* for any level:

» What is the goal of the class?

» Which aspects (themes, exercises, content) will lead to the goal?

» What common thread emerges?

» How can the contents be linked?

» How can I simplify/modify the exercises? (Meaning, first breaking them down into partial aspects and then taking them in a coherent order from simple to complex, familiar to unfamiliar, tangible to subtle).

» The content of which themes could be coordinated and combined?

11.4 DESIGNING AND ADVANTAGES OF THEMED CLASSES

With respect to the Asana practice and the progression of a yoga class, Hatha Yoga has different approaches and models. There are traditions based on set exercise sequences, such as the *Rishikesh series* of Sivananda Yoga or the *Ashtanga Vinyasa* series.

Master yogis developed the specified series largely for a broad mass of students around the world. With respect to their focus and logic, they are in line with the philosophical content of the respective master tradition and largely used worldwide. A student of a respective system is able to do the same practice at schools or Ashrams in India, New York, or Berlin.

Set series have the advantage of always being the same. The practitioner doesn't have to think about the progression, and the series themselves follow a logical order. The student is able to reexperience himself each time he practices the specified series and is able to track his progress over the course of the practice sequence. The "one-series-for-all" system thus has many advantages, but also doesn't or only somewhat takes into account the practitioner's individual theme.

Another and very common approach is the open class content, whereby the emphasis on a specific theme is based on the participant makeup. Here the content can be customized to the individual wants and needs of participants and spiritual themes.

The Hatha Yoga system is very complex and includes many major subject areas. Not all of these areas can be addressed and taught equally during every 90-120 minute yoga class. The wealth of content is simply too great. Moreover, beginners require different content and themes than experienced or advanced participants. The advantage of themed classes lies in the fact that specifically chosen content remains the focus of the practice for a while. It changes (in keeping with *Vinyasa Krama*) whenever the participant group has internalized it.

Themed classes always focus on an overriding theme. It can be a philosophical theme, a particular aspect to be taught, an Asana or a group of Asanas, a Pranayama, an energy- and anatomy-related topic from the area of chakra theory, or introduction to meditation.

Themed classes have the advantage that the content can be taught in a participant-focused manner. The particular class focus provides the participants with the opportunity to become familiar with new aspects while also being able to learn something about themselves. Individual aspects can be taught and experienced at length since the focus is specifically placed on an experience. The goal is to gradually recognize and implement these themes in every day life as well.

11.5 BUILDING A YOGA CLASS

A yoga class consists of:

Introduction – main part – conclusion

a) **Introduction (approx. 15-20% of class time)**
    Greeting/information phase
    » Brief lecture: intro to class theme (explanation of class goal and focus areas or information about the yoga philosophy background).
    » Possibly sounding of a mantra to get attuned to the class.

    Attunement/getting collected (seated or reclined position)
    » Body awareness.
    » Breath awareness.
    » Possibly brief PME (progressive muscle relaxation).
    » Possibly visualization (abbreviated form) that matches the class theme.
    » Breath control -> introduction to full belly breathing.
    » Breath control combined with simple movements (preparation to breath flow).
    » Possibly introduction of Ujjayi breath.

b) **Main part/class focus areas (50-60% of class time)**
    » Preparatory exercises like loosening up joints, pre-stretching, stabilization, and strengthening in preparation for the Asana practice.
    » Introduction of simple Asanas and Karanas that warm the body and prepare for more complex Karanas such as Surya Namaskar (dynamic before static).

» The working phase follows the Vinyasa Krama principle: from simple to complex, from familiar to unfamiliar, from tangible to subtle, from outside to inside.
» The teaching process is divided into preparation, guided introduction, and execution.
» Rest and reflection phases are integrated in accordance with the class theme.
» The goal of the class is also the high point of the class.
» Once the class high point has been reached, balancing exercises follow that also begin to prepare for the relaxation phase. Depending on the class theme, these can include, for instance, sustained cooling Asanas such as forward bends and inversions.

c) **Conclusion (20-25% of class time)**
The conclusion can be designed in different ways. It should include a guided whole-body relaxation component, and can also be filled with different building blocks:

» Guided deep or final relaxation in supine position.

» Possibly visualization related to the theme of the class.

» Possibly meditation in a seated upright posture.

» Possibly a *Pranayama*.

» Possibly sounding of a mantra.

» Possibly ending the class with a quote related to the class theme.

» Possibly issuing "homework", an incentive for an exercise that can be done in everyday life.

» Possibly a handout.

The listed time percentages are a rough estimate. The division of class time can vary based on the class theme and focus.

11.6 PLANNING CLASS CONTENT: GUIDE TO CREATING A LESSON PLAN

Below is a sample pattern for creating a lesson plan based on the example listed under goal setting.

11.6.1 THEME: "IMPROVING BREATH AND BODY AWARENESS"

Rationale: At the beginning of a yoga class for beginners, I often find that a large portion of participants is very outward-focused during the class. They practice Asanas as well as simple Karanas with lots of joy, but many of them do not have a well-developed awareness of their breathing and body as well as the many energy-related aspects of a yoga practice. The participants still associate yoga with physical training. They only become aware of relaxation after they have physically exhausted themselves.

Since I originally came to the yoga practice form a very athletics- and training-focused background, I can relate to the difficulty in understanding the switch from "training" to an awareness- and breath-focused practice. Since one doesn't know what is missing when one doesn't know something, I want to teach participants the positive aspects and effects of improved breath- and body awareness so they are able to gradually integrate these experiences into their practice, and also feel the effects in their everyday life as a gain in vital energy and harmony.

11.6.2 CLASSROOM CONDITIONS

The class is 60 minutes long. The class name is "Hatha Yoga for stress prevention & management". The class is held as part of a workplace health promotion program in the conference room of a large company. The room is square and measures approx. 80 sq. meters (861 sq. feet). The company employees push the conference room tables and chairs against the walls. The floor is covered with a needle felt carpet typically found in offices. There is air conditioning, but it is quite noisy and therefore occasionally disrupts the class. However, it cannot be turned off since it cools the entire floor. The system is also set at a very cold temperature; so I ask participants to bring something warm to cover themselves with during the relaxation and slower phases.

There is no natural light, but the individual light fixtures on the ceiling and walls can be dimmed. Mats are provided, but are of limited suitability for yoga as they are very thick and the feet sink into the mat during standing poses. Some participants bring their own yoga mats. No additional aids are available. There is no music system.

The participants are company employees. The class is held in the late afternoon. Participants come to the class directly from their desks. It is a mixed group of 12 individuals; eight women and four men between the ages of 25-60. Some are very athletic, others have exercised very little or not at all in years. Only a few have practiced yoga before.

Communication before and after the class and group interaction is friendly and outgoing.

11.6.3 GENERAL PREPARATION

This is the third class unit. During the previous two units the focus was on joint mobility, simple stretches, and stabilization. The theme of the first unit was "Meru Danda – the axis of the world", and the spine's directions of movement were explained and practiced, which was repeated during the second class with the addition of the rest- and relaxation aspect. Each class ended with a deep relaxation/whole-body relaxation component.

Simple Asanas like *Apanasana*, *Eka Pada Apanasana* (Wind-relieving poses), *Marjary Asana* variations, *Setu Bhanda Sarvangasana*, *Makarasana* variations, and easy *Karanas* (breath flow and Small Sun Salutation to warm up) were introduced. Also a few standing poses like *Uttanasana*, *Ardha Uttanasana*, and *Padottanasana* to understand the function and straightening of the spine.

Breath and body awareness are part of every unit, however, participants were still very focused on the physical aspects.

11.6.4 LEARNING OBJECTIVES

The goal of this class unit is "Improving breath- and body awareness". Since this is a theme that requires a greater amount of time for implementation and is also selected as a theme again and again in subsequent classes, the goals were as follows:

Long-term goals

» Experiencing a definite increase in energy and vitality through conscious breathing.

» Being able to more clearly feel and experience the body or parts of the body.

» Early recognition of signs of possible tension in the body.

» Recognizing signs of abnormal (unconscious) breath flow.

» Refining the breath and the entire breathing process.

» Integrating conscious breathing into everyday life.

» Learning to synchronize breath and movement during simple Karanas/flows.

Short-term goals

» Being able to feel the body's points of contact with the floor.

» Feeling the difference between physical relaxation and tension.

» Knowing the difference between breath awareness and breath control.

» Being aware of the different breathing spaces through supporting practice.

» Being aware of and observing the breath during Asana practice.

11.6.5 DIDACTIC CONSIDERATIONS

WHAT is being taught WHY?

At the beginning of class, the theme of oneness is explained during a brief lecture. First the link between improved awareness and early recognition of stress symptoms (like tight neck muscles, shallow and irregular breathing, poor posture) is explained. The breathing concept is repeated in summary (first and second class unit: the aspects of energy uptake (Prana) as well as the relationships between exhalation with respect to deacidification and letting go of mental or physical tension). An overview of the etheric energy system (*Nadis*) is given to elucidate the energy- and anatomy-related background.

The practice begins with participants collecting themselves in a supine position during which first the entire body and then the individual points of contact are felt, so the participants move into awareness. Awareness of the breath moving in the body follows to deepen the experience. Here the participant is invited to become an observer to consciously perceive the difference between breath awareness and breath control, which follows.

The flow of the breath linked to movement should be felt through simple movements like arm raises, Apanasana, and Eka Pada Apanasana. Participants practice at their own pace so they can calmly enter the flow of the breathing movement.

This is followed by seated exercises, exercises on hands and knees and knees only for joint mobilization and pre-stretching to prepare the body for the subsequent Asanas.

The Asanas being practiced should focus on the flow of the breath to encourage a deeper understanding of the relationship between breath and movement. The exercises are also selected to facilitate awareness of the breathing spaces. Since most participants are not yet accustomed to focusing their attention continuously on awareness, the in-between physical dynamic practice is slightly more intensive, to subsequently turn the focus inward again during the rest and relaxation phases.

Rest and relaxation phases are integrated after every block of exercise, so the participants can experience the aspects of breath- and body awareness.

At the end of the class, a deep-relaxation component based on body awareness allows the participants to experience that just focusing on different parts of the body, from head to toe, can lead them into a state of deep relaxation.

11.6.6 METHODOLOGICAL CONSIDERATIONS

HOW to teach and WHY?

I am choosing a circular mat arrangement for this class because I find it more conducive to a joint practice. I spread out a cloth with decorations (stones, candles, flowers, etc.) in the center of the circle to reduce the conference room's austere atmosphere. To muffle the sound of the air conditioner, I bring along a Bluetooth speaker and choose a kind of tapestry of sound as subdued background music.

For the short lecture at the beginning of the class, I bring along a chart with an illustration of the Nadi system for a better understanding of the yogic aspects.

In the run-up to the class I made an agreement with the participants that I would address them by their first names.

I teach the content based on the *Vinyasa Krama* principle: from simple to complex, familiar to unfamiliar. With respect to the degree of difficulty, the content is designed so each exercise prepares for the subsequent one.

The teaching method is primarily verbal, so the participants remain focused on themselves and become more aware. For exercises that are more complex I choose the "demonstrate-imitate" method or, depending on the type of exercise, "demonstrate-participate".

To interfere as little as possible with the development of self-awareness, I make primarily verbal corrections or suggestions. I want to give participants the opportunity to focus completely on themselves. I therefore choose only familiar exercises for this class, exercises that have been practiced during previous classes.

At the end of the class, I give participants a "homework assignment" to be done by the next unit, which is intended as an incentive. They are invited to observe their breath on a daily basis without changing it.

11.6.7 PRACTICE PROGRESSION BASED ON THE PRINCIPLE OF VINYASA KRAMA

Theme: Improving breath- and body awareness

Duration: 60 minutes
IH: Inhalation
EH: Exhalation

Dura-tion	Phase	Content, outline	Goal, effect, method	Comments and possible error sources
4 min	Start	Brief lecture	Explain class theme "Improving breath & body awareness"	Circle, show chart
4 min	Start	Collection	Body awareness by feeling contact areas. Breath awareness by feeling breath movements, coming and going of the breath. Being aware of the breath wave. Breath control: intro to complete yogic breathing.	Offering info re. breathing phases, like absorbing energy as you inhale, release spent energy as you exhale.

3 min		Arm raises	IH: extend entire body. Inner focus is on energy absorption EH: Vertically lower arms. Inner focus is on aspects of letting go, deacidification of the body and becoming empty inside.	The breath guides the movement. Find own breathing rhythm linked to the movement.
2 min	Main part	Loosen up hips	Circular movements with thighs (internal and external rotation) to loosen up hips and pre-stretch inside of legs.	Participants all sit at work, which is why loosening up the hips is a good choice here.
2 min	Main part	*Apanasana*	Wind-relieving pose IH: Push legs away from body. EH: Pull legs towards body.	Consciously experiencing the feeling of vastness and narrowness Preparation for *Eka Pada Apansana* Flow of breath is practiced with movement.
4 min	Main part	*Eka Pada Apanasana*	Single-leg, wind-relieving pose combined with whole-body extension and added abdominal muscle contraction/trunk flexion. IH: whole-body extension EH: *Eka Pada Apanasana* Intensification: forehead to knee.	Participants practice with the breath, movements get larger. Here the focus should be shifted to the feeling of energy flowing until lungs are filled, and the pouring out of energy until the lungs are empty.

1 min	Main part	Rest & reflect	Breathe naturally. Observe the free-flowing breath.	The conscious transition from breath control to awareness should be experienced here.
3 min		*Setu Bandha* variation	Dynamic Shoulder Bridge IH: Lift the pelvis and allow the breath to flow in as you raise arms. EH: Roll down the spine. Repeat in time with the breath	Loosen up the spine. Prepare for the subsequent backbends. Open the breathing spaces. Participants should get a feel for the expanse and opening of the chest area, which results from the movement.
No photo Transition to a seated posture: loosening of the shoulder girdle and wrists with circular movements.				
2 min	Main part	*Marjary Asana*	Neutral all-fours position. EH: Marjary Asana/rounded back (cat), while firmly pulling the stomach in for support. IH: extend the back/arch	Loosen up the spine. Preparation for small breathing flow. Make sure not to hyperextend the cervical spine in the backbend and keep shoulders stable.

3 min	Main part	Small breathing flow	EH: Utthita Balasna (Extended Child's pose) IH: All-fours position EH: Marjary Asana/ round the back and IH: arch the back. EH: return to Utthita Balasana (Extended Child's pose)	The breath leads the movement. The body warms up.
3 min	Main part	On knees *lunge*	From kneeling position move into the hip-flexor stretch. Hold 8-10 long breaths per side. Emphasis on letting go during exhalation phase.	Hip flexors (iliopsoas muscles) are stretched in preparation for the *Small Sun Salutation* and backbends.
3 min	Main part	*Ustrasana* modification	Stabilize starting position on knees with lower abdomen and pelvis. Place hands on iliac blade for support; pull elbows towards each other. IH: move into backbend. Only go as far as current mobility level allows. EH: Return to kneeling position. Do several dynamic repetitions.	Preparation for *small Sun Salutation* Gently stretch the chest If thoracic spine mobility is still rather limited, modify backbend. Lift the sternum and pull shoulder blades and elbows together. Keep the back of the neck long during the backbend.

| 5 min | Main part | *Small sun salutation* | EH: *Tadasana/Anjali Mudra*: Preparatory collection and grounding in upright standing position.

IH: *Urdhva Hastasana with backbend*

EH: *Uttanasana/forward bend*

IH: *Anjaney Asana/backbend in lunge*

EH: *Uttanasana/forward bend*

IH: *Urdhva Hastasana with backbend*

EH: *Tadasana/Anjali Mudra* | The class goal is the progression of the *Small Sun Salutation*

The breath should be practiced in combination with the individual poses.

The progression is first taught to the entire group. After that, participants can practice at their own pace.

The experience of stretching and expansion should be felt as a natural inhalation phase.

Participants can experience how forward bends support exhalation.

The following alternatives can be practiced in place of deep back and forward bends:

Anjaney Asana without backbend

Uttanasana with bent knees |

3 min	Conclusion	*Dandasana, Paschimottasana*	Forward bend with straight or rounded back as a gentle counterpose. Begin with several dynamic repetitions in time with the breath. IH: Straighten up. EH: Forward bend. The emphasis is on experiencing the breath during the forward bend. Create space as you exhale and feel the breath in your flanks and back.	Knees can be bent if muscles at the back of the body are severely shortened.
3 min	Conclusion	*Makarasana*	Relaxed form (wide leg position) of *Makarasana* IH: Supine starting position, feet are planted on the ground. EH: Sink into the twist. Alternate sides several times in time with the breath, then hold for several breaths on each side. *Apanasana* as a counterpose.	Gentle release of tightness; gently dynamic. The spine rotates around its vertical axis, which gently massages the internal organs and allows body and mind to rest.
12 min	Conclusion	*Shavasana*	Whole-body relaxation based on body awareness. (See directions for relaxation in chapter 10).	Here participants can once more notice the possible differences between the points of contact at the start of the practice and at the end. The breath flows freely.
3 min	Conclusion	Upright-seated posture	Joint OM to close. "Homework"/incentive for daily practice until the next class: Observe the breath in various everyday situations.	After the class, I make myself available to participants for 10 more minutes to answer questions or address concerns.

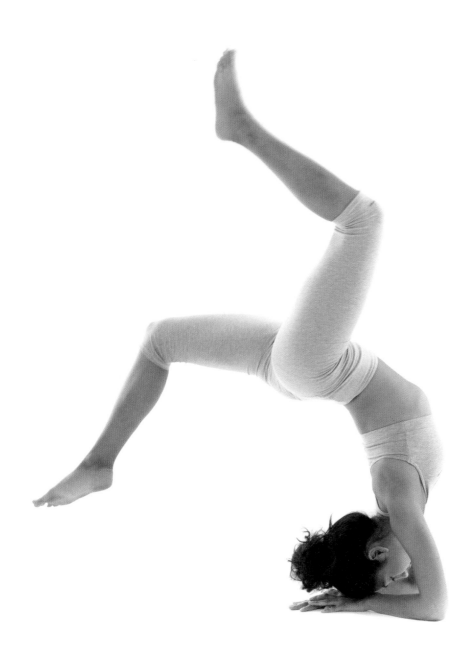

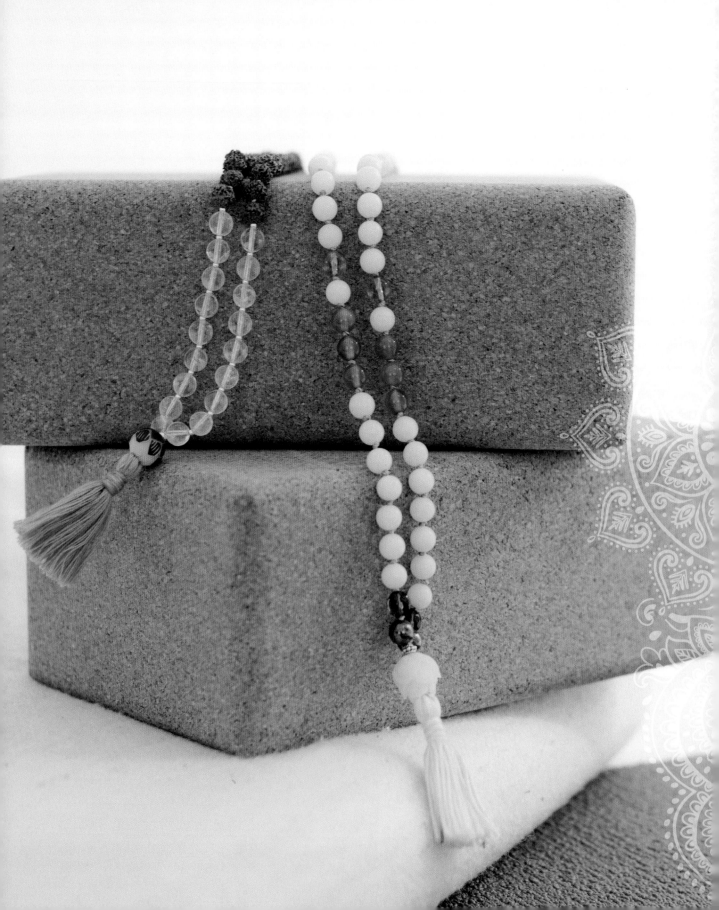

12 THEMED SAMPLE CLASSES

12 THEMED SAMPLE CLASSES

The following themed classes build on each other with respect to their content. First, the focus is on breath and body awareness. Then basic forms of movement are added and expanded upon with each lesson plan.

Every lesson plan takes up new content but also repeats themes (exercise and movement sequences) from previous lesson plans.

Each class unit in turn builds on itself. Each individual class focuses on preparatory introduction. Every lesson plan emphasizes and teaches specific Asana categories based on the basic theme. Lesson plans can be simplified or shortened any time without detracting from the basic theme of a class.

Every lesson plan requires sufficient time in the form of repetitions to internalize the content. If the content is modified slightly, the individual lesson plans can be repeated at least 10-15 times before moving on to the next theme. It is possible to create 10-20 variations from each of the eight lesson plans introduced here, each emphasizing another partial aspect. There are many possibilities and approaches for developing a certain theme.

12.1 LESSON PLAN 1: FINDING YOUR OWN PACE

In our daily lives, we are often subject to rhythms and timing that we have little or no control over. This includes work schedules, as well as the pace at which certain processes must be handled and that are usually predetermined. Within this rigid structure it is often difficult to find or live at one's own pace. Consequently, we can develop a tendency to unconsciously rush through our daily life, even when it isn't necessary to do so, like, for instance, in our free time.

There is a nautical term, hull speed, which means that the length of the hull determines the maximum speed a ship can reach. In Stan Nadolny's seafaring novel "Discovery of Slowness" he takes up this topic with respect to humans. It is ultimately about the right to discover the world at one's own pace.

The goal of the class theme "Finding one's own pace" is an invitation to feel the individual pace and to find the pace that feels good, which can vary from day to day. The participant is taught that synchronizing breath and movement speed makes good sense.

The participants should first experience the breath and develop a feel for the breathing spaces over the course of the practice. During the practice, they will learn what it feels like to move in time with the breathing rhythm. For this reason the entire unit is awareness-focused and consists of small steps.

FINDING YOUR OWN PACE

- In time with the breath: The exercises are repeated several times in time with the inhalation and exhalation rhythm.
- IH: Inhalation
- EH: Exhalation
- See chapter 7 for detailed descriptions of the individual Asanas and their modifications.

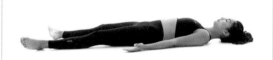	**Shavasana/arriving on the mat:** • Notice the external space with eyes closed. • Next shift your awareness to the internal space. • Notice your body. • Feel the ground beneath you; feel the body's points of contact.
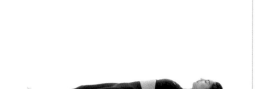	**Breath awareness and observation** • Notice your natural breath without forcing it. • Notice the coming and going of the breath. • Feel the vibration of the breathing movement. • What is your breathing rhythm? • How long does your breath flow? • Where does your breath flow? • Where in your body can you feel the movement of the breath? • Notice the undulation of the breath. • Offer tips on breathing pauses, e.g. absorb energy as you inhale and release spent energy as you exhale.

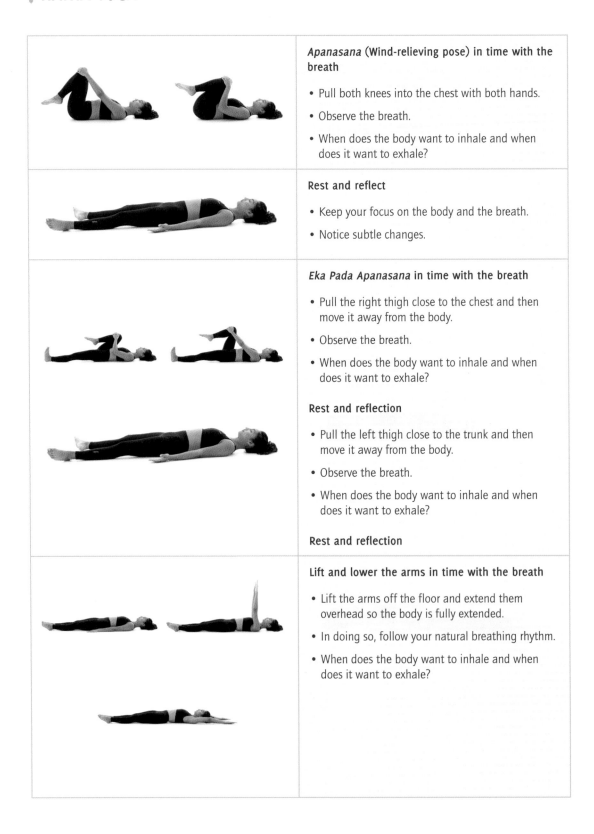

Apanasana (Wind-relieving pose) in time with the breath

- Pull both knees into the chest with both hands.
- Observe the breath.
- When does the body want to inhale and when does it want to exhale?

Rest and reflect

- Keep your focus on the body and the breath.
- Notice subtle changes.

Eka Pada Apanasana in time with the breath

- Pull the right thigh close to the chest and then move it away from the body.
- Observe the breath.
- When does the body want to inhale and when does it want to exhale?

Rest and reflection

- Pull the left thigh close to the trunk and then move it away from the body.
- Observe the breath.
- When does the body want to inhale and when does it want to exhale?

Rest and reflection

Lift and lower the arms in time with the breath

- Lift the arms off the floor and extend them overhead so the body is fully extended.
- In doing so, follow your natural breathing rhythm.
- When does the body want to inhale and when does it want to exhale?

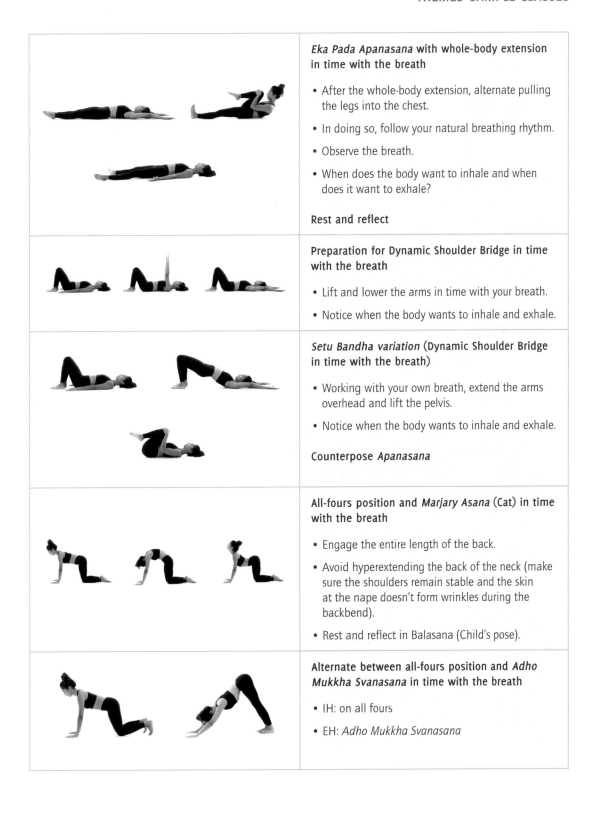

Eka Pada Apanasana with whole-body extension in time with the breath

- After the whole-body extension, alternate pulling the legs into the chest.
- In doing so, follow your natural breathing rhythm.
- Observe the breath.
- When does the body want to inhale and when does it want to exhale?

Rest and reflect

Preparation for Dynamic Shoulder Bridge in time with the breath

- Lift and lower the arms in time with your breath.
- Notice when the body wants to inhale and exhale.

Setu Bandha variation (Dynamic Shoulder Bridge in time with the breath)

- Working with your own breath, extend the arms overhead and lift the pelvis.
- Notice when the body wants to inhale and exhale.

Counterpose *Apanasana*

All-fours position and *Marjary Asana* (Cat) in time with the breath

- Engage the entire length of the back.
- Avoid hyperextending the back of the neck (make sure the shoulders remain stable and the skin at the nape doesn't form wrinkles during the backbend).
- Rest and reflect in Balasana (Child's pose).

Alternate between all-fours position and *Adho Mukkha Svanasana* in time with the breath

- IH: on all fours
- EH: *Adho Mukkha Svanasana*

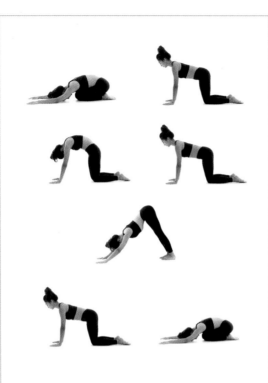

Flow "Cat-Cow pose combined with Adho Mukkha Svanasana"

- EH: *Balasana*
- IH: All-fours pose
- EH: *Marjary Asana*
- IH: All-fours pose
- EH: *Adho Mukkha Svanasana*
- IH: All-fours pose
- EH: *Balasana*

Practitioners can choose to practice IH/EH in a specified breathing rhythm. Or they can choose to let the breath flow freely and observe how the breath wants to flow without conscious breath control.

Repeat the *Karana* several times and rest and reflect in *Balasana*.

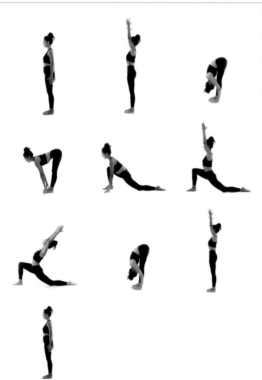

Karana from a standing posture in time with the breath

- EH: *Tadasana*
- IH: *Urdhva Hastasana*
- EH: *Uttanasana*
- IH: *Ardha Uttanasana*
- EH: *Lunge*
- IH: *Anjaney Asana* (with optional backbend)
- EH: *Uttanasana*
- IH: *Urdhva Hastasana*
- EH: *Tadasana*

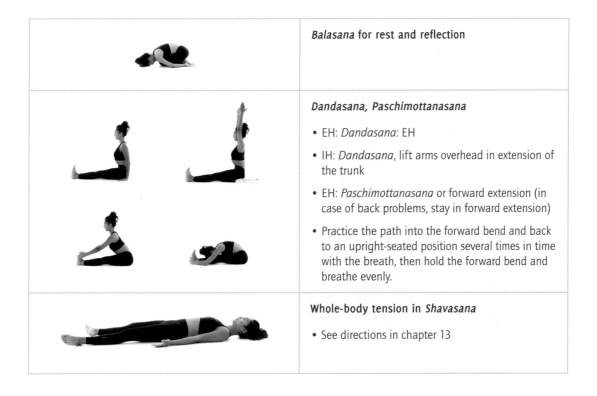

	Balasana for rest and reflection
	Dandasana, Paschimottanasana • EH: *Dandasana*: EH • IH: *Dandasana*, lift arms overhead in extension of the trunk • EH: *Paschimottanasana* or forward extension (in case of back problems, stay in forward extension) • Practice the path into the forward bend and back to an upright-seated position several times in time with the breath, then hold the forward bend and breathe evenly.
	Whole-body tension in *Shavasana* • See directions in chapter 13

12.2 LESSON PLAN 2: THE MULADHARA CHAKRA – GROUNDING AND STABILITY

The Muladhara chakra (root chakra) is located in the lower pelvic region at the lower end of the spine.

Being grounded in oneself and having both feet firmly on the ground requires a certain amount of stability. Particularly the trunk-erecting muscles, the muscles of the feet and legs, and the pelvic floor muscles give us support and carry us upright through life. An erect trunk combined with solid grounding provides the foundation for all standing poses, side- and backbends, as well as twists. In the Asana practice, we need that support as well as energy-related permeability to be able to continuously feel, to perceive.

Before the start of the practice unit, show the lotus symbol of the Muladhara chakra and explain it via the individual symbols (see chapter 5). With respect to the class progression, explain the function and position of the pelvic floor, how to control the pelvic floor to contract it, or rather how to set Mula Banda. The activation of the pelvic floor travels like a common thread through the entire class and is integrated into the Asana practice in all trunk-erecting exercises. This also serves as preparation for the more subtle aspects of energy control, which however do not yet come to bear in this lesson plan since we are first creating -meaning sensing, feeling, and controlling- the foundation on the physical level.

The following lesson plan offers different options for developing the grounding and trunk-stabilizing theme providing the basic postures have been practiced beforehand.

CLASS THEME: THE ROOT CHAKRA – MULADHARA CHAKRA

- In time with the breath: Each of the exercises is repeated several times in time with inhalation and exhalation.
- IH: Inhalation / EH: Exhalation / PF: Pelvic floor
- See chapter 7 for a detailed description of the Asanas.

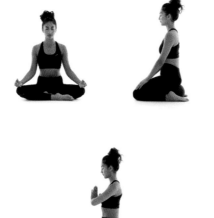

Arriving/grounding

- Find an upright-seated posture, either with legs crossed or in hero pose. If necessary support your bottom with a folded blanket or a pillow.
- Lift the spine so the lower pelvic area and the crown of the head are lined up vertically.
- Notice your body and the breath.
- Shift your attention to the lower pelvic region; become aware of the lower pelvic area.
- Connect to the Muladhara chakra: How does energy flow in that area?
- Create a sense of grounding by visualizing vigorous roots reaching from the pelvic region deep into the earth, lending support and forging a connection with the earth.

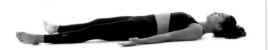

Supine position/activating the pelvic floor

- Shift your focus deeper into the lower pelvic region, contracting and releasing the individual layers one-by-one (see "Exercises to contract the pelvic floor", chapter 6).
- Rest and reflect.

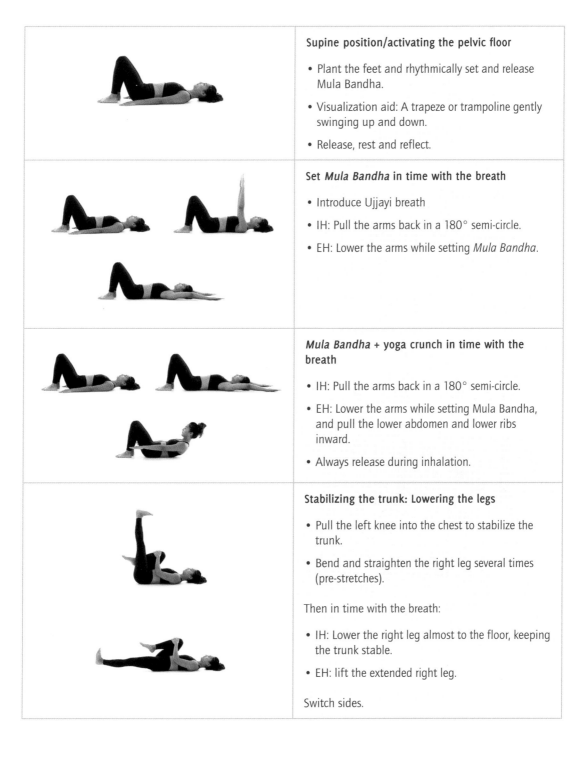

Supine position/activating the pelvic floor

- Plant the feet and rhythmically set and release Mula Bandha.
- Visualization aid: A trapeze or trampoline gently swinging up and down.
- Release, rest and reflect.

Set *Mula Bandha* in time with the breath

- Introduce Ujjayi breath
- IH: Pull the arms back in a 180° semi-circle.
- EH: Lower the arms while setting *Mula Bandha*.

Mula Bandha + yoga crunch in time with the breath

- IH: Pull the arms back in a 180° semi-circle.
- EH: Lower the arms while setting Mula Bandha, and pull the lower abdomen and lower ribs inward.
- Always release during inhalation.

Stabilizing the trunk: Lowering the legs

- Pull the left knee into the chest to stabilize the trunk.
- Bend and straighten the right leg several times (pre-stretches).

Then in time with the breath:

- IH: Lower the right leg almost to the floor, keeping the trunk stable.
- EH: lift the extended right leg.

Switch sides.

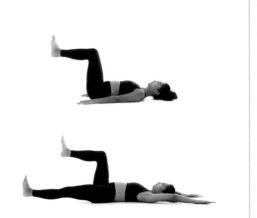

Stabilizing the trunk: Legs in tabletop pose

- Move your legs into tabletop and press the low back into the floor several times without moving your legs. Then hold your lower ribs down on the floor, or rather hold your back steady during the exercise.

In time with the breath:

- EH: Tabletop legs
- IH: Extend the right leg along the floor.
- EH: Tabletop legs
- IH: Extend the left leg along the floor.

To make the exercise more intense, you can move the arms overhead during inhalation after a few repetitions.

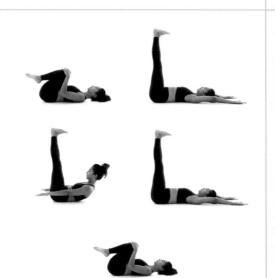

Flow *Apanasana*, *Prasarita Padasana*, Crunch

- EH: *Apanasana*
- IH: *Prasarita Padasana* (table)
- EH: Crunch
- IH: *Prasarita Padasana* (table)
- EH: *Apanasana*

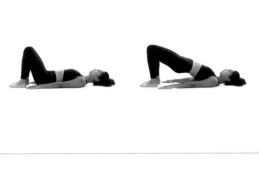

Dwi Pada Pitham – Shoulder Bridge

- IH: Shoulder Bridge
- EH: Roll down vertebrae by vertebrae

Practice a few times in time with breathing, then hold Shoulder Bridge for several breaths.

- Rest and reflect

Counter pose: *Apanasana*

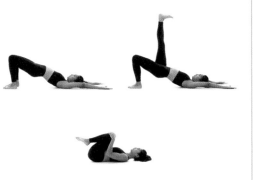

Dwi Pada Pitham with leg lift

Grounding and stabilization of the trunk muscles by alternately lifting the legs while the trunk is stabilized (grounded) by the pelvic floor and the trunk muscles.

- IH: Lift the pelvis, move the arms overhead and remain there for the duration of the exercise.
- EH: Alternate extending your legs to the ceiling.

After finishing the exercise, roll back down vertebrae by vertebrae and do *Apanasana* as a counter pose.

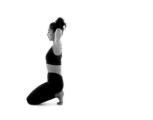

Stretch your toes and plantar fasciae along with loosening up the shoulders

- Various variations of upper arm circles
- Circle the wrists (no photos)
- Make fists and then spread your fingers wide in preparation of support poses (no photo).

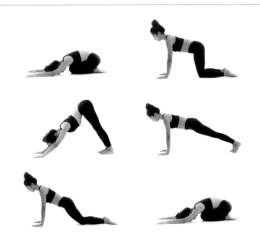

Flow "Introduction to *Adho Mukha Svanasana* and *Phalakasana*"

- *Balasana* EH
- All-fours pose IH
- *Marjary Asana* EH
- All-fours pose IH
- *Adho Mukkha Svanasana* EH
- All-fours pose IH
- *Balasana* EH

Repeat the Karana several times and rest and reflect in Balasana.

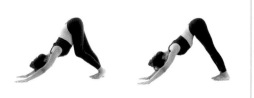

"Walking Dog"

Alternate pedaling the feet in *Adho Mukkha Svanasana*, then hold in *Adho Mukkha Svanasana*.

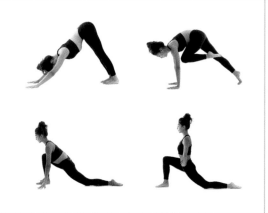

Hip-flexor stretch and introduction to
Anjaney Asana

- Preparation for the subsequent standing flow; set Mula Bandha as you lift the trunk and watch your body alignment (joint position) and grounding of feet and legs in the deep lunge.

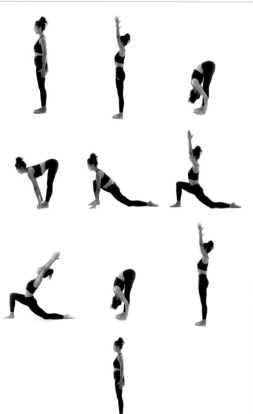

***Karana* from a standing position in time with the breath**

- EH: *Tadasana*
- IH: *Urdhva Hastasana*
- EH: *Uttanasana*
- IH: *Ardha Uttanasana*
- EH: *Lunge*
- IH: *Anjaney Asana*
- EH: *Uttanasana*
- IH: *Urdhva Hastasana*
- EH: *Tadasana*

The flow is practiced in a calm breathing rhythm; set Mula Bandha with every inhalation (trunk erection).

The emphasis of the flow is on the trunk erection.

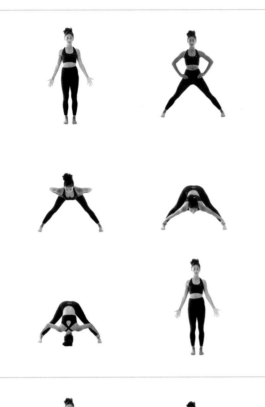

Prasarita Padottanasana – Straddle Forward Bend

- Here the emphasis is on grounding the feet, as well as hip- and knee alignment.

- The backs and insides of the legs are being stretched.

- The difference between the forward bend and forward extension should be experienced here.

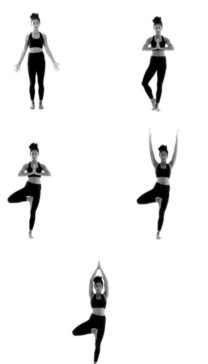

Vriksasana – Tree

- The pose is built with various modifications, depending on hip flexibility and current sense of balance.

- Even if you sway and wobble a lot in the pose, it ultimately helps you experience grounding.

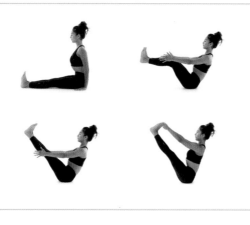

Navasana – Boat

- Here the emphasis is on experiencing the grounding trunk erection.

- The Boat is built with the modification "Half Boat" with knees bent.

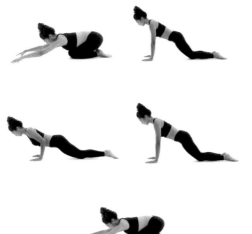

Preparatory introduction to *Chaturanga Dandasana* (Four-link Staff pose)

Flow with small steps to build arm- and shoulder strength combined with trunk stability.

- EH: Utthita Balasana

- IH: Half plank

- EH: triceps pushup*

- IH: Half plank

- EH: Utthita Balasana

*If shoulders and arms are not yet strong enough for half pushups, bend the elbows slightly less.

Trunk and pelvic floor muscles are engaged during the flow.

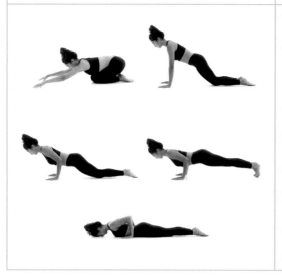

Phalakasana – High Plank

- The high plank prepares for *Chaturanga Dandasana*. Here, too, the trunk and pelvic floor muscles are engaged.

- Transition to the floor can be done via *Half Plank*.

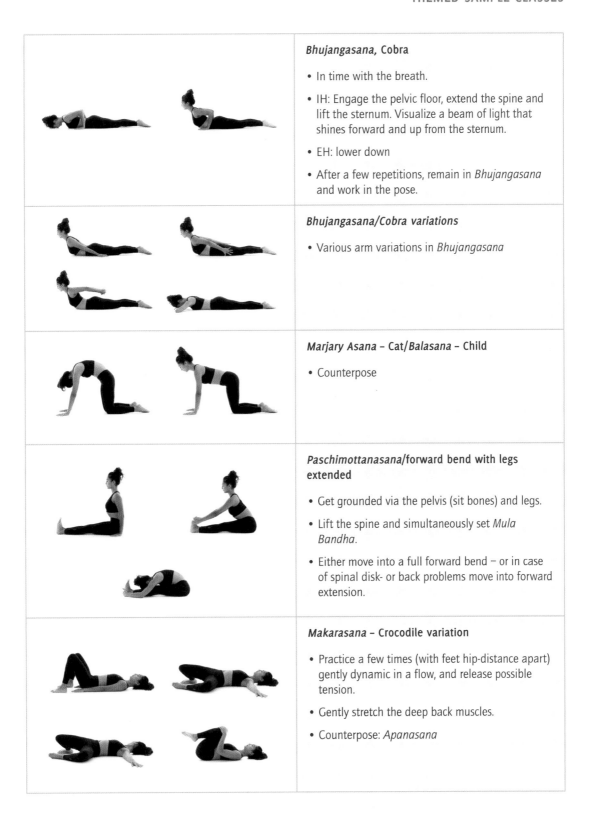

Bhujangasana, Cobra

- In time with the breath.
- IH: Engage the pelvic floor, extend the spine and lift the sternum. Visualize a beam of light that shines forward and up from the sternum.
- EH: lower down
- After a few repetitions, remain in *Bhujangasana* and work in the pose.

Bhujangasana/Cobra variations

- Various arm variations in *Bhujangasana*

Marjary Asana – Cat/*Balasana* – Child

- Counterpose

Paschimottanasana/forward bend with legs extended

- Get grounded via the pelvis (sit bones) and legs.
- Lift the spine and simultaneously set *Mula Bandha*.
- Either move into a full forward bend – or in case of spinal disk- or back problems move into forward extension.

Makarasana – Crocodile variation

- Practice a few times (with feet hip-distance apart) gently dynamic in a flow, and release possible tension.
- Gently stretch the deep back muscles.
- Counterpose: *Apanasana*

	Whole-body relaxation in *Shavasana* • See instructions in chapter 13.
	Visualization exercise – • "Tree" • See instruction in chapter 13

12.3 LESSON PLAN 3
THE SVADHISTHANA CHAKRA – WATER, FLOW OF MOVEMENT, LETTING GO

The *Svadhisthana chakra* is located in the sacral-bladder region at a level with the internal genitalia. Areas of the body associated with this chakra are low back, genitalia, kidneys, bladder, as well as the cardiovascular system.

The associated element is water. Water represents the changeability of feelings. Water represents cooling and especially the flow of energy in the different density and aggregation states.

The following class theme is intended to direct the focus to the pelvic area, lower back, and hips. The physical emphasis of the praxis is on opening the hips. The energy-related emphasis of the class is on letting go (allowing flow), which is initiated with the prolonged forward- and side bends. The class intensity is rather more calm, gentle, and measured with the inner focus on sensing and feeling. Becoming aware of the changeability within us, and allowing solidified energy to gently begin to flow again. Often it is the calm, awareness-oriented meditative yoga classes that trigger internal processes and allow us to experience on a deeper level.

Before starting the unit, show the Svadhisthana chakra lotus symbol and explain it via the different symbols (see chapter 5).

CLASS THEME: THE SACRAL CHAKRA – SVADISTHANA CHAKRA

- In time with the breath: The exercises are repeated several times in time with the inhalations and exhalations.
- IH: Inhalation / EH: Exhalation / PF: Pelvic floor
- See chapter 7 for a detailed description of the Asanas.

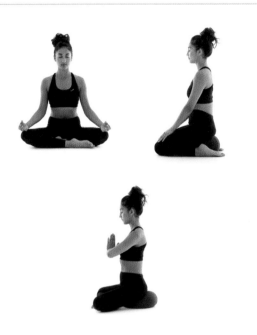

Arriving/introduction

- Find the upright-seated posture with legs crossed or hero pose. Support your bottom with a folded blanket or a pillow.
- Lift the spine so the lower pelvic area and the crown of the head are lined up vertically.
- Gather yourself and attune yourself to the class.

Supine position

- Notice the body (e.g. via its points of contact).
- Notice your natural breath without forcing or changing it.
- Direct your focus to the flow within the body. The flow of the blood, the lymph, the flow of the breath that supports the flow on all planes.
- Direct your focus to the flow of energy in the body. Where does the energy flow? Where do I feel energized? Where is the energy backed up? Are there areas of the body I currently feel less or not at all?
- Gently direct the breath to the lower abdomen; feel the movement of the breath in the lower abdomen and become aware of the energy center in the lower abdomen.

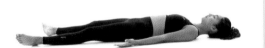

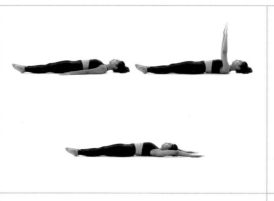

Synchronization of breath- and movement flow

- Notice the undulation of the breath inside the body and connect with it; follow the natural rhythm of the breath.

- Gently initiate *Ujjayi breath**, allow breaths to get longer, letting them gently flow.

- Combine the flow of the breath with the exercise "arm raises".

*See chapter 9

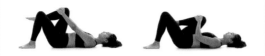

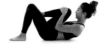

Eka Pada Apana Asana – one-legged, Wind-relieving pose

- EH: Pull the playing leg into the chest.
- IH: Release

To deepen the effect, after several repetitions also lift the upper body as you exhale (nose to knee) and pull in the lower abdomen for support.

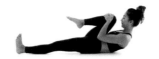

Eka Pada Apanasana with whole-body extension in time with the breath

- After the whole-body extension, alternate pulling the knees into the chest.

- As you do so, follow your natural breathing rhythm.

- EH: Consciously pull your lower abdomen in during *Eka Pada Apana Asana*. Consciously let go as you exhale.

- IH: release and allow the energy to flow into the body.

Rest and reflect

- Notice the energy in the body.

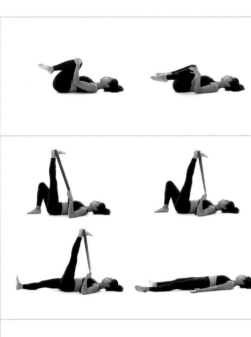

Loosening up the hips

- Use your hands to move your thighs in circles from the hip joint in both directions.
- Notice your hip mobility.
- Gently pre-stretch the inner-thigh muscles.

Stretching the ischiocrural muscles – back of the legs

- Gentle dynamic stretches of the back of the legs, first with the supporting leg propped, then deeper with the supporting leg extended on the floor and holding the stretch.
- Rest and reflect and compare both sides of the body before stretching the other leg.

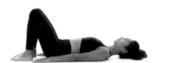

Pelvic tilts in time with the breath

- EH: Gently press the low back into the floor.
- IH: Arch the low back.

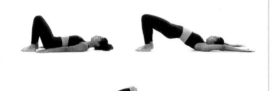

Dwi Pada Pitham – Shoulder Bridge

- IH: Shoulder Bridge with arms extended overhead.
- EH: Roll down vertebrae by vertebrae.

Practice several times in time with the breath.

Rest and reflect.

- Counterpose: *Apanasana*

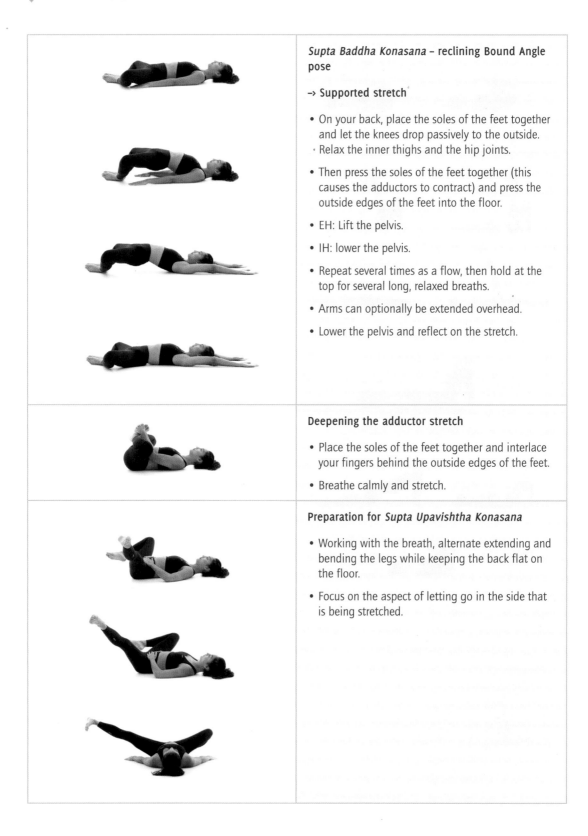

Supta Baddha Konasana – reclining Bound Angle pose

–> Supported stretch

- On your back, place the soles of the feet together and let the knees drop passively to the outside. Relax the inner thighs and the hip joints.

- Then press the soles of the feet together (this causes the adductors to contract) and press the outside edges of the feet into the floor.

- EH: Lift the pelvis.

- IH: lower the pelvis.

- Repeat several times as a flow, then hold at the top for several long, relaxed breaths.

- Arms can optionally be extended overhead.

- Lower the pelvis and reflect on the stretch.

Deepening the adductor stretch

- Place the soles of the feet together and interlace your fingers behind the outside edges of the feet.

- Breathe calmly and stretch.

Preparation for *Supta Upavishtha Konasana*

- Working with the breath, alternate extending and bending the legs while keeping the back flat on the floor.

- Focus on the aspect of letting go in the side that is being stretched.

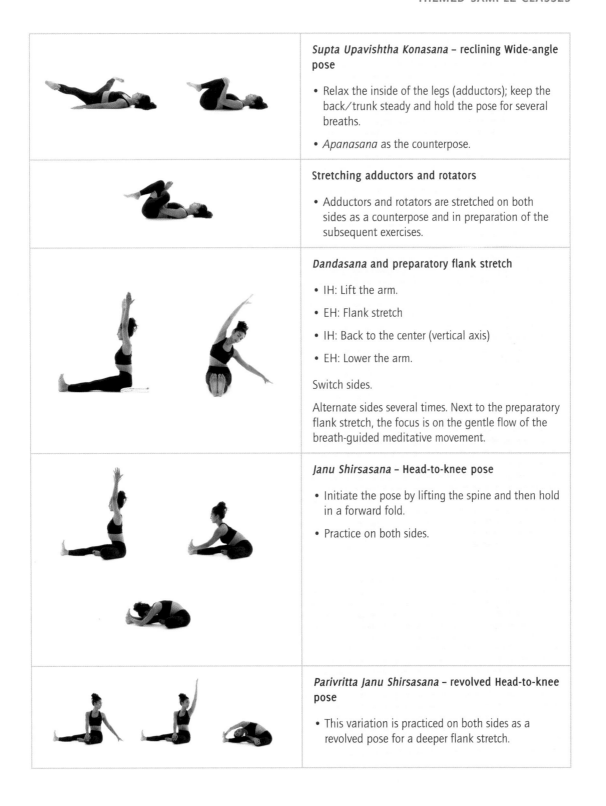

Supta Upavishtha Konasana – reclining Wide-angle pose

- Relax the inside of the legs (adductors); keep the back/trunk steady and hold the pose for several breaths.
- *Apanasana* as the counterpose.

Stretching adductors and rotators

- Adductors and rotators are stretched on both sides as a counterpose and in preparation of the subsequent exercises.

Dandasana and preparatory flank stretch

- IH: Lift the arm.
- EH: Flank stretch
- IH: Back to the center (vertical axis)
- EH: Lower the arm.

Switch sides.

Alternate sides several times. Next to the preparatory flank stretch, the focus is on the gentle flow of the breath-guided meditative movement.

Janu Shirsasana – Head-to-knee pose

- Initiate the pose by lifting the spine and then hold in a forward fold.
- Practice on both sides.

Parivritta Janu Shirsasana – revolved Head-to-knee pose

- This variation is practiced on both sides as a revolved pose for a deeper flank stretch.

353

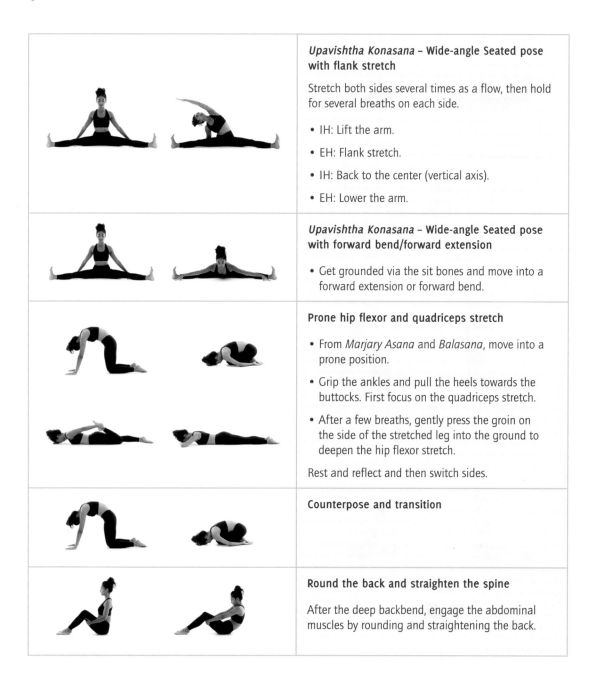

Upavishtha Konasana – Wide-angle Seated pose with flank stretch

Stretch both sides several times as a flow, then hold for several breaths on each side.

- IH: Lift the arm.
- EH: Flank stretch.
- IH: Back to the center (vertical axis).
- EH: Lower the arm.

Upavishtha Konasana – Wide-angle Seated pose with forward bend/forward extension

- Get grounded via the sit bones and move into a forward extension or forward bend.

Prone hip flexor and quadriceps stretch

- From *Marjary Asana* and *Balasana*, move into a prone position.
- Grip the ankles and pull the heels towards the buttocks. First focus on the quadriceps stretch.
- After a few breaths, gently press the groin on the side of the stretched leg into the ground to deepen the hip flexor stretch.

Rest and reflect and then switch sides.

Counterpose and transition

Round the back and straighten the spine

After the deep backbend, engage the abdominal muscles by rounding and straightening the back.

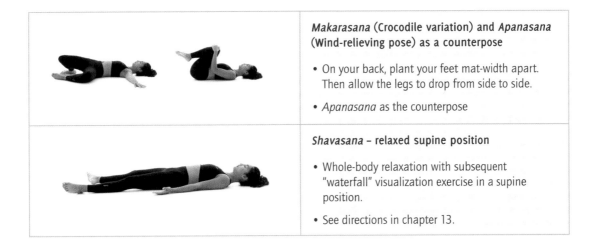

	Makarasana (Crocodile variation) and *Apanasana* (Wind-relieving pose) as a counterpose
	• On your back, plant your feet mat-width apart. Then allow the legs to drop from side to side.
	• *Apanasana* as the counterpose
	Shavasana – relaxed supine position
	• Whole-body relaxation with subsequent "waterfall" visualization exercise in a supine position.
	• See directions in chapter 13.

12.4 LESSON PLAN 4: THE MANIPURA CHAKRA – FIRE, TRANSFORMATION, WILLPOWER

The *Manipura chakra* is also called *"City of Jewels"*, which refers to the brightness and radiance of the sun's energy. It is located not directly in the navel area but in the region between the solar plexus and the navel. The associated areas of the body are the upper and middle stomach area, the digestive system, and the vegetative nervous system.

The chakra's main themes are transformation on all planes, the awakening of the inner fire, and the development of willpower. Traveling on the spiritual path sometimes requires lots of willpower to reach loftier goals. The associated element is fire. It contributes the necessary energy to initiate and halt processes.

The practice linked to the element fire is heat building, stimulating, and requires a certain amount of willpower during some of the yoga unit's phases. The Asanas affect the belly area and include primarily forward and backbends, as well as the classic *Rishikesh* Sun Salutation to stimulate energy and promote its flow. Here practitioners can experience warmth and heat in the body and their transformation.

Show the *Manpipura chakra's* lotus symbol before the start of the practice unit and explain it via the individual symbols (see chapter 5).

CLASS THEME: THE MANIPURA CHAKRA – THE NAVEL CHAKRA

- In time with the breath: Each of the exercises is repeated several times in time with the inhalations and exhalations.
- IH: Inhalation / EH: Exhalation / PF: Pelvic floor
- See chapter 7 for a detailed description of the Asanas.

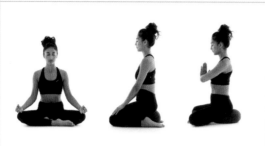

Arriving/Introduction

- Find an upright-seated pose, either with legs crossed or hero pose. Support your bottom with a folded blanket or a pillow.
- Lift the spine so the lower pelvic area and the crown of the head are lined up vertically.
- Mentally gather yourself and get attuned to the class.

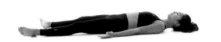

Body and breath awareness

- Notice your body, for instance via its points of contact.
- Notice your natural breath without forcing it.
- Feel how the energy is distributed in the body. Are there areas that feel particularly warm or vibrant? Are there areas you perceive less vividly?
- Focus your attention on the belly, notice the undulation of the breath and gradually lengthen the breath, use Ujjayi breath.

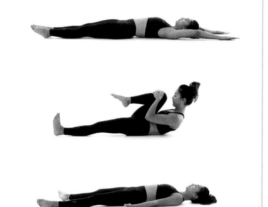

Eka Pada Apanasana (one-legged, Wind-relieving pose) with whole-body extension in time with the breath

- IH: Lift the arms and extend the body completely.
- EH: Alternate pulling the knees to the chest; as you do so, pull the lower and upper abdomen as well as the lower ribs in and up.
- Repeat several times and reflect.

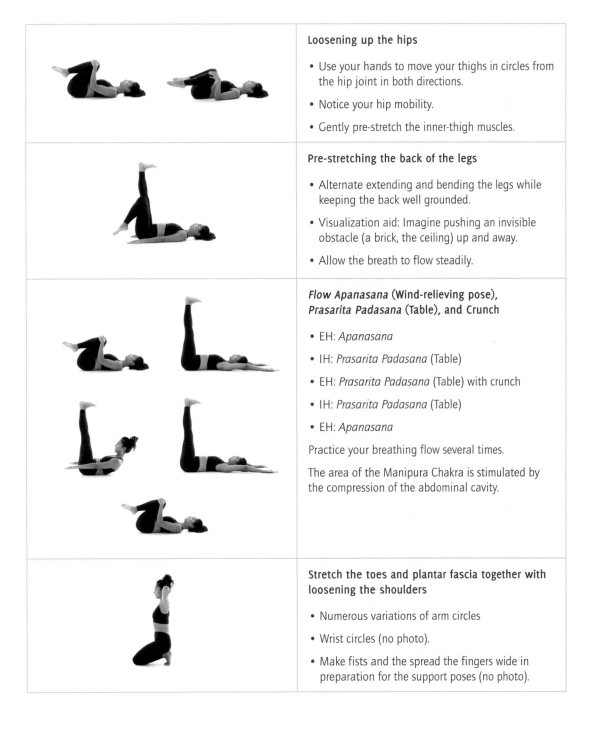

Loosening up the hips

- Use your hands to move your thighs in circles from the hip joint in both directions.
- Notice your hip mobility.
- Gently pre-stretch the inner-thigh muscles.

Pre-stretching the back of the legs

- Alternate extending and bending the legs while keeping the back well grounded.
- Visualization aid: Imagine pushing an invisible obstacle (a brick, the ceiling) up and away.
- Allow the breath to flow steadily.

Flow Apanasana (Wind-relieving pose), *Prasarita Padasana* (Table), and Crunch

- EH: *Apanasana*
- IH: *Prasarita Padasana* (Table)
- EH: *Prasarita Padasana* (Table) with crunch
- IH: *Prasarita Padasana* (Table)
- EH: *Apanasana*

Practice your breathing flow several times.

The area of the Manipura Chakra is stimulated by the compression of the abdominal cavity.

Stretch the toes and plantar fascia together with loosening the shoulders

- Numerous variations of arm circles
- Wrist circles (no photo).
- Make fists and the spread the fingers wide in preparation for the support poses (no photo).

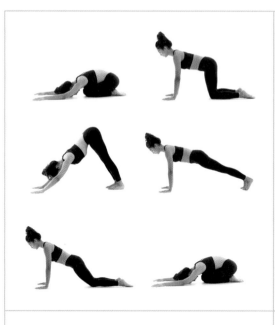

Flow "Introduction to *Adho Mukkha Svanasana* (Downward-facing Dog) and *Phalakasana* (Plank)"

- *Balasana*: EH
- All-fours pose: IH
- *Marjary Asana*: EH
- All-fours pose: IH
- *Adho Mukkha Svanasana*: EH
- All-fours pose: IH
- *Balasana*: EH

Repeat this *Karana* several times and rest and reflect in *Balasana*.

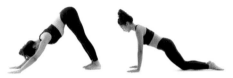

"*Walking Dog*" – pedal the feet

In *Adho Mukkha Svanasana* alternate pedaling the feet, then hold in *Adho Mukkha Svanasana*.

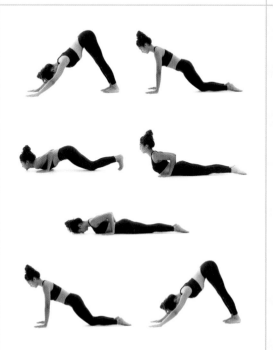

Flow "*Floor Vinyasa/prostration*" in preparation for the *Rishikesh* Sun Salutation

- EH: Adho Mukkha Svanasana
- IH: Half plank
- EH: Knee-chest-chin pose
- IH: Small Cobra
- EH: From a supine position to Half Plank (or All-fours pose) to *Adho Mukkha Svanasana*.

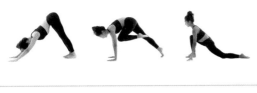

Hip flexor stretch and transition to Lunge

Preparation for *Rishikesh Sun Salutation*

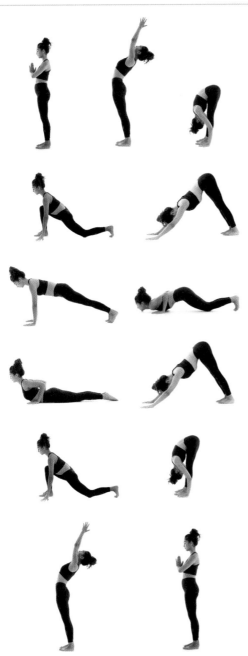

Rishikesh Sun Salutation

- IH/EH: *Tadasana/Anjali Mudra*, gather yourself, prayer hands.

- IH: *Tadasana* with backbend, open up to the light.

- EH: *Uttanasana*, bow to the sun.

- IH: Lunge, get grounded and lift the heart to the higher sun.

- *Adho Mukkha Svanasana*

- IH/EH: Fluid movement via Plank (*Phalakasana*) to Eight-angle pose.

- IH: *Bhujangasana* (Cobra), lift the higher heart towards the sun.

- EH: *Adho Mukkha Svanasana*

- IH: Forward Lunge

- EH: *Uttanasana*, bow to the sun.

- IH: *Tadasana* with backbend

- EH: Gather in *Tadasana*

Repeat everything on the other side for 6-12 repetitions.

Afterwards, rest and reflect and notice the pulsation and warmth in the body. Observe the breath and the breathing rhythm.

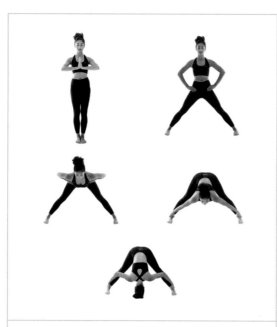

Prasarita Padottanasana (Straddle Forward Bend)

- Straighten the spine and pre-stretch the inner thigh muscles (adductors).

- Particular emphasis is placed on the transition from Forward Bend to Forward Extension (and vice-versa).

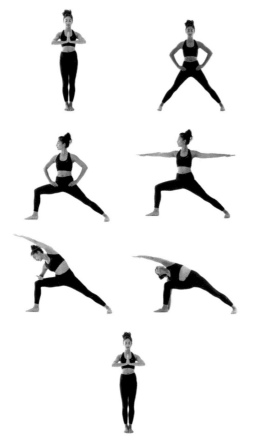

Virabhadrasana II (Kriegerhaltung II) and Parsvakonasana (Extended Side Angle)

- Long, calm breaths while assuming the poses.

- Hold for a few breaths in *Virabhadrasana II* and *Parsvakonasana* and align body and mind.

- Combining both poses prepares for *Trikonasana* (Triangle).

- Set *Mula Bandha* for all trunk-erecting poses.

- Rest and reflect after the first side, then practice on the other side.

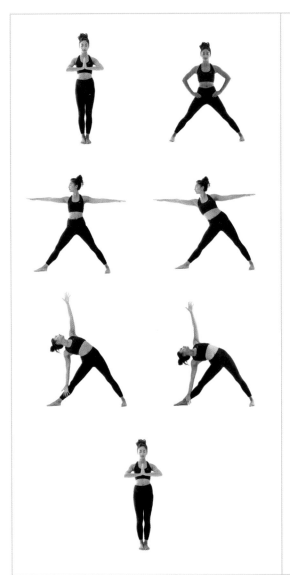

Trikonasana – Triangle

- Bring the length of *Prasvakonasana* into *Trikonasana*.

- Breathe calmly and evenly in *Trikonasana*.

- Rest and reflect and repeat on the other side.

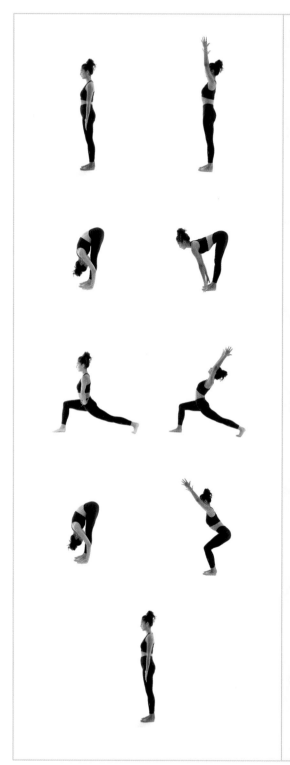

Alanasana-Flow – deep hip flexor stretch

- *Alanasana* (modification of *Virabhadrasana I*) deeply stretches the hip flexor muscles in preparation of the backbends. Practice *Utkatasana* on the way back to standing to stabilize the trunk muscles again after the deep backbend/lunge.

- EH: *Tadasana*

- IH: *Urdhva Hastasana*

- EH: *Uttanasana*

- IH: *Ardha Uttanasana*

- EH: Lunge

- IH: *Alanasana* with backbend

- EH: *Uttanasana*

- IH: *Utkatasana*

- EH: *Tadasana*

Set *Mula Bandha* every time you lift the trunk or when you inhale.

Rest and reflect and repeat on the other side.

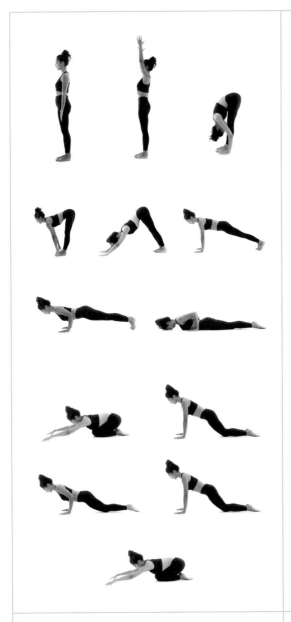

Transition to prone position via *Chaturanga Dandasana*

- EH: *Tadasana*
- IH: *Urdva Hastasana*
- EH: *Uttanasana*
- IH: *Ardha Uttanasana*
- EH: *Adho Mukkha Svanasana*

Either practice the fluid transition from standing to the prone position or practice a dynamic transition to Chaturanga Dandasana several times via Half Plank:

- EH: *Utthita Balasana*
- IH: *Half Plank*
- EH: *Triceps pushup*
- IH: *Half Plank*
- EH: *Utthita Balasana*
- IH: *Phalakasana*
- EH: *Chaturanga Dandasana* to move into a prone position.

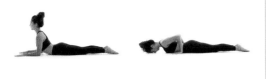

Sphinx

- *Sphinx* is practiced in preparation of the subsequent backbends with emphasis on stabilizing the pose and activating the pelvic floor muscles (set *Mula Bandha*) and lower abdominal muscles.

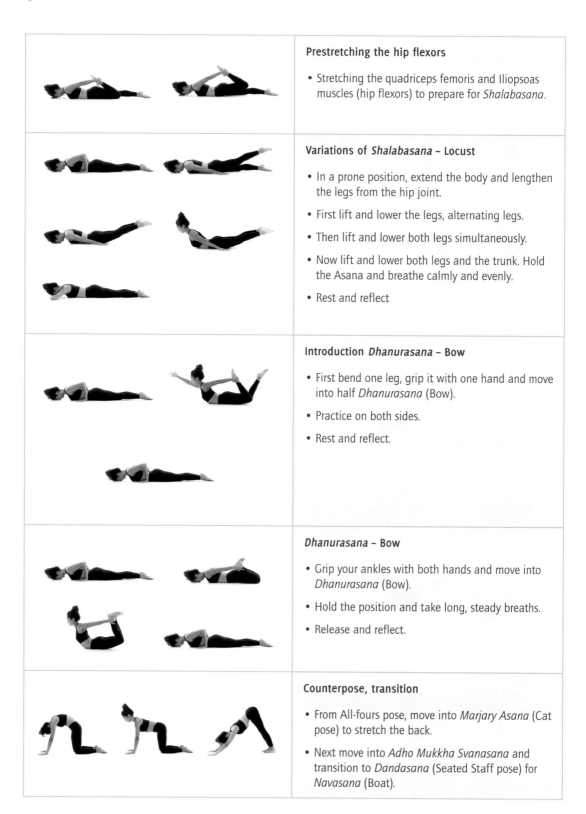

Prestretching the hip flexors

- Stretching the quadriceps femoris and Iliopsoas muscles (hip flexors) to prepare for *Shalabasana*.

Variations of *Shalabasana* – Locust

- In a prone position, extend the body and lengthen the legs from the hip joint.
- First lift and lower the legs, alternating legs.
- Then lift and lower both legs simultaneously.
- Now lift and lower both legs and the trunk. Hold the Asana and breathe calmly and evenly.
- Rest and reflect

Introduction *Dhanurasana* – Bow

- First bend one leg, grip it with one hand and move into half *Dhanurasana* (Bow).
- Practice on both sides.
- Rest and reflect.

Dhanurasana – Bow

- Grip your ankles with both hands and move into *Dhanurasana* (Bow).
- Hold the position and take long, steady breaths.
- Release and reflect.

Counterpose, transition

- From All-fours pose, move into *Marjary Asana* (Cat pose) to stretch the back.
- Next move into *Adho Mukkha Svanasana* and transition to *Dandasana* (Seated Staff pose) for *Navasana* (Boat).

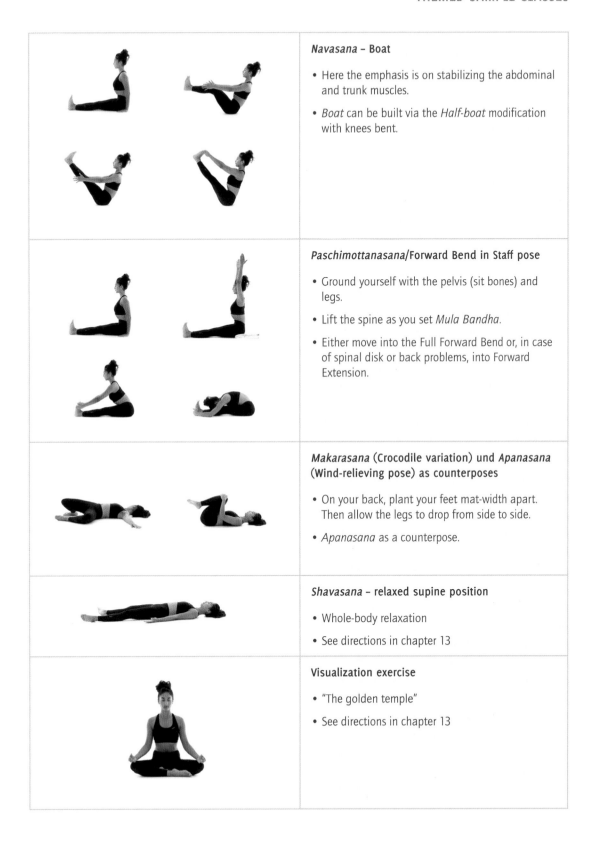

Navasana – Boat

- Here the emphasis is on stabilizing the abdominal and trunk muscles.
- *Boat* can be built via the *Half-boat* modification with knees bent.

Paschimottanasana/Forward Bend in Staff pose

- Ground yourself with the pelvis (sit bones) and legs.
- Lift the spine as you set *Mula Bandha*.
- Either move into the Full Forward Bend or, in case of spinal disk or back problems, into Forward Extension.

Makarasana (Crocodile variation) und *Apanasana* (Wind-relieving pose) as counterposes

- On your back, plant your feet mat-width apart. Then allow the legs to drop from side to side.
- *Apanasana* as a counterpose.

Shavasana – relaxed supine position

- Whole-body relaxation
- See directions in chapter 13

Visualization exercise

- "The golden temple"
- See directions in chapter 13

12.5 LESSON PLAN 5: THE ANAHATA CHAKRA – AIR, EXPANSE, SPIRITUAL CENTER

The *heart chakra* is located at a level with the physical heart, behind the sternum. The associated areas of the body are the ribcage, upper back, heart, lungs, arms, and hands. The *Anahata chakra's* dominant element is air.

The heart chakra is our spiritual center. When our heart feels heavy, and worry and hardship dominate mental and emotional wellbeing, it often manifests itself in a protective stance. The shoulders pull forward and the upper back is rounded. A wide and open chest cavity also creates an inner feeling of openness and freedom. Since the chakras don't just open to the front, but also to the back, the upper back, the area between the shoulder blades, is particularly important. We are not able to see this very sensitive part of the body, only feel it. Many people have painful muscle tension there that is caused by muscle imbalances on the physical plane. The upper back is too weak while the front of the ribcage is shortened.

The following lesson plan will shift the focus to the higher heart space, combined with exercises and poses that stretch the chest to create a feeling of openness, and strengthen the upper back. Since the heart often needs protection on the emotional plane, the chosen exercises include the opening and closing of the heart space to facilitate a flexible inner posture for these processes.

The polarity of Shiva and Shakti, of descending and rising energy, of the power of consciousness and energy express themselves in the heart.

Before the start of the unit, show the lotus symbol of the *Anahata chakra* and explain it via the individual symbols (see chapter 5).

THEMED SAMPLE CLASSES

- In time with the breath: Each of the exercises is repeated several times in time with the inhalation and exhalation.
- IH: Inhalation / EH: Exhalation / PF: Pelvic floor
- See chapter 7 for a detailed description of the Asanas.

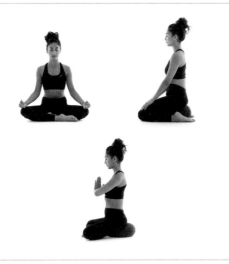

Arriving/introduction

- Find an upright-seated position either with legs crossed, or hero pose. If necessary, support your bottom with a folded blanket or a pillow.
- Lift the spine so the lower pelvic area and the crown of the head are lined up vertically.
- Gather yourself and attune yourself to the class.
- For support, place your hands in Anjali Mudra or lay both hands over the higher heart space and breathe into the heart space to become aware of the higher heart.

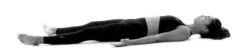

Body and breath awareness

- Notice your body, e.g. via its points of contact.
- Notice your natural breath without forcing it.
- Place one hand on your stomach and the other hand on the higher heart space and connect to the breathing wave.

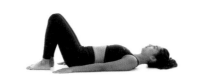

Pelvic tilt

- Plant your feet and practice the pelvic tilt in time with the breath.
- EH: Gently press the lower back into the floor.
- IH: Tilt the lumbar spine upward.

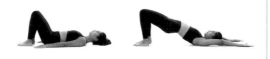

Dwi Pada Pitham – Dynamic Shoulder Bridge in time with the breath

- IH: Move into Shoulder Bridge while lifting the arms.
- EH: Roll back down vertebrae by vertebrae.

	Dwi Pada Pitham and _Apanasana_ variation in time with the breath • IH: Move into Shoulder Bridge while lifting the arms. • EH: _Apanasana_ and roll the body up. Experience the polarity of expanse and narrowness.
	Loosen up the hips • Use your hands to move your thighs in circles from the hip joint in both directions. • Notice your hip mobility; gently pre-stretch the inner-thigh muscles. Preparation for the upright seated exercises.
	Pre-stretching of the back of the legs • Alternate extending and bending the legs while keeping the back well grounded. • Visualization aid: Imagine pushing an invisible obstacle (a brick, the ceiling) up and away. • Allow the breath to flow steadily.
	Shoulder circles Loosening up the shoulders. • EH: Rest your fingertips on your shoulders, then move the elbows forward until they touch. • IH: Lift the elbows and keep circling the arms back. As you do so, either tuck the toes (stretches toes and plantar fascia) or rest on the tops of the toes. Keep the trunk steady during the exercise.

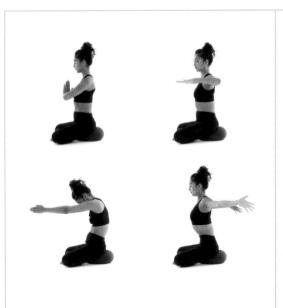

"Flap your wings" in time with your breathing

- IH: Short wing beat. Pull the elbows back at shoulder-level while lifting the sternum and squeezing the shoulder blades together.

- EH: Extend the arms forward to stretch the upper back.

- IH: Long wing beat. Move the extended arms far back with the palms facing out to stretch the muscle chain between fingertips and ribcage.

- EH: Long forward wing beat until hands touch.

- IH: Short wing beat.

Feel the connection between the chest and upper back. Experience expanse and narrowness.

Keep the trunk (lumbar spines and pelvis) steady during the exercise.

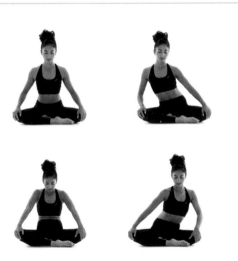

Sufi grinds

Experience flexibility and suppleness in the thoracic spine area. During the exercise the pelvis remains stable while the ribcage moves in fluid circles forward, to the side, back, and to the side.

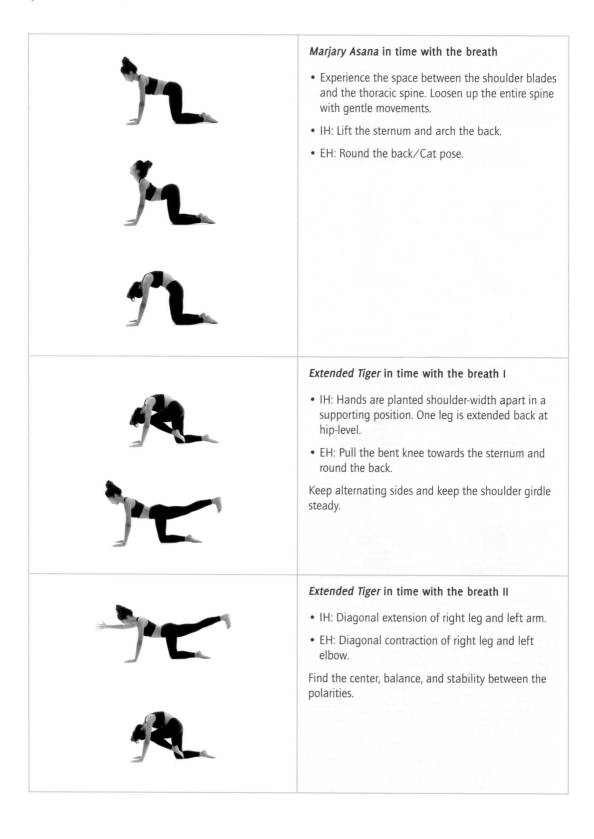

Marjary Asana in time with the breath

- Experience the space between the shoulder blades and the thoracic spine. Loosen up the entire spine with gentle movements.
- IH: Lift the sternum and arch the back.
- EH: Round the back/Cat pose.

Extended Tiger in time with the breath I

- IH: Hands are planted shoulder-width apart in a supporting position. One leg is extended back at hip-level.
- EH: Pull the bent knee towards the sternum and round the back.

Keep alternating sides and keep the shoulder girdle steady.

Extended Tiger in time with the breath II

- IH: Diagonal extension of right leg and left arm.
- EH: Diagonal contraction of right leg and left elbow.

Find the center, balance, and stability between the polarities.

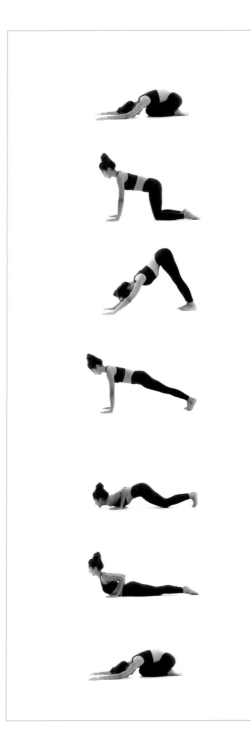

Flow in preparation of subsequent backbends

- EH: *Balasana*
- IH: All-fours pose
- EH: *Adho Mukkha Svanasana*
- IH: *Phalakasana*
- EH: Eight-angle pose (knee-chest-chin)
- IH: *Bhujangasana*
- EH: *Balasana*

The heart space leads the movement with the mental image of a spotlight shining straight ahead from the sternum.

Repeat the *Karana* several times and reflect in *Balasana*.

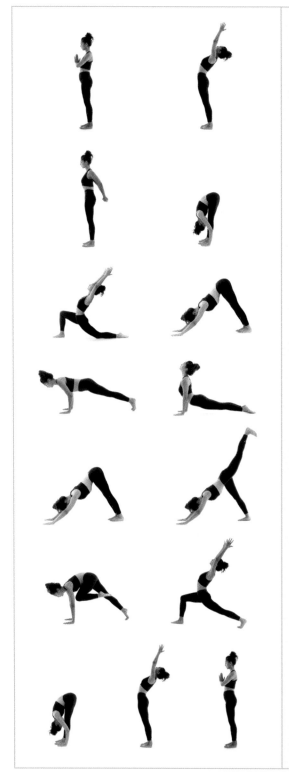

Flow "heart-space opener"

- EH: Tadasana *"Anjali Mudra"*

- IH: Standing backbend

- EH: Lower the arms and interlace your fingers behind your back.

- IH: Squeeze the shoulder blades together and lift the sternum.

- EH: Release the hands and move into *Uttanasana.*

- IH: *Anjaney Asana*

- EH: *Adho Mukkha Svanasana*

- IH: Transition *Chaturanga Dandasana* to *Urdhva Mukkha Svanasana* (or *Bhujangasana* as an alternative).

- EH: *Adho Mukkha Svanasana*

- IH: *Eka Pada Adho Mukkha Svanasana*

- EH: Transition to Lunge.

- IH: *Alanasana*

- EH: *Uttanasana*

- IH: *Standing backbend*

- EH: *Tadasana "Anjali Mudra"*

Repeat everything on the other side.

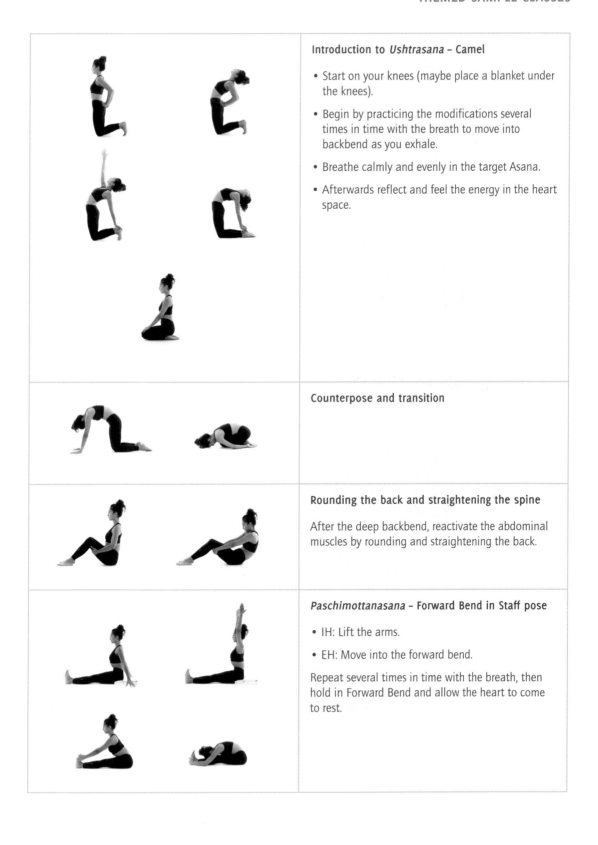

Introduction to *Ushtrasana* – Camel

- Start on your knees (maybe place a blanket under the knees).
- Begin by practicing the modifications several times in time with the breath to move into backbend as you exhale.
- Breathe calmly and evenly in the target Asana.
- Afterwards reflect and feel the energy in the heart space.

Counterpose and transition

Rounding the back and straightening the spine

After the deep backbend, reactivate the abdominal muscles by rounding and straightening the back.

Paschimottanasana – Forward Bend in Staff pose

- IH: Lift the arms.
- EH: Move into the forward bend.

Repeat several times in time with the breath, then hold in Forward Bend and allow the heart to come to rest.

	Makarasana variations – Crocodile variations Practice one of the variations based on your flexibility, and shift the focus to the chest/heart space.
	Counterpose *Apanasana*
	***Shavasana* – relaxed supine position** • Whole-body relaxation • See directions in chapter 13.
	Visualization exercise • "Light in the higher heart" • See directions in chapter 13.

12.6   LESSON PLAN 6: THE VISHUDDHA CHAKRA – SPACE, VIBRATION, SOUND, VOICE, COMMUNICATION

The *Vishuddha chakra*, also called the *throat chakra*, is located in the middle of the throat. The associated parts of the body are neck and nape, throat, vocal cords, voice apparatus, thyroid, and esophagus.

A large percentage of the population is familiar with painful tightness in the neck area. As the connection between head and body (intellect and emotion), this narrow passage between the two is usually the target organ for all sorts of stressors. The *Vishuddha chakra's* associated element is space. The following lesson plan is intended to create space on the physical level via gently releasing movements for neck and nape to get the energy to flow again in that area.

The sounding of vowels (vowel space exercise) creates subtle vibrations in the body that can release muscle tension. Focusing on the neck area during the flows will make it easier to experience the head- and neck movements in combination with the breath.

The target Asana in this yoga unit is *Viparita Karani, Half Shoulder stand*. The introduction via *Shoulder Bridge* (*Setu Bandha*) will train the feel for the neck- and nape area.

Before the start of the practice unit, show the lotus symbol of the *Vishuddha chakra* and explain it via the individual symbols (see chapter 5).

CLASS THEME VISHUDDHA CHAKRA

- Moving with the breath: The exercises are repeated several times in time with the breath.
- IH: Inhalation / EH: Exhalation / PF: Pelvic floor
- See chapter 7 for a detailed explanation of the Asanas.

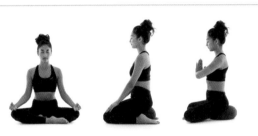

Arriving/introduction

- Find an upright-seated position either with legs crossed, or Hero pose. If necessary, support your bottom with a folded blanket or a pillow.
- Lift the spine so the lower pelvic area and the crown of the head are lined up vertically.
- Gather yourself and attune yourself to the class.

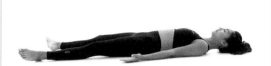

Body and breath awareness

- Notice the body (e.g. via its points of contact).
- Notice your natural breath without forcing or changing it.
- Connect to the breathing wave.
- Direct the breath and your focus to the neck space (larynx and nape) and feel how the energy flows there. What sensations does this trigger? Vastness? Narrowness, permeability, sturdiness, the feeling of a lump in the throat?

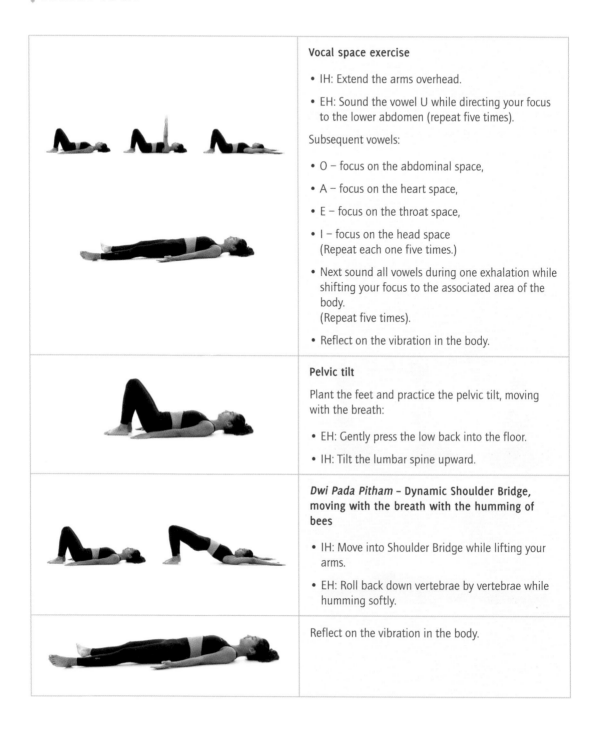

Vocal space exercise

- IH: Extend the arms overhead.
- EH: Sound the vowel U while directing your focus to the lower abdomen (repeat five times).

Subsequent vowels:

- O – focus on the abdominal space,
- A – focus on the heart space,
- E – focus on the throat space,
- I – focus on the head space
  (Repeat each one five times.)
- Next sound all vowels during one exhalation while shifting your focus to the associated area of the body.
  (Repeat five times).
- Reflect on the vibration in the body.

Pelvic tilt

Plant the feet and practice the pelvic tilt, moving with the breath:

- EH: Gently press the low back into the floor.
- IH: Tilt the lumbar spine upward.

Dwi Pada Pitham – **Dynamic Shoulder Bridge, moving with the breath with the humming of bees**

- IH: Move into Shoulder Bridge while lifting your arms.
- EH: Roll back down vertebrae by vertebrae while humming softly.

Reflect on the vibration in the body.

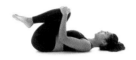
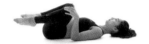

Loosening up the hips

- Breath-guided circles with the thighs from the hip joint in both directions.
- Feel your hip mobility; gently pre-stretch the inner thigh muscles.

Preparation for upright-seated exercises.

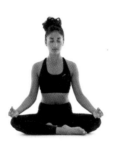

Neck-nape flow

- Center the head over the shoulders; lengthen the neck (visualization aid: suggested double-chin).
- Next gently turn your head right to left (cervical spine rotation).
- Reflect.
- Tilt the head from right to left (visualization aid: resting the right ear on the right shoulder, and vice-versa).
- Reflect.

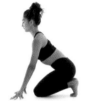

Loosening up the spine

Loosening up the spine while sitting back on the heels. In doing so the neck-nape-head area is consciously integrated.

- IH: Slightly lift the sternum and the chin, lengthen the spine, and open up the larynx.
- EH: Round the back, pull the chin towards the chest, and stretch the back of the nape.

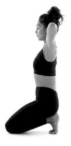

Shoulder circles

Loosening up the shoulders.

- EH: Rest your fingertips on your shoulders, then move the elbows forward until they touch.
- IH: Lift the elbows and make a big backward circle.

The toes can either be tucked (stretches toes and plantar fascia) or you can rest on the tops of the toes. Keep the trunk steady during the exercise.

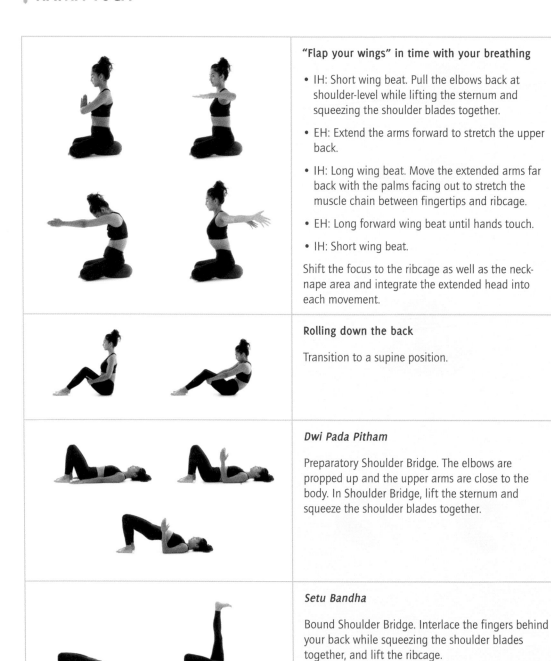

"Flap your wings" in time with your breathing

- IH: Short wing beat. Pull the elbows back at shoulder-level while lifting the sternum and squeezing the shoulder blades together.

- EH: Extend the arms forward to stretch the upper back.

- IH: Long wing beat. Move the extended arms far back with the palms facing out to stretch the muscle chain between fingertips and ribcage.

- EH: Long forward wing beat until hands touch.

- IH: Short wing beat.

Shift the focus to the ribcage as well as the neck-nape area and integrate the extended head into each movement.

Rolling down the back

Transition to a supine position.

Dwi Pada Pitham

Preparatory Shoulder Bridge. The elbows are propped up and the upper arms are close to the body. In Shoulder Bridge, lift the sternum and squeeze the shoulder blades together.

Setu Bandha

Bound Shoulder Bridge. Interlace the fingers behind your back while squeezing the shoulder blades together, and lift the ribcage.

To prepare for *Viparita Karani*, first lift one leg and hold for several breaths, then repeat on the other side.

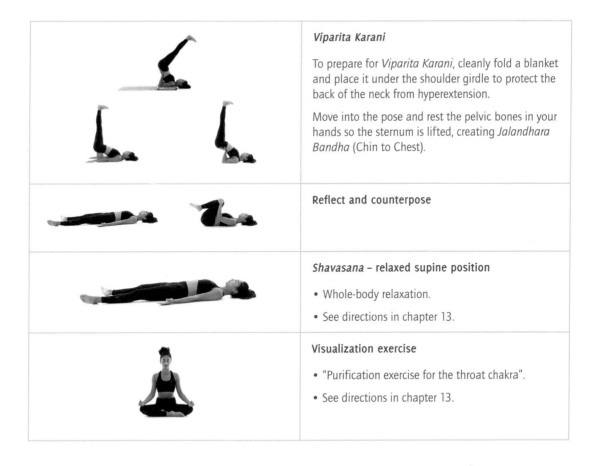

	Viparita Karani To prepare for *Viparita Karani*, cleanly fold a blanket and place it under the shoulder girdle to protect the back of the neck from hyperextension. Move into the pose and rest the pelvic bones in your hands so the sternum is lifted, creating *Jalandhara Bandha* (Chin to Chest).
	Reflect and counterpose
	***Shavasana* – relaxed supine position** • Whole-body relaxation. • See directions in chapter 13.
	Visualization exercise • "Purification exercise for the throat chakra". • See directions in chapter 13.

12.7 LESSON PLAN 7: THE AJNA CHAKRA – INTUITION, SUPERIOR WISDOM, POLARITIES, INNER CENTER, LIGHT

This chakra is located at the center of the head, slightly above the eyes between the eyebrows, and can be perceived via *Bhrumadhya* (*eyebrow center*). That is why it is also called the third eye or eyebrow center. The associated body parts are the forehead region, eyes, ears, nose, sinuses, and nervous system.

The main theme of the following lessons about the *Ajna chakra* is twists. Twists require a strong center, the vertical axis that is created in the inner space when one is aligned to it. We will rotate in both directions around this vertical axis. We turn to the right side, which is associated with the energy of the sun and represents our active, resourceful, joyful, and fiery side. We turn to the left side, which is associated with the moon and connects us to our emotional, cooing, and intuitive side. So as we twist we steadily look with our inner eye, the eyes of perception, at the polar aspects in us. The unifying aspect between them is the center.

Before the start of the practice unit, show the lotus symbol of the *Ajna chakra* and explain it via the individual symbols (see chapter 5).

LESSON PLAN: AJNA CHAKRA

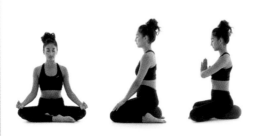

Arriving/introduction

- Sit upright, either with legs crossed or hero pose. If necessary, support your bottom with a blanket or a pillow.
- Lift the spine so the lower pelvic area and the crown of the head are lined up vertically.
- Gather yourself and attune yourself to the class.
- Focus your attention on the vertical axis in the inner space.

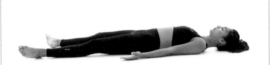

Body and breath awareness

- Notice the body. Notice your natural breath without forcing it.
- Starting from the inner axis, first shift your awareness to the left, and then to the right side of the body.
- Notice whether the two sides feel identical or if there are differences. Can you feel one side of the body more vividly?

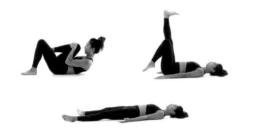

Loosening up the hips and pre-stretching the back of the legs

- EH: Pull the bent right knee in while doing a crunch.
- IH: Lower the upper body and extend the left leg.

Repeat several times, working with the breath.

Reflect and then repeat on the other side.

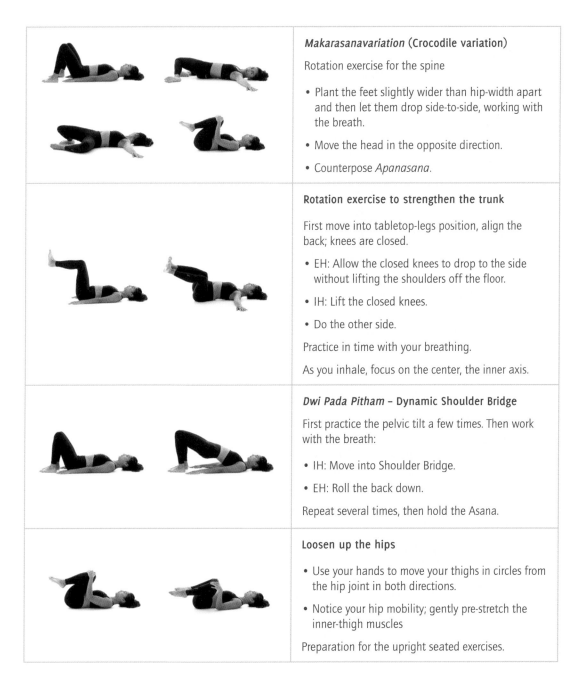

Makarasanavariation (Crocodile variation)

Rotation exercise for the spine

- Plant the feet slightly wider than hip-width apart and then let them drop side-to-side, working with the breath.
- Move the head in the opposite direction.
- Counterpose *Apanasana*.

Rotation exercise to strengthen the trunk

First move into tabletop-legs position, align the back; knees are closed.

- EH: Allow the closed knees to drop to the side without lifting the shoulders off the floor.
- IH: Lift the closed knees.
- Do the other side.

Practice in time with your breathing.

As you inhale, focus on the center, the inner axis.

Dwi Pada Pitham – Dynamic Shoulder Bridge

First practice the pelvic tilt a few times. Then work with the breath:

- IH: Move into Shoulder Bridge.
- EH: Roll the back down.

Repeat several times, then hold the Asana.

Loosen up the hips

- Use your hands to move your thighs in circles from the hip joint in both directions.
- Notice your hip mobility; gently pre-stretch the inner-thigh muscles

Preparation for the upright seated exercises.

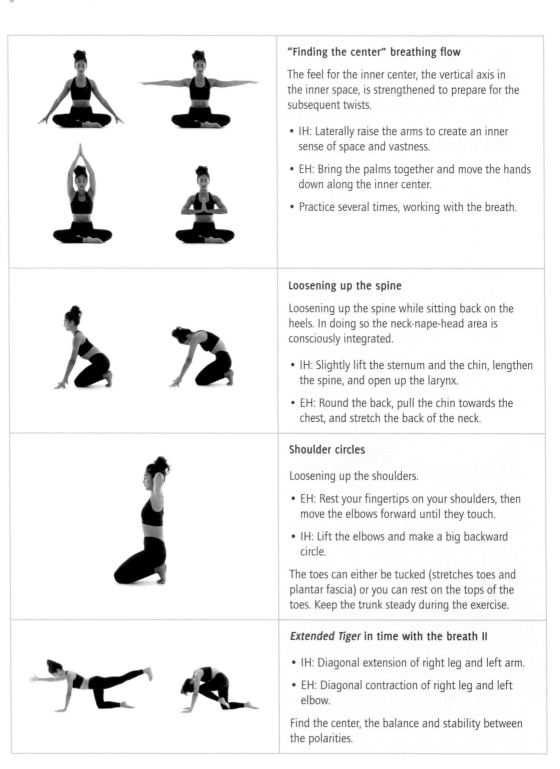

"Finding the center" breathing flow

The feel for the inner center, the vertical axis in the inner space, is strengthened to prepare for the subsequent twists.

- IH: Laterally raise the arms to create an inner sense of space and vastness.
- EH: Bring the palms together and move the hands down along the inner center.
- Practice several times, working with the breath.

Loosening up the spine

Loosening up the spine while sitting back on the heels. In doing so the neck-nape-head area is consciously integrated.

- IH: Slightly lift the sternum and the chin, lengthen the spine, and open up the larynx.
- EH: Round the back, pull the chin towards the chest, and stretch the back of the neck.

Shoulder circles

Loosening up the shoulders.

- EH: Rest your fingertips on your shoulders, then move the elbows forward until they touch.
- IH: Lift the elbows and make a big backward circle.

The toes can either be tucked (stretches toes and plantar fascia) or you can rest on the tops of the toes. Keep the trunk steady during the exercise.

Extended Tiger in time with the breath II

- IH: Diagonal extension of right leg and left arm.
- EH: Diagonal contraction of right leg and left elbow.

Find the center, the balance and stability between the polarities.

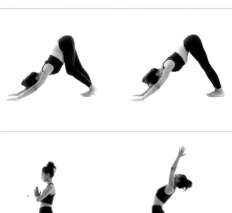

Walking Dog

Alternate pedaling the feet in *Adho Mukkha Svanasana*, then hold in *Adho Mukkha Svanasana* and transition to standing.

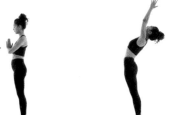

Utkatasana flow

- EH: Gather yourself in Tadasana *"Anjali Mudra"*
- IH: *Tadasana* with backbend
- EH: *Uttanasana*
- IH: *Anjaney Asana*
- EH: *Uttanasana*
- IH: *Utkatasana*
- EH: Gather yourself in *Tadasana "Anjali Mura"*

Repeat on both sides; the focus is on core stability.

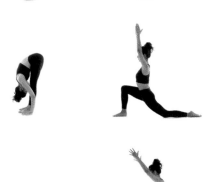

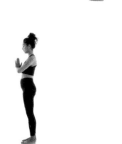

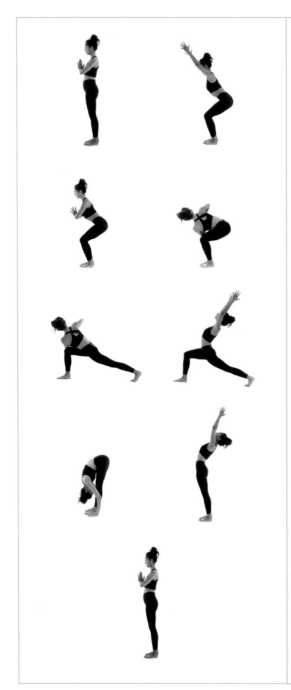

Parivritta Utkatasana/Parivritta Parsva Konasana

- EH: Gather yourself in *Tadasana "Anjali Mudra"*
- IH: *Utkatasana*
- IH: *Utakatasana/Anjali Mudra*
- EH: *Parivritta Utkatasana*
- IH: Lunge back into *Parivritta Parsva Konasana*
- EH: Hold
- IH: *Alanasana*
- EH: *Uttanasana*
- IH: *Tadasana* with backbend
- EH: Gather yourself in *Tadasana "Anjali Mudra"*

And repeat on the other side.

This sequence can be practiced in time with breathing or by holding each pose for several breaths.

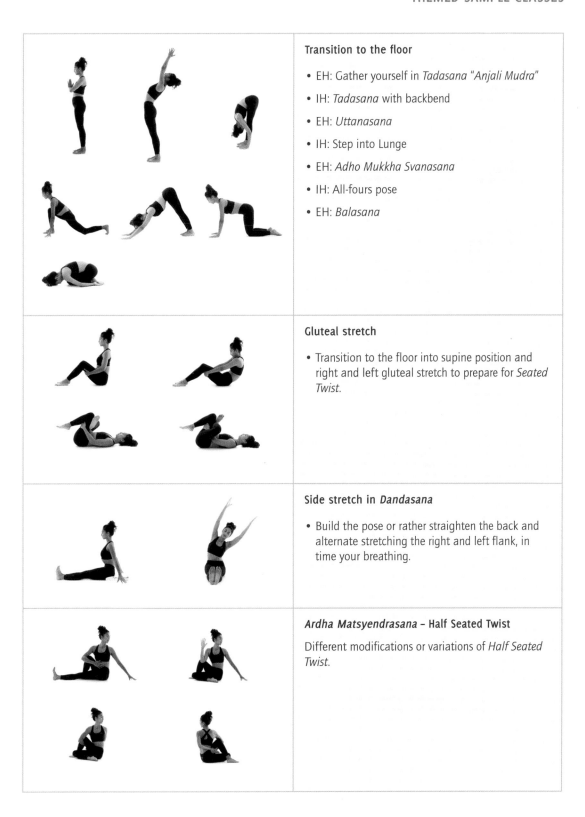

Transition to the floor

- EH: Gather yourself in *Tadasana "Anjali Mudra"*
- IH: *Tadasana* with backbend
- EH: *Uttanasana*
- IH: Step into Lunge
- EH: *Adho Mukkha Svanasana*
- IH: All-fours pose
- EH: *Balasana*

Gluteal stretch

- Transition to the floor into supine position and right and left gluteal stretch to prepare for *Seated Twist*.

Side stretch in *Dandasana*

- Build the pose or rather straighten the back and alternate stretching the right and left flank, in time your breathing.

***Ardha Matsyendrasana* – Half Seated Twist**

Different modifications or variations of *Half Seated Twist*.

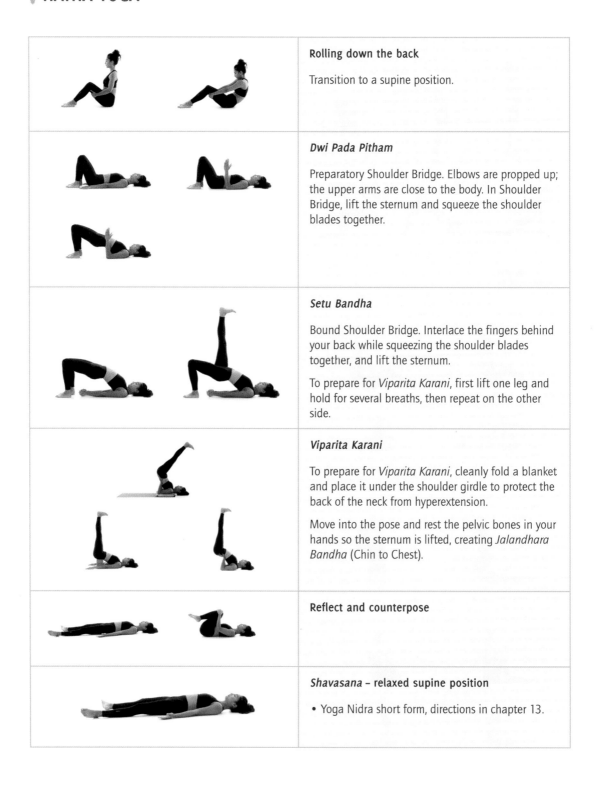

	Rolling down the back Transition to a supine position.
	Dwi Pada Pitham Preparatory Shoulder Bridge. Elbows are propped up; the upper arms are close to the body. In Shoulder Bridge, lift the sternum and squeeze the shoulder blades together.
	Setu Bandha Bound Shoulder Bridge. Interlace the fingers behind your back while squeezing the shoulder blades together, and lift the sternum. To prepare for *Viparita Karani*, first lift one leg and hold for several breaths, then repeat on the other side.
	Viparita Karani To prepare for *Viparita Karani*, cleanly fold a blanket and place it under the shoulder girdle to protect the back of the neck from hyperextension. Move into the pose and rest the pelvic bones in your hands so the sternum is lifted, creating *Jalandhara Bandha* (Chin to Chest).
	Reflect and counterpose
	***Shavasana* – relaxed supine position** • Yoga Nidra short form, directions in chapter 13.

12.8 LESSON PLAN 8: THE SAHASRARA CHAKRA – SUPERIOR KNOWLEDGE, SUPERIOR CONSCIOUSNESS

The *Sahasrara chakra* is located in the center of the highest point of the head, which is why it is also called *crown chakra*. The associated parts of the body are the skullcap, fontanel, and cerebral cortex.

The goal of this lesson plan is a visualization exercise in an upright-seated position that travels through all of the energy centers starting with alignment to the vertex. All of the previously practiced exercises serve as internal and external preparation for the seated meditation pose (*Shukasana*).

Before the start of the practice unit, show the lotus symbol of the *Sahasrara chakra* and explain it via the individual symbols (see chapter 5).

CLASS THEME SAHASRARA CHAKRA	
	Arriving/introduction • Body and breath awareness.
	***Apanasana* (Wind-relieving pose) in time with your breathing** • As you exhale pull the knees into the chest, as you inhale extend the legs away from the body.
	***Eka Pada Apanasana* with whole-body extension in time with your breathing** • Enhanced *Apanasana* with whole-body extension and crunch and deepened breaths.
	Loosening up the hips • Use your hands to move your thighs in circles from the hip joint in both directions. • Notice your hip mobility; gently pre-stretch the inner-thigh muscles. Preparation for the upright seated exercises.

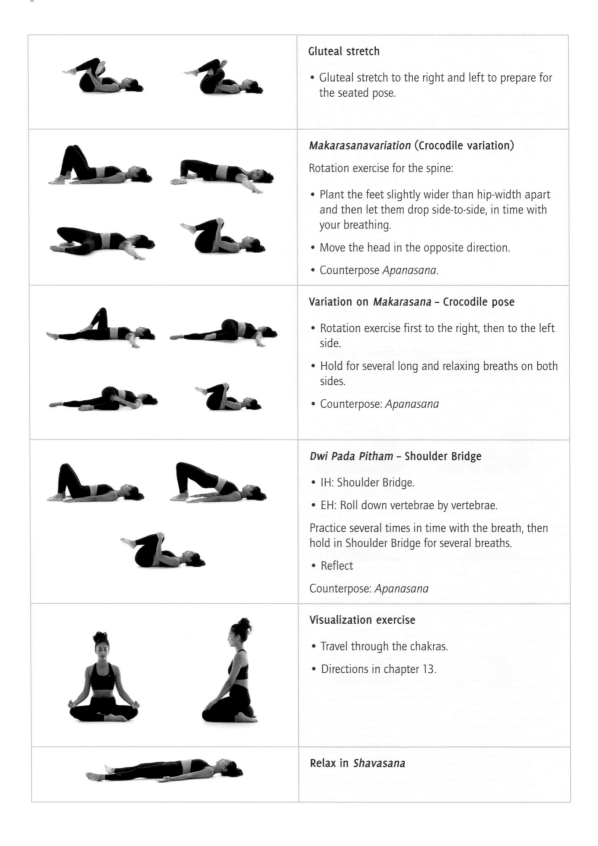

Gluteal stretch

- Gluteal stretch to the right and left to prepare for the seated pose.

Makarasanavariation (Crocodile variation)

Rotation exercise for the spine:

- Plant the feet slightly wider than hip-width apart and then let them drop side-to-side, in time with your breathing.
- Move the head in the opposite direction.
- Counterpose *Apanasana*.

Variation on *Makarasana* – Crocodile pose

- Rotation exercise first to the right, then to the left side.
- Hold for several long and relaxing breaths on both sides.
- Counterpose: *Apanasana*

Dwi Pada Pitham – Shoulder Bridge

- IH: Shoulder Bridge.
- EH: Roll down vertebrae by vertebrae.

Practice several times in time with the breath, then hold in Shoulder Bridge for several breaths.

- Reflect

Counterpose: *Apanasana*

Visualization exercise

- Travel through the chakras.
- Directions in chapter 13.

Relax in *Shavasana*

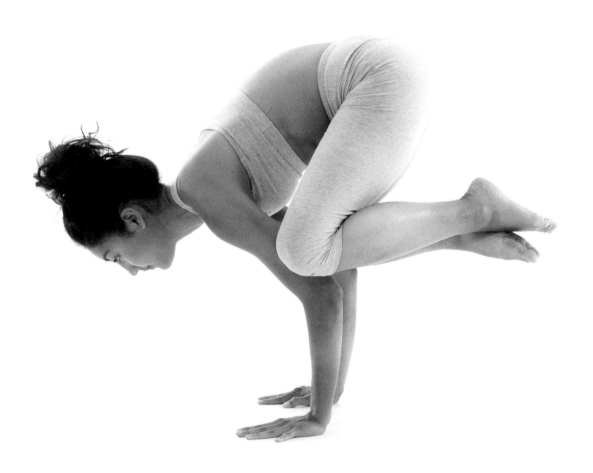

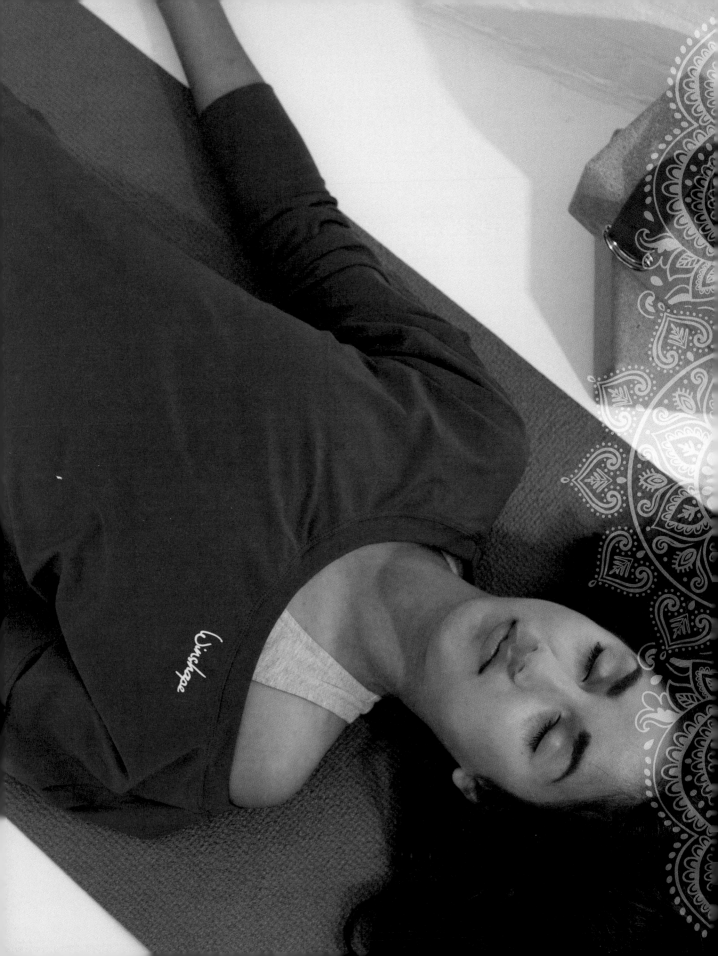

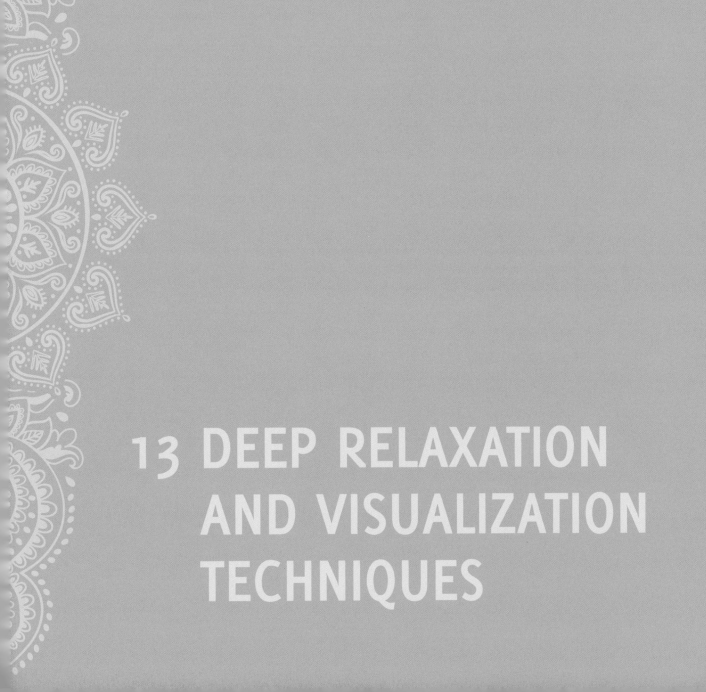

13 DEEP RELAXATION AND VISUALIZATION TECHNIQUES

13 DEEP RELAXATION AND VISUALIZATION TECHNIQUES

13.1 SUGGESTIVE AND NON-SUGGESTIVE FORMS OF RELAXATION

Guiding relaxation can be divided into two topics: suggestive and non-suggestive forms of relaxation. The difference between the two forms is primarily the kind of phrasing, the verbal instructions.

13.1.1 NON-SUGGESTIVE FORMS OF RELAXATION

Non-suggestive forms of relaxation are exclusively perception-oriented. These forms of instruction are beneficial particularly at the beginning of a class as well as during the course of the class. The participant arrives to class from his everyday life and first is able to experience how he feels. Non-suggestive instructions ask the participant How?, What?, and Where?, or indirectly name these topics.

A yoga class is primarily about being able to look inward and to perceive the genuine current status quo. Examples:

» How is the body positioned on the mat? (Feel the body's contact points and surfaces!)

» Where in the body does the energy flow? (Which areas of the body do you currently feel really vividly, and which do you feel less vividly?)

» How does the breath flow? (Notice the natural rhythms of your breathing without forcing it.)

The type of instruction does not just train and improve perception ability. The participant is also taught that he is permitted to accept himself just the way he feels at that moment. No one has to arrive on the mat smart, cheerful, or deeply relaxed. There are days when we arrive at a yoga class exhausted, frustrated, or tense. And we can initially give space to precisely these aspects. First we accept what is before the practice can gradually change the state.

Imagine a person who has experienced massive tension and time pressure the entire day, may be was even criticized by a superior or a colleague, was stuck in traffic on the way to yoga class, then took forever to find a parking spot, and arrives on the yoga mat in the last second, completely exhausted. In this case well-intended, suggestive instructions like: "You are completely relaxed", or "Your heart is open and full of love for all of creation", would most likely cause frustration or resistance.

Practicing yoga always means perceiving through observation. That is why suggestive and autosuggestive forms of instruction only make sense within the context of deep relaxation. Anything that happened before that, such as the Asana practice, reflection phases, and *Pranayama* should be led in a way that allows the participant to enter a state of observing self-experience.

Here it is important to differentiate between *instructions* and *suggestions*. *Suggestions* always intervene in the immediate state of mind, while *instructions* like: "Arrive in the moment and gradually let the issues of daily life fade away", or: "Allow the breath to flow long and softly", or: "Feel the energy in the pelvic area", either build bridges or offer information about the type of practice.

13.1.2 SUGGESTIVE FORMS OF RELAXATION

Suggestion means *influence*. In everyday life, the term *suggestive* has a rather negative connotation, because it sounds like unwanted or emotional manipulation. But in terms of the relaxation process, suggestion/autosuggestion is a method used to move from a performance state to a resting state.

Suggestive and autosuggestive forms of relaxation affect the participants' physical, mental, and emotional experience. This methodology is controversial amongst yoga instructors. The "opponents" of these methods claim that suggestion interferes with participants' experience. Proponents emphasize the relaxation effect of this form of instruction.

As described in chapter 10, under the topic "Distress", *"Stress reactions can also be triggered without external causes, meaning just by imagining a calamitous situation, e.g. extreme mental-emotional stress like test anxiety or fear of all sorts of failures".*

Suggestive forms of relaxation take advantage of the fact that the mind possesses a great power of imagination. Here the process actually works in the opposite way. Instead of visualizing emotionally threatening situations, definite relaxation characteristics (of the relaxation state) such as heaviness, warmth, calm, and comforting coziness are suggested, usually in combination with calming images (smooth forest lake), and terms such as clarity, expanse, tranquility, lightness, openness, or permeability.

The most common form of the suggestive method is *autogenic training*, which is based on autosuggestion and referred to as a *concentrated self-relaxation* or *self-hypnosis*. The practitioner learns so-called short and very concise formulas that are mentally repeated.

During a deep relaxation or final relaxation phase in yoga it is certainly common to work with suggestive formulas (see sample text "Whole-body relaxation based on autosuggestion").

13.2 IMAGINATION TECHNIQUES

Imagination Techniques are *visualization exercises*. This type of relaxation method uses the imagination, our visual thinking, the power of imagination, in a positive way to create a state or inner serenity. The spectrum stretches from relaxation exercises to fantasy travel, dream vacations, to suggestions in the form of mental imagery or metaphors.

Integrating the senses makes imagination techniques particularly effective:

Visually: "You discover a big, vigorous tree that magically draws you to it, and you settle down at its base."

Auditory: "You can hear the gentle rustling of the leaves in the wind."

Kinesthetically: "You trustingly lean against the tree's trunk and feel its strength against your back."

Olfactory: "You breathe in the fresh mountain air."

Gustatory: "You can taste the salty ocean breeze on your lips."

In behavioral and trauma therapy imagination techniques are successfully used to treat various disorders.

With respect to yoga classes, imagery and imagination in the form of visualization exercises or –travel, serve to teach more in depth content. They contain archetypical content and symbols that make yoga-relevant groups of topics much more experienceable.

For instance, the subtle energy body (*Pranamaya Kosha*) can be visualized by imagining a complex network of countless glowing energy pathways in which vitalizing vital energy flows. Themes from chakra theory, such as grounding and stability (*Muladhara chakra*) can be experienced and internalized on a deep level by visualizing a mountain or a tree. Visualizing colors can have a stimulating and healing effect on the entire experience (physical and mental), as well as imagining characteristics like flowing, streaming, purifying, invigorating, etc.

Some participants put pressure on themselves at the beginning of the imagination process because they may expect something unusual. These participants sometimes say that they don't have the talent for visualization or it doesn't work for them.

In fact, we all continuously visualize in our daily lives. For example, when we think about whether we'd like to wear the red or the blue t-shirt, or whether we'd prefer to eat strawberries or blueberries, whether we prefer to vacation on a beach with turquoise water, or rather hike in the mountains. During all of these contemplations we visualize in one way or another. One person may see the turquoise-colored ocean, another person can feel the water on their skin, or in their mind can even smell the salty sea air. It is therefore beneficial to integrate the senses into the practice (seeing, smelling, hearing, tasting, feeling), so the instructions can reach every type equally.

13.3 YOGA NIDRA – YOGA'S HEALING SLEEP

The origin of the *Yoga Nidra* is the *Tantras*. *Nidra* means *sleep*. It is a technique that is supposed to systematically lead to a state of deep consciousness. *Yoga Nidra* was developed by Swami Satyananda Saraswati (1923-2009), the founder of the "Bihar School of Yoga".

Yoga Nidra is based on a systematic process that is primarily perception-oriented and guides the practitioner into a state between wakefulness and sleep. In this state the practitioner is supposed to get in touch with subconscious and unconscious planes.

The exercise takes about 20-40 minutes and leads from the outside to the inside. Formulating a *Sankalpas*, a positive inner intention or goal, as well as the subsequent rapid circling of the consciousness through the entire body, is typical for *Yoga Nidra*. Next is awareness of breathing (mental Pranayama in advanced classes), imagining feelings and sensations (heaviness, warmth, and later for experienced practitioners feelings like cold, pain, pleasure, sorrow) and the flash-like visualization of different archetypical images in rapid succession.

In some advanced forms of *Yoga Nidra*, visualizing unpleasant feelings or images is supposed to give the practitioner practice in looking at themes from a superior plane without identifying with them. This is meant to nurture the qualities of *Vairagya* (non-attachment) and *Viveka* (faculty of discrimination, spiritual insight).

Swami Satyananda Saraswati's work by the same name includes detailed descriptions of five classes that build on each other as well as additional examples.[84]

A short form of *Yoga Nidra* will be introduced later as part of the relaxation directions.

---

84 Swami Satyananda Saraswati (1992).

13.4 GUIDE TO RELAXATION AND VISUALIZATION TECHNIQUES

Leading or practicing relaxation and visualization exercises require proper preparation beforehand. The relaxation or visualization text supplements and deepens the respective theme of a yoga unit.

When visualization exercises are led, it is a good idea to do them in an upright-seated position because participants tend to fall asleep in a supine position. If a visualization exercise or imagination technique is planned at the end of the yoga unit, it might be good to first do some deep relaxation based on body awareness or an autosuggestive form of instruction in supine position.

The following points are intended to help make relaxation an enriching experience for participants:

» Prior to relaxation, explain to participants what it is about, what the theme of the relaxation will be, and to what extent it will enhance the class theme.

» Since new participants (yoga novices) are sometimes not open to deep relaxation, or may even be resistant or timid, it helps to tell a group beforehand that they can mentally back out and disconnect when the content of a respective relaxation theme triggers uneasiness or resistance. The advice to lie on the side and ignore the instructor's voice or words gives participants the freedom of choice and removes the pressure of "having to relax".

» It is a good idea to leave adequate time for the transition from the Asana practice to the deep relaxation phase. Is the light appropriate? Is everyone in a comfortable position? Does someone require aids (a pillow under the head or a bolster under the knees)? If a visualization exercise or seated meditation is planned afterwards, ask participants to have any aids ready beforehand for a smooth transition.

» Allow participants sufficient time to settle down.

» In a circular arrangement, people who have trouble hearing should position themselves with the head to the center (or ask to form an inward-facing circle) to better hear the instructor.

» In case of background noises, address them (e.g.: First pay attention to all the noises in the room and outside the room without judging them. Listen with your ears wide open. As you do so, move from one noise to the next. Then take your awareness deeper and deeper inside, notice the inner noises, the breath ...). ·

» When working with music, make sure the music isn't too loud. A subtle tapestry of sound in the background is ideal for relaxation. Music with lyrics or with major highs and lows or rather "loud-quiet phases" is unsuitable. It is best to take the time to do a sound check before class because every room has different acoustics.

» Your voice should be friendly, neutral, and clear. Neither too empathetic nor too authoritarian. The voice is merely a device and ideally should not divert the participant's attention from himself.

» A "You" or "We" address is unsuitable for relaxation (e.g. "We relax our right leg", is grammatically incorrect since we don't have one mutual right leg).

» Speak neither too loudly nor too softly. It helps to ask participants for feedback like, for example: "If I speak at this volume, can you hear me?"

» Leave sufficiently long pauses between individual instructions. During relaxation, participants are exclusively attuned to listening. It takes time for the message to reach them and for them to implement it.

» A tip for instructing with text: First read a sentence silently, then recite it, then repeat it in your mind and feel the content of the spoken words yourself or mentally reflect on them.

» Choose an instruction method and stick with it, meaning no "colorful" mix of autosuggestive forms of relaxation, suggestive forms, perception-oriented, etc. It would only confuse the participants.

» Plan at least 15-20 minutes for relaxation. If that amount of time is not available, shorten relaxation accordingly. Definitely do not speak faster to "fit everything in" in less time. Here less is often more.

» A spoken text is followed by a period of rest. Inform participants beforehand that they can rest quietly until the sound of a cymbal (OM or your voice) brings them back.

» Bringing them back is done with an appropriate signal (cymbal, singing bowl, OM, etc.). Attention is then gently directed back to the breath, then the body (fingertips, move the toes, then the arms and legs, stretch out). Some participants love to vigorously rub their hands to come back to the present moment.

» Plan at least five minutes for the conclusion of the class, more is better.

» Since participants have rested during relaxation, it is generally not a good idea to make them speak (e.g. asking for feedback). The *Vrittis*, the mental movements should not be immediately stimulated.

» After relaxation, a small ritual like sounding an OM, reciting a mantra, a quote, or a short story are an ideal way to conclude a yoga class.

13.5 RELAXATION TEXTS

The heading "Preparation, main part, and conclusion" is not spoken. It is merely for orientation purposes.

13.5.1 WHOLE-BODY RELAXATION BASED ON BODY AWARENESS

Duration approx. 15 minutes

a) Preparation

Get in a comfortable position. The feet are slightly more than hip-width apart and the feet gently fall open. The spine rests on the mat in its natural curve; the tailbone and the back of the head form a straight line. The arms rest on the floor at a slight angle to the body, the palms face the ceiling.

Gently close your eyes. Take a few relaxed breaths through the nose and exhale through the slightly open mouth. As you do so, you can let go of anything that currently still occupies you mentally or emotionally.

Now allow the breath to flow naturally without forcing it. Notice the natural flow of your breath.

b) Main part

Now notice all of the body's contact points and surfaces. Notice how the body rests on the floor. Feel which areas of the body have large contact areas on the floor and which areas only have points of contact. Also shift your awareness to the areas that currently don't touch the floor. Allow an image of your body landscape on the mat to form before your mind's eye.

Now direct your attention to your feet. Really notice your feet. Feel your toes, the soles of the feet, the arches, the heels, and the ankles. Feel both feet. Now feel the calves, the knees, and the thighs. Feel both feet and legs.

Feel your bottom, the entire lower pelvic area, the low back, the middle back, the shoulder blades, and the space between the shoulder blades. Feel how your entire body rests on the floor. Feel your belly and your ribcage. Feel the movement of the breath in your belly and your ribcage.

Feel the shoulder girdle, the upper arms, the forearms, the wrists, the palms, the back of the hands, and every single finger. Feel both shoulders and both arms.

Feel the neck and nape, the entire head, the scalp, feel the height and width of the forehead. Feel the temples, the ears, the cheeks, the lower jaw, the lips, the nose, the bridge of the nose. Feel the eyebrows, the eyelids, and the eyes. Feel the space behind the eyes.

Feel yourself breathing, notice the movement of the breath. Feel yourself get immersed in your own breathing.

(A few minutes break)

c) Conclusion

Now once more, notice your body's contact surfaces and points. Allow your breath to flow a little deeper again and gently move your fingers and toes. Now let the breath flow more vigorously, and when you're ready, stretch luxuriously. Then lie on your side for a few moments longer. Then move from your side to an upright-seated position.

13.5.2 WHOLE-BODY RELAXATION (AUTOSUGGESTIVE GUIDANCE)

Duration approx. 20 minutes

Prior to the start of the class, the instructor tells the participants that beginning with the main part they will switch to the first-person address, because it is easier for the subconscious mind to implement autosuggestions in the first person.

a) Preparation

Lie on your back in a relaxed position. The feet are slightly more than hip-width apart and the feet gently fall open. The spine rests on the mat in its natural curve; the tailbone and the back of the head form a straight line. The arms rest on the floor at a slight angle to the body, the palms face the ceiling.

Gently close your eyes. Take a few relaxed breaths through the nose and exhale through the slightly open mouth. As you do so you can let go of anything that currently still occupies you mentally or emotionally.

Now allow the breath to flow naturally without forcing it. Notice the natural flow of your breath.

During the following exercises you will create a feeling of relaxation. Please repeat the following statements in your mind:

b) Main part

I am relaxing the toes, the soles of the feet, the arches, the heels, and the ankles. Both feet and both legs are heavy, warm, and relaxed.

I am relaxing my bottom. I am relaxing the entire lower pelvic region and the external and internal genitalia. I am relaxing my lower back, my middle back, the shoulder blades and the space between the shoulder blades. My entire back is heavy, warm, and relaxed on the mat.

I am relaxing my belly and ribcage. I am relaxing all of the organs in the belly and the ribcage. I am relaxing the stomach, the digestive organs, the liver, the pancreas, the kidneys, the gall bladder, and the lungs. My heart beats calmly and evenly.

I am relaxing the shoulder girdle, the upper arms, the elbows, the forearms, the wrists, the palms, the back of the hands, and every single finger. Both shoulders and arms are pleasantly heavy, warm, and relaxed.

I am relaxing neck and nape, the head, the scalp, and every follicle.

I am relaxing my forehead, which feels pleasantly cool and clear. I am relaxing my temples, ears, cheeks, lower jaw, lips, nose, and the bridge of the nose. My entire face is loose, soft, and relaxed.

I am relaxing my eyebrows, eyelids, and eyes. I am relaxing the space behind the eyes all the way deep inside my head.

I am relaxing into the most powerful silence of my innermost being.

(A few minutes break)

c) Conclusion

Now let your breath flow slightly deeper again and gently move your fingers and toes. Gently resurface and bring that soothing feeling of relaxation into your waking consciousness. Now allow the breath to flow more vigorously, and when you are ready, stretch luxuriously. Then lie on your side for a few moments longer. Then move from your side to an upright-seated position.

13.5.3 WHOLE-BODY RELAXATION (SUGGESTIVE GUIDANCE)

Duration approx. 15 minutes

a) Preparation

Lie on your back in a relaxed position. The feet are slightly more than hip-width apart and the feet gently fall open. The spine rests on the mat in its natural curve; the tailbone and the back of the head form a straight line. The arms rest on the floor at a slight angle to the body, the palms face the ceiling.

Gently close your eyes. Take a few relaxed breaths through the nose and exhale through the slightly open mouth. As you do so you can let go of anything that currently still occupies you mentally or emotionally.

Now allow yourself to breathe naturally without forcing it. Notice the natural flow of your breath.

b) Main part

Now direct your attention to your feet. Really notice your feet. Relax the toes, the soles of the feet, the arches, the heels, and the ankles. Both feet are relaxed. Relax the calves, the knees, and the thighs. Both feet and both legs are heavy, warm, and relaxed.

Relax your bottom, your entire lower pelvic area, and the external and internal genitalia. Relax the lower back, the middle back, and the shoulder blades. Relax the space between the shoulder blades. The entire back is heavy, warm, and relaxed on the mat.

Relax the belly and the ribcage. Relax all of the organs in the belly and ribcage. Relax the stomach, the digestive organs, the liver, the pancreas, the kidneys, the gall bladder, and the lungs.

Relax the shoulder girdle, the upper arms, the elbows, the forearms, the wrists, the palms, the back of the hands, and every single finger. Both shoulders and both arms are heavy, warm, and relaxed.

Relax neck and nape, the head, the scalp, and every follicle.

Relax the forehead, the temples, the ears, cheeks, lower jaw, lips, nose, and bridge of the nose.

Relax the eyebrows, eyelids, and eyes. Relax the space behind your eyes all the way deep inside your head.

Relax into the powerful silence of your innermost being. Cheerful tranquility and dynamic calm penetrate every cell in your body.

(A few minutes break)

c) Conclusion

Now let your breath flow slightly deeper again and gently move your fingers and toes. Gently resurface and bring that soothing feeling of relaxation into your waking consciousness. Now allow the breath to flow more vigorously, and when you are ready, stretch luxuriously. Then lie on your side for a few moments longer. Then move from your side to an upright-seated position.

13.5.4 BREATHING RELAXATION

Duration approx. 12-15 minutes

a) Preparation

Lie on your back in a relaxed position. The feet are slightly more than hip-width apart and the feet gently fall open. The spine rests on the mat in its natural curve; the tailbone and the back of the head form a straight line. The arms rest on the floor at a slight angle to the body, the palms face the ceiling.

Gently close your eyes. Take a few relaxed breaths through the nose and exhale through the slightly open mouth. As you do so you can let go of anything that currently still occupies you mentally or emotionally. Now allow the breath to flow naturally without forcing it. Notice the natural flow of your breath.

b) Main part

Now notice the subtle whiff of the breath in your nose. Notice how your inhaled breath gently flows in through your two nostrils and touches the lining of the nose. Feel the two streams of air combine into one stream at the bridge of the nose.

Feel the breath flow, and notice the abdominal wall gently rise as you inhale and drop as you exhale. Completely let go as you exhale until a small, natural breathing pause occurs. Imagine all along your exhalation a small stone sinking to the bottom of an alpine lake. Notice the breath automatically streaming back into your body, that it rises up inside you as light as a cosmic haze.

Imagine the breath flowing through you like a gentle, drawn-out ocean wave. The inhaled wave permeates you with freshness, vitality, with cosmic vital energy, with *Prana*. The exhaled wave carries with it everything the body wishes to let go of, everything that is used up, metabolic waste, contaminants and toxins, unnecessary baggage, all that is past.

Feel this wave coming and going inside you. The more consciously, subtly, and evenly the breath flows, the more energy you absorb, the more intensely and comprehensively do you experience letting go.

Every breath is an immersion in the present, in the timeless moment. The breath connects you to the universe; it is the bridge between you and the universe. With every breath, immerse yourself deeper in the powerful calm of being.

(A few minutes break)

c) Conclusion

Now let your breath flow slightly deeper again and gently move your fingers and toes. Gently resurface and bring that soothing feeling of relaxation into your waking consciousness. Now allow the breath to flow more vigorously, and when you are ready, stretch luxuriously. Then lie on your side for a few moments longer. Then move from your side to an upright-seated position.

13.5.5 TREE (MULADHARA CHAKRA)

Duration approx. 15-20 minutes

Whole-body relaxation in a supine position can be practiced beforehand.

The visualization exercise "Tree" is intended to make it possible to experience the element earth and the qualities of the *Muladhara chakra* (root chakra), such as grounding, rootedness, trust, stability, and the experience of being profoundly nurtured.

a) Preparation

Come into an upright and relaxed seated position of your choice. Lend your posture the quality of *Sukha-Sthira*: solid, stable, comfortable, and permeable. Move the spine into an upright position along it natural curvature. The vertex and the lower pelvic area are on a vertical axis so the energy can flow freely. Now gently close your eyes. Spread your awareness once more across the entire body, from head to toes, and release all tension. Notice the natural flow of the breath.

b) Main part

In a moment, a tree will appear in front of your mind's eye. If several trees should appear right away, choose the first tree you saw. Look closely to see what kind of tree it is. Look to see if it is big or small, if it is a mature or a young tree. Also notice the tree's surroundings. Does it stand in a meadow or a clearing? In the mountains or are the sea? Are there other plants in the vicinity? Maybe you can hear birdsong or the rush of water nearby.

Once you have carefully looked at everything, slowly walk towards the tree. Once you have reached it, mentally ask it for permission to lean against its trunk. Then you settle in and lean with your back against its trunk. You are in a very meditative, internally alert state of mind and completely relaxed as you listen to the subtle rustling of the leaves in the breeze. You are aware of the smell of the earth beneath your feet and can sense the tree's aromatic woodsy scent in your nose.

You look deeper inside yourself and suddenly notice that you are connecting with the tree's core. You can feel the tree's invitation to merge with it and its energy for a while.

You feel yourself becoming the tree's trunk and your roots are reaching deep into the earth, the tree being securely anchored in the earth via its many, countless, big and small roots, drawing energy through them from the earth. You can feel how the earth nurtures the tree.

You feel the tree's strong trunk and now direct your attention to its crown, which is as big and expansive as its root system. You feel how the tree receives light energy through its foliage, converts it, and releases oxygen to its environment.

In your mind's eye you can see the tree through the years and decades. You see it through the change of the seasons, see its leaves change color in the fall and finally drop; see it covered in snow and thaw out again; see it weather storms and rain showers, the wind raking its crown with its rough fingers; and how it buds again in the spring, and may be even bears fruit in summer.

You feel this deep connection with and rootedness to the earth, and feel completely resilient yourself, faithfully held, carried, and nurtured. Now immerse yourself in this experience a few minutes longer and vividly feel your inner calm and the tree's grounded strength carry you.

(A few minutes break)

c) Conclusion

Now slowly resurface from the tree experience and notice your body. Feel your feet and legs, gently move your fingers and toes. Breathe slightly more vigorously and deeply, stretch luxuriously and arrive back in this room.

13.5.6 WATERFALL (SVADHISTHANA CHAKRA)

Duration approx. 15-20 minutes

Whole-body relaxation in a supine position can be practiced beforehand.

The visualization exercise "The waterfall" is intended to make it possible to experience the qualities of the *Svadhisthana chakra* (sacral chakra) associated with the dominant element water (flowing, purification, the quick variability of the emotional experience).

a) Preparation

Come into an upright and relaxed seated position of your choice. Lend your posture the quality of *Sukha-Sthira*: solid, stable, comfortable, and permeable. Move the spine into an upright position along it natural curvature. The vertex and the lower pelvic area are on a vertical axis so the energy can flow freely. Now gently close your eyes. Spread your awareness once more across the entire body, from head to toes, and release all tension. Notice the natural flow of the breath.

b) Main part

In a moment, a waterfall will appear before your mind's eye. Carefully look at the waterfall as well as the waterfall's surroundings. You notice that an idyllic lake is located at the foot of the waterfall. Find a spot at the lake a safe distance from the waterfall, where you can settle down. Maybe you will discover an inviting log or a round rock to sit on.

You sit down and immediately feel with all your senses the special clear and purifying atmosphere surrounding this place. You close your eyes and feel the delicate, refreshing mist that is blowing over from the waterfall onto your skin. You inhale the clean air and with every breath you feel the vital energy flowing through you. You go deeper into yourself and notice how you are beginning to internally flow with the waterfall. At first you are cautious, but after a while, you joyfully and playfully plunge into the lake along with the waterfall, flow around rocks and form eddies, and for a while enjoy the unbridled joy of being.

After a while, you feel your consciousness spread across the entire path of the water. Before your mind's eye you can see the water's source, you follow a creek that flows through meadows and fields, and gradually gets bigger and becomes a river, until it finally reaches the waterfall.

From there you continue to flow, become increasingly powerful and rapid, until you finally reach the ocean. And then you can feel that you are the ocean, but also the drop within the ocean. You are an ocean wave and at the same time feel your connection with all the waves. You experience yourself as a gently rolling swell, as an angry, stormy ocean, and as a smooth sea.

You feel yourself rise as evaporated water, form clouds that travel around the globe, and experience yourself as the complete water cycle. You fall down as rain and find your way back to the source, where the entire cycle starts all over again.

Now spend a few more minutes in the purifying and clarifying energy of the water. Realize that all of the flowing and streaming inside you comes from the healing power of water.

(A few minutes break)

c) Conclusion

Now slowly resurface from the water-cycle experience and notice your body. Feel your feet and legs, gently move your fingers and toes. Breathe slightly more vigorously and deeply, stretch luxuriously and arrive back in this room.

13.5.7 GOLDEN TEMPLE (MANIPURA CHAKRA)

Duration approx. 15-20 minutes

Whole-body relaxation in a supine position can be practiced beforehand.

The visualization exercise "The golden temple" is intended to make it possible to experience the qualities of the *Manipura chakra* (solar plexus chakra) associated with the dominant element fire (light, heat, radiance, inner strength, and the power to bring about positive change).

a) Preparation

Come into an upright and relaxed seated position of your choice. Lend your posture the quality of *Sukha-Sthira*: solid, stable, comfortable, and permeable. Move the spine into an upright position along it natural curvature. The vertex and the lower pelvic area are on a vertical axis so the energy can flow freely. Now gently close your eyes. Spread your awareness once more across the entire body, from head to toes, and release all tension. Notice the natural flow of the breath.

b) Main part

In a moment, a desert landscape will appear before your mind's eye. You stand with both feet in the desert sand, it is early morning and the temperature is pleasantly warm. Look around carefully. You spy a kind of building in the distance and start to walk towards it. As you get closer, you can see that it is a golden temple. You inspect it carefully. It seems to radiate a special purity and brilliance. After you reach it you feel a silent invitation and also the intense desire to enter the temple because you know that something special is waiting for you inside.

Inside the temple you are also met with golden-yellow splendor. In the center of the temple a place has been prepared for you, a thick, gold-colored pillow on which you now sit down. You close your eyes and absorb the temple's concentrated, powerful atmosphere with your breath and every pore in your body.

You feel the temple's energy nurture you with light, with inner warmth and with a powerful inner strength. You can feel how this strength is stored in your solar plexus region, the navel center, and from there spreads throughout your entire body. You are flooded by the radiant glow, and with your mind's eye you can see a small light shining in every cell of your body. And you notice that this glow extends beyond your body's physical borders, that an aura of brilliant light surrounds your body.

With each breath you notice how this light gives you the inner power to kick-start or change things in your life that will allow you to continue to grow inside.

Now spend a few more minutes in the temple's powerful energy and allow it to course through you.

(A few minutes break)

c) Conclusion

Now slowly resurface from the golden-temple experience and notice your body. Feel your feet and legs, gently move your fingers and toes. Breathe slightly more vigorously and deeply, stretch luxuriously and arrive back in this room.

13.5.8 LIGHT IN THE HEART (ANAHATA CHAKRA)

Duration approx. 12-15 minutes

Whole-body relaxation in a supine position can be practiced beforehand.

The visualization exercise "Light in the heart" is intended to make it possible to experience the qualities of the *Anahata chakra* (heart chakra) associated with the dominant element air (open heart space, love, empathy, connectedness with the Self).

a) Preparation

Come into an upright and relaxed seated position of your choice. Lend your posture the quality of *Sukha-Sthira*: solid, stable, comfortable, and permeable. Move the spine into an upright position along it natural curvature. The vertex and the lower pelvic area are on a vertical axis so the energy can flow freely. Now gently close your eyes. Spread your awareness once more across the entire body, from head to toes, and release all tension. Notice the natural flow of the breath.

b) Main part

Now focus your attention on the space of the higher heart. It is located behind the sternum at a level with the physical heart. This energy center is your spiritual home.

In a moment a tiny point of light will appear before your mind's eye. This point of light is the symbol of the center of the higher heart. Now direct your breath towards this inner light and watch what happens. Maybe you can feel your inner light grow larger.

Now you notice a brilliant light energy flowing into you from above the crown of your head. How the higher light flows into your neck via the middle of your head, and on to the space of the higher heart. Feel how the light of the heart stretches towards the higher light, and how the two energies merge.

Notice a feeling of openness, peace, and love spreading inside you. How this energy first spreads across the entire heart and chest area, and then fills your entire being.

You may notice a feeling of all-encompassing connectedness with existence grow inside you.

Now spend a few more minutes in the light of your heart and allow it to course through you.

(A few minutes break)

c) Conclusion

Now slowly resurface from the light-of-the-heart experience and notice your body. Feel your feet and legs, gently move your fingers and toes. Breathe slightly more vigorously and deeply, stretch luxuriously and arrive back in this room.

13.5.9 CLEANSING EXERCISE FOR THE THROAT CHAKRA (VISHUDDHA CHAKRA)

Duration approx. 15-20 minutes

Whole-body relaxation in a supine position can be practiced beforehand.

The visualization exercise "Cleansing exercise for the throat chakra" is intended to make it possible to experience the qualities of the *Vishuddha chakra* (throat chakra) associated with the dominant element expanse (expansion, clarity, verbal expression).

a) Preparation

Come into an upright and relaxed seated position of your choice. Lend your posture the quality of *Sukha-Sthira*: solid, stable, comfortable, and permeable. Move the spine into an upright position along it natural curvature. The vertex and the lower pelvic area are on a vertical axis so the energy can flow freely. Now gently close your eyes. Spread your awareness once more across the entire body, from head to toes, and release all tension. Notice the natural flow of the breath.

b) Main part

Focus your attention on the neck space, on your *Vishuddha chakra*. Let your awareness circle there for a few moments, feel the larynx, the back of the neck, the entire space of the neck.

In a moment, a building will appear before your mind's eye, which will symbolize your throat chakra. Look closely to see what type of building it is. It can be a small hut, a cave, a modern design temple, an ornate palace, a tenement, or whatever appears before your mind's eye. If several choices appear, choose the one you thought of first and stick with it.

Now enter the building and look around. If it is dark, find a light switch. Then carefully look around the room of your throat. Does the room communicate expanse or does it feel oppressive or tight? Is it comfortable? Do you feel good there? Is it clear and orderly? Or is it filled with all sorts of junk; are the windows covered with spider webs and dust, preventing clarity?

If that is the case, or you would like to change something, then get to work and tidy up. A thought or an inspiration from your heart is enough to change the room the way you imagine it.

Get rid of the things that are tough to swallow and prevent clear verbal communication. Symbolically liberate yourself from all the things that are breathing down your neck. In the process of tidying up and changing things around you might discover this or that detail you may not have noticed before. Take all the time you need!

Maybe you would like to completely redo something and express things or possibilities that have long been dormant inside you. Be brave and design the room of your throat according to your present mood and situation.

When you have designed everything according to your wishes and ideas, find a place in the room, your power place, where you can settle down.

Now take some time to enjoy the luxury of silence and allow the room, the mood, and the clarity of the atmosphere to take effect on you.

c) Conclusion

Now slowly resurface from the light-of-the-heart experience and notice your body. Feel your feet and legs, gently move your fingers and toes. Breathe slightly more vigorously and deeply, stretch luxuriously and arrive back in this room.

After this experience, it helps to write down what you have seen and experienced. Also beneficial is a group discussion about the symbolism and what has been experienced.

13.5.10 YOGA NIDRA (SHORT FORM)

Duration approx. 15-20 minutes

This short form of *Yoga Nidra* is geared to participants who have not yet gotten accustomed to staying awake while lying down for an extended period of time. The significant thing about *Yoga Nidra* is that during the first part, the focus changes very rapidly from one area of the body to the next.

It helps to address *Sankalpa* (positive intentions, wishes, goals) before the start of the unit so participants don't have to spend a lot of time during the practice thinking about which *Sankalpa* is most appropriate to their current circumstances and needs. It should be positive, brief, concise, and formulated in the present tense.

The following images should be viewed like a slide show. No associations should be formed between the individual images, meaning no stories should be created from them. The images are intended to help participants learn, to observe without mentally engaging with their content.

a) Preparation

Lie on your back in a relaxed position with your feet planted slightly wider than hip-width apart and feet gently falling open. The spine rests on the mat in its natural curvature. The tailbone and the back of the head form a straight line. The arms rest on the floor at an angle to the body; palms face the ceiling.

Now gently close your eyes. Take a few languid breaths through the nose and exhale through your slightly open mouth. As you do so, let go of anything that currently still occupies you mentally or emotionally.

Now allow your breath to come and go naturally without forcing it. Notice the natural flow of your breath.

Now listen for a while to all the noises you hear. First listen with relaxed ears to just the noises here in this room. Then gradually expand your awareness to the noises outside of this room. As you do so, allow your perception to become increasingly sensitive. How deeply can you listen?

Now bring your awareness back to this room and listen to my voice. Focus all your attention on my voice and stay awake. Now mentally repeat three times: "I will stay awake!"

Allow the breath to continue to flow calmly and mentally formulate your Sankalpa, your goal, your intention. Make it brief, concise, positive, and phrased in the present tense. Repeat your Sankalpa three times and trust that your intention will embed itself in your consciousness like a seed, and will unfold when the time is right.

c) Main part

We now come to the rapid circling of your consciousness in your body. In the process your awareness jumps from one area of the body to the next. Direct your attention to your right hand, the right thumb, index finger, middle finger, ring finger, pinky, palm, back of the hand, wrist, right forearm, elbow, upper arm, right shoulder, armpit, right side of the ribcage, right side of the waist, right hip, thigh, knee, calf, ankle, sole of the foot, instep, right big toe, second toe, third toe, fourth toe, and little toe. Feel the entire right side of your body.

Now shift your attention to the left hand, the left thumb, index finger, middle finger, ring finger, pinky, palm, back of the hand, wrist, right forearm, elbow, upper arm, right shoulder, armpit, left side of the ribcage, left side of the waist, left hip, thigh, knee, calf, ankle, sole of the foot, instep, left big toe, second toe, third toe, fourth toe, and little toe. Feel the entire left side of your body.

Now feel the soles of both feet, the calves, back of the knees, back of the thighs, your bottom, low back, shoulder blades, the entire back, the nape, the back of the head, the vertex, forehead, eyebrows, the eyebrow center, the eyes, temples, ears, cheeks, nose, mouth, chin, the laryngeal area, the ribcage, belly, and navel. Feel the navel lifting and lowering with the flow of the breath. As you inhale the navel lifts, as you exhale the navel drops.

Now calmly count in your head:

"10, the navel lifts, 10, the navel drops."

"Nine, the navel lifts, nine, the navel drops.'

"Continue counting backwards in your head until you arrive at "one". Stay awake!"

I will now name images in quick and unrelated succession that will appear and disappear lightning-fast before your mind's eye: a spiral staircase, sunflower, white sand beach, galloping horse, pitch-black night, dust particles dancing in the sunlight, snow-covered mountains, volcanic eruption, an iceberg, campfire, Indian temple, clouds traveling across the sky, wheat field in the summer breeze, full moon, fall leaves, smiling Buddha, a clear starry night, lotus flower on a lake, blue sky, sunrise, smooth lake surface, smooth lake surface, smooth lake surface.

(A few minutes break)

c) Conclusion

We now come to the end of *Yoga Nidra*. Once more, repeat your *Sankalpa* three times in your mind, and trust that your intention will embed itself in your consciousness like a seed, and will unfold when the time is right.

Become aware of your entire body and allow the breath to flow slightly deeper and more vigorously again. Gently move your fingers and toes. When you are ready, stretch luxuriously. Then lie on your side for a few moments longer. Then move from your side to an upright-seated position.

13.5.11 JOURNEY THROUGH THE CHAKRAS

Duration approx. 15-20 minutes

This guided visualization through the energy centers is intended to deepen participants' awareness of the position and qualities of the individual chakras on the experience level.

a) Preparation

Come into an upright and relaxed seated position of your choice. Lend your posture the quality of *Sukha-Sthira*: solid, stable, comfortable, and permeable. Move the spine into an upright position along its natural curvature. The vertex and the lower pelvic area are on a vertical axis so the energy can flow freely. Now gently close your eyes. Spread your awareness once more across the entire body, from head to toes, and release all tension. Notice the natural flow of the breath.

b) Main part

Now direct your attention to the vertex, the crown of your head. If possible, take your awareness beyond the vertex and notice the space above your head. The crown chakra, *Sahasrara*, is the doorway to the cosmic consciousness. Allow yourself to be permeable there, to connect with the higher parts of yourself. Visualize a diamond-colored, healing light that gently streams through your vertex into your head and clears it out and purifies you.

Now take your awareness to the center of the head, to the *Ajna chakra*, the center of your intuition. As you do so, you may notice subtle movement between and slightly above the eyebrows. The Ajna chakra connects you to higher knowledge and the ability to intuitively understand things and coherences. Imagine a violet light in the forehead area at the center of the head that gives you inner peace.

Now take your awareness to the throat area, the *Vishuddha chakra*. The neck connects head and body, mind and emotion. Circle there with your perception and consciously notice the laryngeal area and the nape. Immerse the entire neck area in a clear and calming blue that gives you the quality of freedom and openness. Feel how potential blocks in the throat gently dissolve in the light of the purifying blue.

Now shift your attention to the higher heart in the middle of the ribcage, behind the sternum, at a level with the physical heart. The *Anahata chakra* is your spiritual center and connects you to the qualities of love, warmth, and empathy. Feel your heart space being drenched with the verdant green of spring and feel the healing power of the light in your heart.

Now take your awareness to the solar plexus area, to your *Manipura chakra*, and allow your awareness to circle there. Mentally connect to the golden-yellow power of the light and feel how the transforming power of the light purifies and nurtures you.

Now take your awareness to the low abdomen, to your sacral chakra, the *Svadisthana chakra*. *Sacral* means *holy*. This is a sacred space. Feel an invigorating orange gently circling in your low abdomen, regenerating and stimulating and connecting you to deep joy.

Now enter your lower pelvic region, the *Muladhara chakra*. *Mula* means *root* and *Adhara* means *support*. This energy center connects you to the qualities of grounding, inner resilience, and complete faith in the flow of life. Feel a warming, nurturing red in the lower pelvic area and let yourself be suffused on all levels of your being with the nurturing and healing qualities of the red light.

Before your mind's eye, see all the colors of the energy centers you just experienced one more time: the warming, nurturing red in the lower pelvic region; the vitalizing, joyful orange in the lower abdomen; the radiant, cheerful golden-yellow in the solar plexus region; the calming and healing green in the ribcage; the clarifying and purifying blue in the throat; the calming and intuitive power of violet; the radiant and penetrating power of the diamond-colored light in the vertex area.

c) Conclusion

Gradually return to a state of waking consciousness. Notice your feet and legs, gently move the fingers and toes. Breathe deeper and more vigorously, stretch luxuriously and arrive back in this room.

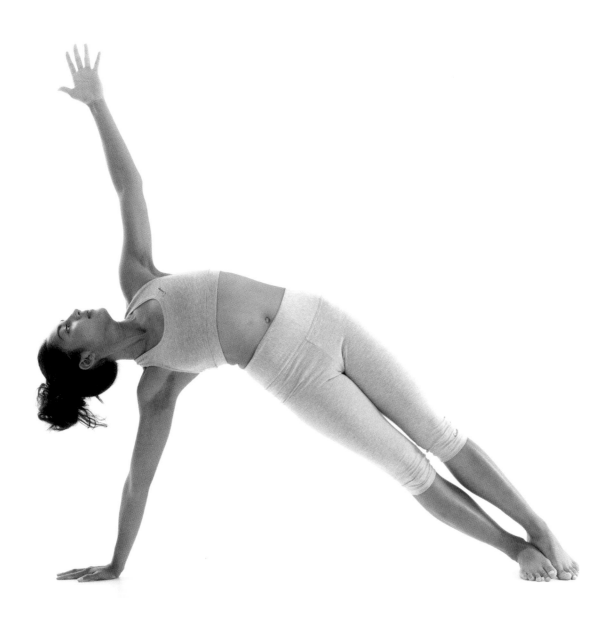

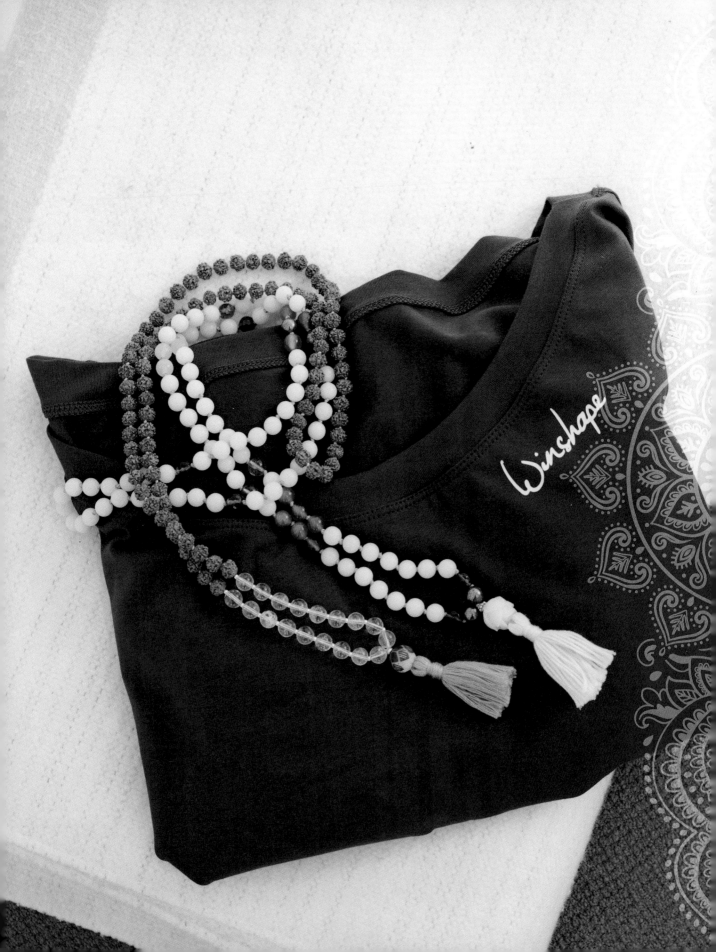

APPENDIX

APPENDIX

1 REFERENCES

Anodea, J. (2004). *Lebensräder. Das große Chakren-Lehr- und -übungsbuch*. Goldmann Arkana.

Aurobindo, S. (1972, 5. Unveränderte Auflage 2008). *Die Synthese des Yoga*. Gladenbach. Verlag Hinder + Deelmann.

Aurobindo, S. (1981, unveränderte Auflage 2005). *Bhagavadgita*. Gladenbach. Verlag Hinder + Deelmann.

Bäumer, B. (3. Auflage 2013). *Vijnana Bhairava. Das göttliche Bewusstsein*. Frankfurt. Insel Verlag. Verlag der Weltreligionen.

Bäumer, B. & Deshpande, P. Y. (1976, sechste Auflage 1990). *Patanjali. Die Wurzeln des Yoga*. Bern, München Wien Schwerz Verlag für Otto Wilhelm Barth Verlag.

Berufsverband Deutscher Yogalehrer (BDY). (4. Auflage 2003). *Der Weg des Yoga. Handbuch für Übende und Lehrende*. Petersberg. Verlag Via Nova.

Broad, W. J. (2013). *The science of yoga. Was es verspricht – und was es kann*. Freiburg im Breisgau. Herder Verlag GmbH.

Cope, S. (2007). *Die Weisheit des Yoga. Auf der Suche nach einem freien, erfüllten und glücklichen Leben*. München. Goldmann Arkana.

Easwaran, E. (2008, 4. Auflage). *Die Upanishaden*. München, Goldmann Arkana.

Emotu, M. (2001). *Die Antwort des Wassers*. Band 1. Burgrain. Koha-Verlag.

Frawley, D. & Summerfield Kozak, S. (2003). *Yoga für Ihren Typ. Das große Yoga-Praxisbuch. Asanas im Einklang mit Ayurveda*. Aitran. Windpferd Verlagsgesellschaft mbH.

Huchzermeyer, W. (2006, 6. Auflage 2015). *Das Yoga-Wörterbuch. Sanskrit-Begriffe, Übungsstile, Biographien*. Karlsruhe, Verlag W. Huchzermeyer.

Irmer, B. & Mager, C. (2009). *Nada Yoga. Hinwendung zum inneren Klang*. Bielefeld. Theseus Verlag,

Kruse, P. Pavlekovic, B. & Haak, K. (1992). *Autogenes Training*. Niederhausen. Falken Verlag.

Long, R. (2015). *Yoga Anatomie 3D, Band 1. Vinyasa Flow und Standhaltungen*. München. Riva Verlag.

Long, R. (2015). *Yoga Anatomie 3D, Band 2. Hüftöffner und Vorbeugen*. München. Riva Verlag.

Long, R. (2015). *Yoga Anatomie 3D, Band 3. Rückbeugen und Drehhaltungen*. München. Riva Verlag.

Long, R. (2015). *Yoga Anatomie 3D, Band 4. Armgestützte Haltungen und Umkehrhaltungen*. München. Riva Verlag.

Michel, K. P. & Wellmann, W. (2003). *Das Yoga der Fünf Elemente*. Bern, Scherz Verlag, O. W. Barth.

Paramahansa Yogananda (1993, 19. deutschsprachige Auflage). *Autobiografie eines Yogi*. Bern und München. Scherz Verlag für O. W. Barth Verlag.

Selye, H. (1976). *Stress in health and disease*. USA. Butterworth-Heinemann.

Skuban, R. (2011, zweite Auflage). *Patanjalis Yogasutra. Der Königsweg zu einem weisen Leben*. München. Arkana.

Srimad. Swami Sivananda (1998). *Bhagavadgita*. Lautersheim. Mangalam Verlag s. Schang & Sita Devi B. Gottschalk.

Swami Svatmarama (2009). *Hatha-Yoga-Pradipika. Die Leuchte des Hatha Yoga*. Hamburg. Phänomen-Verlag Norina Ebele.

Swami Satyananda, S. (zweite Auflage 1992). *Yoga Nidra*. Satyananda Yoga Zentrum e. V. Ananda Verlag.

Thode, E. (2015). *Die göttliche Shakti. Die Kraft des Weiblichen im Yoga*. Bielefeld. Theseus.

Trökes, A. (2004). *Pranayama, BDY Studienbegleitung in der Yogalehrausbildung*. Göttingen. Geschäftsstelle des BDY e. V.

Trökes, A. (2013). *Die kleine Yoga Philosophie. Grundlagen und Übungspraxis verstehen*. München. O. W. Barth Verlag.

Yesudian S. & Haich, E. (1972, 29. Auflage 1984). *Sport + Yoga*. München. Drei Eichen Verlag.

Zhuang Z. (2016, vierte Auflage, Berliner Ausgabe. Durchgesehener Neusatz, bearbeitet und eingerichtet von Holzinger M.). *Das wahre Buch vom südlichen Blütenland*. Düsseldorf/Köln. Eugen Diederichs Verlag.

ADDITIONAL:

Broad, W. J., *New York Times Magazine*, 2012, How yoga can wreck your body, http://www.nytimes.com/2012/01/08/magazine/how-yoga-can-wreck-your-body.html?mcubz=3

J. H. Schultz (1932). Oberstufe des autogenen Trainings und Raya Yoga. *Zeitschrift für die gesamte Neurologie und Psychiatrie*. Band 139, 34.

Stangl, W. http://psychologie.stangl.eu/definition/Stress.shtml

Viveka. Hefte für Yoga. http://www.viveka.de/pdf/viveka_22_Asanas_und_Druesen.pdf

Zitat Gautama Buddha: www.aphorismen.de/zitat/190559

Zitat Vivekananda: https://www.aphorismen.de/zitat/19586

Kapitel 4, Grafiken Gunas: Kirti Peter Michel, unveröffentlicht

Kapitel 8, Surya Namaskar, Die meditative Erfahrung des Sonnengrußes von Kirti Peter Michel, unveröffentliches Manuskript.

Kapitel 9, Zitat, Kirti P. Michel, Bildunterschrift zur Collage „The Final Curtain".

Animierte Yoga Anatomie Lehrvideos:

https://muscleandmotion.net/m&m/

https://www.youtube.com/watch?v=DZlZ4MsQQk8 (Lehrvideos von Ray Long)

ttps://www.bandhayoga.com/DailyBandha.html (Website von Ray Long)

2 CREDITS

Cover design: Sannah Inderlest, Annika Naas

Interior layout: Sannah Inderlest, Annika Naas

Typesetting: Falcon Oast Graphic Art Ltd

Managing editor: Elizabeth Evans

Interior photos: Sonja Lesinski Photography, www.sonjalesinski.com

Model: Sara Lyn Chana

Handmade mala beads (yoga meditation necklaces): www.chandra-gems.de

Interior illustrations:

Adobe Stock:

Pg. 49, 50, 51, 52, 53, 63, 68, 122, 285, 297, 317

Pg. 47: http://rapunzelturm.blogspot.de/2016/06/der-weltenbaum-teil-2-kabbala-ashwatta.html: Holder of rights cannot be ascertained.

Pg. 74, 77, 80, 83, 86, 89, 91: Chakras: *Energy Centers of Transformation* by Harish Johari © 1987. Reprinted by permission of Inner Traditions International and Bear & Company. www.innertraditions.com

Page 21: Wikipedia Creative Commons (CC BY 2.0)

Page 30: Wikipedia Creative Commons (CC BY 2.0)

Page 64: https://www.flickr.com/photos/39453315@N04/3750430764/ (CC BY 2.0)

Page 66: http://media.tumblr.com/884fde2495055a2cc961d8d8affca68a/tumblr_inline_muo0m7KAbj1rmxgp4.jpg

3   PORTRAIT: SARA LYN CHANA (YOGA MODEL)

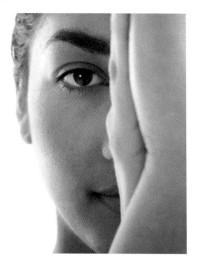

Sara Lyn Chana is a passionate yoga instructor, ambitious Pilates instructor, and inquisitive trade journalist. Her degree in social science as well as her extensive travels across the Asian continent reinforced her desire to make the world a better place. During her nearly 20-year ballet career she developed an interest in the human body and esthetic movement sequences. She first began to seriously practice yoga during a nine-month trip across the Asian continent. She quickly realized that instructor training would have to follow. As part of an effort to reconcile her biggest passions, she completed her first yoga instructor training in Southern India while doing a correspondence course in journalism. The multi-style training gave her deeper insights into the Hatha-, Astanga-, and Vinyasa yoga practice.

"Self-study is the prerequisite for achieving a better understanding of one's own wellbeing. The in-depth engagement with the body and the deeper essence of being requires patience, time, and discipline. For me the time I spent in Asia was an important step in my ongoing personal development. I hope to pass these experiences on to others on the yoga trips I organize. Only letting go of material things and everyday habits will give you the necessary space to get closer to yourself."

Her Asian roots let her add a touch of Far Eastern spirituality to her European work ethic. In doing so, she places great value on maintaining the balance between the scientific findings of Western medicine and the alternative healing powers of Asian traditions. She finds the interplay between body, mind, and social interactivity so fascinating that she has made it her goal to improve general awareness of physical and mental wellbeing. Implementation ultimately takes place through practical work with people and via published texts on the topics of yoga health, and fitness.

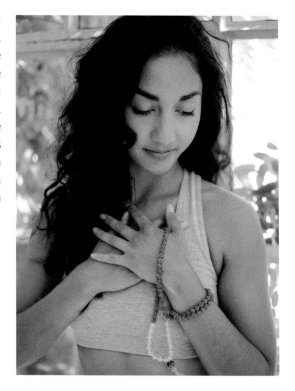

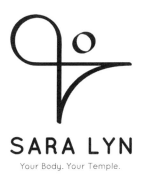

On her blog Sara Lyn regularly publishes articles about all things pertaining to a healthy and mindful lifestyle. Whether you have tight neck muscles or metabolic problems, you are sure to find the appropriate yoga sequence here. She also eagerly reports on newly gained knowledge during her regular trips to Asia, be it in Far Eastern healing methods, Asian massage techniques, or traditional martial arts.

"I hope to reach lots of people through my work and enable them to live a carefree life long-term!"

All current workshop dates, yoga trips, as well as her blog articles can be found at:

www.saralyn.de

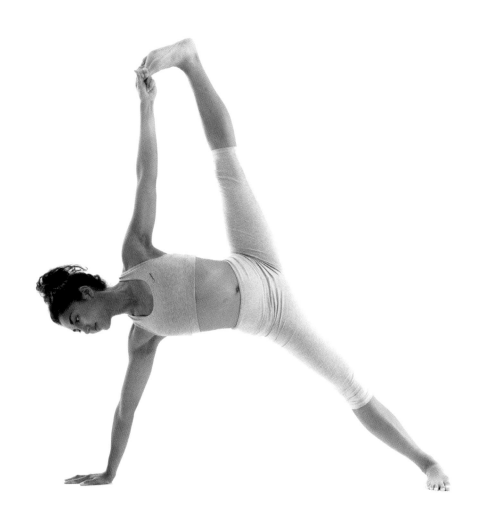

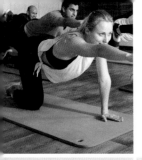

YOGA & PILATES

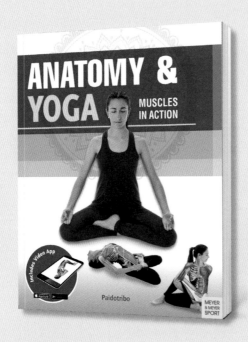

ANATOMY & YOGA
Muscles in Action

This book introduces the yoga tradition from a practical and scientific point of view. It is aimed at students, teachers, and others who practice yoga. Combining science and tradition, this book explains the history of yoga, 50 classical asanas as well as variations and adaptations for safe practice, proper breathing, and the important yoga aspect of inner development. Each asana is accompanied by images illustrating the exercise and anatomical drawings which show the main muscles used in each posture.

144 p., in color
250 photos + illus.
Paperback, 8.3" x 10.8"
ISBN: 978-1-78255-152-2
$22.95 US

All information subject to change © Adobe Stock

MEYER & MEYER SPORT

MEYER & MEYER Sport
Von-Coels-Str. 390
52080 Aachen
Germany

Phone   +49 02 41 - 9 58 10 - 13
Fax   +49 02 41 - 9 58 10 - 10
E-Mail   sales@m-m-sports.com
Website www.thesportspublisher.com

All books available as E-books.

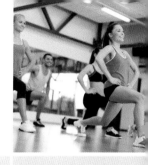

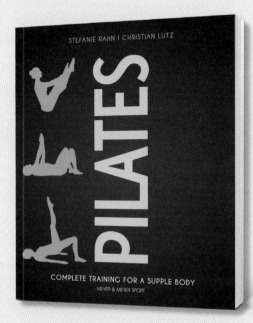

PILATES

Complete Training for a Supple Body

This book provides comprehensive knowledge and contains a variety of exercises as well as professional tips and hints for trainers and exercisers. The exercises are based on strengthening the body's core and supporting muscles, including the pelvic floor, abdominal, and back muscles. The basis of the training is to promote a correct and healthy posture. The main part of the book gives targeted, group-specific exercise programs with and without small equipment. These versatile exercises can be easily integrated into any training program!

384 p., in color
1039 photos + illus.
Paperback, 8.3" x 10"
ISBN: 978-1-78255-186-7
$29.95 US

All information subject to change © Adobe Stock

MEYER & MEYER Sport
Von-Coels-Str. 390
52080 Aachen
Germany

Phone   +49 02 41 - 9 58 10 - 13
Fax   +49 02 41 - 9 58 10 - 10
E-Mail   sales@m-m-sports.com
Website   www.thesportspublisher.com

All books available as E-books.

MEYER & MEYER SPORT